*The Development of*
*Movement Control and Co-ordination*

# WILEY SERIES IN
# DEVELOPMENTAL PSYCHOLOGY

*Series Editor*
**Professor Kevin Connolly**

**The Development of Movement Control and Co-ordination**
*J. A. Scott Kelso and Jane E. Clark*

Further titles in preparation

# The Development of Movement Control and Co-ordination

*Edited by*

**J. A. Scott Kelso**
*Haskins Laboratories, New Haven, Connecticut*
and
*Departments of Psychology and Biobehavioral Sciences,*
*University of Connecticut, USA*

and

**Jane E. Clark**
*University of Maryland, USA*

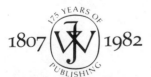

1807 1982

**JOHN WILEY & SONS LTD**
Chichester · New York · Brisbane · Toronto · Singapore

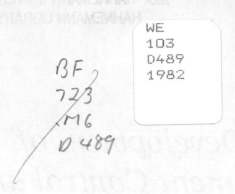
**Library of Congress Cataloging in Publication Data**

Main entry under title:

The Development of movement control and co-ordination.

   (Developmental psychology)
   Includes index.
   1. Motor learning.   2. Child psychology.
I. Kelso, J. A. Scott.   II. Clark, Jane E.
III. Series
BF723.M6D48   1982       155.4'12       81-14690
ISBN 0-471-10048-X                 AACR2

**British Library Cataloguing in Publication Data:**

The Development of movement control and
   coordination. – (Developmental psychology)
   1. Motor learning
   I. Kelso, J. A. Scott     II. Clark, Jane E.
   155.4'2     BF723.M6

   ISBN 0 471 10048 X

Typeset by Pintail Studios Ltd, Ringwood, Hampshire.
Printed in Great Britain by Page Bros. Norwich Ltd.

# List of Contributors

CRAIG R. BARCLAY, *Department of Psychology, University of Michigan, Ann Arbor.*

DENISE C. R. BENEL, *Department of Psychology, University of Illinois, Champaign, Illinois.*

JANE E. CLARK, *Department of Physical Education, University of Pittsburgh, Pittsburgh, Pennsylvania.*

SHARON R. GARBER, *Division of Speech Pathology and Audiology, University of Pittsburgh, Pittsburgh, Pennsylvania.*

NORMA SUE GRIFFIN, *Department of Physical Education, University of Nebraska, Lincoln, Nebraska.*

JOHN HAUBENSTRICKER, *Department of Physical Education, Michigan State University, East Lansing, Michigan.*

BILL JONES, *Department of Psychology, Carleton University, Ottawa, Ontario, Canada.*

J. A. SCOTT KELSO, *Haskins Laboratories, 270 Crown Street, New Haven, Connecticut and Departments of Psychology and Biobehavioral Sciences, University of Connecticut, Storrs, Connecticut.*

JACK F. KEOGH, *Department of Kinesiology, University of California, Los Angeles, California.*

PETER N. KUGLER, *Department of Psychology, University of Connecticut, Storrs, Connecticut and Haskins Laboratories, 270 Crown Street, New Haven, Connecticut.*

KARL M. NEWELL, *Institute for Child Behavior and Development, University of Illinois, Champaign, Illinois.*

HERBERT L. PICK, JR., *Institute of Child Development, University of Minnesota, Minneapolis, Minnesota.*

G. LAWRENCE RARICK, *Department of Physical Education, University of California, Berkeley, California.*

MARY ANN ROBERTON, *Department of Physical Education and Dance, University of Wisconsin, Madison, Wisconsin.*

RICHARD A. SCHMIDT, *Department of Kinesiology, University of California, Los Angeles, California.*

VERN D. SEEFELDT, *Department of Physical Education, Michigan State University, East Lansing, Michigan.*

DIANE C. SHAPIRO, *Department of Kinesiology, University of California, Los Angeles, California.*

G. M. SIEGEL, *Department of Communication Disorders, University of Minnesota, Minneapolis, Minnesota.*

FRANK L. SMOLL, *Department of Kinesiology, University of Washington, Seattle, Washington.*

MICHAEL T. TURVEY, *Department of Psychology, University of Connecticut, Storrs, Connecticut, and Haskins Laboratories, 270 Crown Street, New Haven, Connecticut.*

MICHAEL G. WADE, *Institute for Child Behavior and Development, University of Illinois, Champaign, Illinois.*

CHRISTOPHER D. WICKENS, *Department of Psychology, University of Illinois, Champaign, Illinois.*

# Foreword

At a time when the rate of publication in the behavioural sciences is still increasing, the appearance of a new series of books requires some comment. Psychology covers a truly enormous domain of subject matter and it is perhaps more useful to think of it as a federation of interrelated disciplines than as a single subject. Inevitably, as the knowledge base grows and as new theories and methods of investigation are devised, tensions appear and there is a tendency for the whole to fragment. In some measure this is unavoidable because as new disciplines or subdisciplines emerge special interest groups are formed and special publications appear. However, while psychologists become increasingly specialized in their techniques and their specific area of study, they need at the same time to maintain an intellectual and conceptual approach to their subject matter which is wide and open to new ideas and information. At first sight these two requirements seem quite incompatible: however, some fields of psychology have a unifying quality because they are concerned with almost the whole range of the behavioural and mental sciences. Developmental psychology is one of the best examples of this since it is focussed upon an understanding of how behavioural and mental attributes emerge and change during an individual's life history. It thus involves the whole range of analysis from the biological to the cultural level.

Over the last 20 years interest in developmental psychology, including its applications in clinical, educational, and social contexts, has exploded. The data base has grown prodigiously and continues to do so unabated. New theories and new methods, along with new applications of our knowledge, are introduced each year. A general feature of growth is that it is uneven, some parts grow earlier or at a faster rate than others, and so the overall form changes and shifts. The biological metaphor is appropriate in more ways than one for describing events in developmental psychology. As new ideas emerge and as new techniques and theories are produced, shifts in emphasis and achievement appear; these provide the basis of fashion in science. Problems, theories, and methods become fashionable and tend to be retained until better theories and better methods are developed or until new problems capture the scientists' attention and imagination. As this process unfolds some topics become the subject of not one or a few books but of many, and thus one can see the uneven growth of the literature on development.

This series is aimed at treating issues which have not already been adequately dealt with in book form in recent years. The volumes in this new Wiley series are not intended to be 'one in a million'. Our intention is to select those topics which, for whatever reason, are in need of a book-length treatment. In some cases there may be an extensive literature which has not been pulled together, in others it may be a new critical evaluation which is needed. The aim is ambitious. We hope that these books will arouse new interests and play a significant part in changing the emphases in the study of development. We hope too that they will serve to further the practical use of knowledge for the well-being of children. The series is deliberately eclectic in terms of the subjects on which books are being prepared; it ranges from the biological to the cultural ends of the spectrum. Some of the volumes in preparation will be predominantly of interest to research workers whilst others are likely to have value as texts for undergraduate and graduate courses.

The essays which make up the first volume are all from North America and are based upon a conference held at the University of Iowa. It is easy to overlook fundamental and ubiquitous phenomena; the fact that skilled motor actions are commonplace seems to lead to an implicit assumption that they are perhaps not very important or scientifically exciting. Of course the reverse is true. The study of the development of motor skills and motor control is of great theoretical importance in the behavioural and brain sciences and also of enormous practical significance. These essays which have been collected and edited by Drs. Kelso and Clark deal with new concepts and ideas not yet widely known, with new data bearing on some of the central questions in the control and co-ordination of skilled movement and with the use of this knowledge in physical education and in therapy. Thus theory, methods, data, and the application of this knowledge are all considered. Despite the central importance of skilled action in the achievement of competence and the individual's growing mastery over the environment during childhood there have been few books on this subject in the last decade. The ideas and information discussed in this book will be of interest beyond the customary confines of developmental psychology; psychologists not specifically interested in development and others who are not psychologists will find important ideas and information in these essays.

Professor Kevin Connolly
Series Editor

# Preface

When we watch the growth of motor competence in the developing child it is difficult to imagine that the child's activities are organized arbitrarily. But what are the organizational principles that sit behind the development of motor skill? More fundamentally, what is it that the developmental scientist seeks to explain? It was not too long ago that scientific research on motor development operated at the purely descriptive level of analysis yielding volumes of data on the development of certain basic skills such as crawling, walking, and prehension. This was important work in its own right even if the focus of the problem was probably misguided. Few among us now would spend much time debating the 'nature' versus 'nurture' dichotomy; the issue is one of how to understand the mutuality or synergistic relationship between environmental structure and the developing child.

The last time an integration was attempted of the motor skill development area – a decade ago in Connolly's now classic *Mechanisms of Motor Skill Development* (Academic Press, New York, 1970) – there was a good deal of press given to the need to shift away from so-called 'normative-descriptive' approaches and to ask more 'process-oriented' questions. Mapping the timing of changes in movement behavior across the life span – so it was said – is all very well, but surely at the beginnings of the 70s it was time to move from questions dealing with 'what?' to questions of 'how?' With the advent of increasingly elaborate information-processing models of adult skilled performance, with their partialling up of the system into stages of stimulus detection, perception, short-term memory, response output and so on, the time was ripe for dramatic advances in the developmental sciences. The focus on revealing *mechanisms* is an honorable one for it potentially affords a theoretical approach to issues of practical concern – helping neurologically dysfunctioning children, for example. But mechanism is a strange word indeed if we think about it. What scientists working at one level of inquiry agree to call mechanism, can at a more 'molecular' level be more simply described as a set of interrelated and interacting parts. Moreover, there is always the possibility lurking in the background that the search for mechanisms in complex systems that change, and whose activities change as a function of time, may be premature – particularly if the description of what we are trying to explain is not quite appropriate.

In this collection of papers we see the so-called 'process-oriented' approach to motor skill development well represented. There is little doubt in our minds – though the reader must judge for himself – that the focus on 'process' has served to revitalize and refocus an area that was of limited interest. But it would be a mistake, we believe, in urging a laboratory analysis of skill development (which may or may not tell us anything about process) to ignore the important work on real-life skills. We do not choose to dismiss this work as merely descriptive or atheoretical; rather, we believe the *type* of theorizing to be different but no less relevant.

In bringing together this group of distinguished scientists we had in mind a meshing, as it were, of the so-called descriptive and process-oriented approaches. If nothing else we forced the experimentalists and the ethologists to talk to each other and to recognize each other's problems. We did not expect either group suddenly to switch their paradigmatic allegiances – only to share their thoughts about a common problem. Skill development requires an adaptive response of the system over time to specific aspects of environmental structure. The task is to explore the nature and origin of the fairly slowly changing dynamic constraints that determine motor competence.

With this long-term goal in mind we present the outcome of a conference sponsored by the Big Ten Committee on Institutional Co-operation (CIC) and the University of Iowa, to whom we gratefully extend our appreciation. Numerous individuals aided in the success of this venture. We are especially indebted to Drs Louis Alley and Margaret Fox – Chairs of Departments of Physical Education, Men and Women respectively – for their support in initiating the conference; Drs Dee Norton (Psychology) and William Coffman (Visual Scholars Program and School of Education) for financial support; Dr Wynne Updike, Chairperson of the CIC Executive Committee for his interest and co-operation; and Mary Foster, who took care of many of the administrative details and assured that the conference ran smoothly.

Finally, we express our sincere thanks to the contributors to this volume and the University of Pittsburgh and Haskins Laboratories for their generous support during the final preparation phase. The editorial and production staff of John Wiley in Chichester were also a great help and we thank them.

J. A. SCOTT KELSO
JANE E. CLARK

# Contents

# PART I

# Information, Co-ordination, and Control in Motor Skill Development

The development of motor skill – as a problem – would probably be less interesting to many if it could be shown that the nature of acquisition processes in children and adults was fundamentally the same. While the evidence is hardly conclusive at this point, Jones in a provocative paper makes the strong claim that the above so-called 'developmentalist attitude' is far from justified: comparing the catching behavior of a two-year-old to a fifteen-year-old is like comparing a novice guitar player to Segovia! That the guitar playing of Segovia and the catching behavior of the adult display quite different movement characteristics than those of the novice and the child is hardly surprising, but, according to Jones, hardly warrants a special developmental theory. Of course many of the contributors in this volume might disagree strongly. But whether Jones is correct or not is hardly the issue. What seems to be more important is to understand the similarities (and the differences) between the ways children and adults acquire new skills – a search that leads one to ask many interesting questions.

Jones reviews for us – almost as a 'test case' – his own work as well as others on intersensory integration, specifically the efficiency with which children and adults map one modality onto another. The important outcome is not the putative asymmetry *per se* that might exist between matching visual to proprioceptive information and vice versa, but the efficiency with which information in each mode is picked up in the first place. As emphasized in James Gibson's classic *The Senses Considered as Perceptual Systems*, animals are enormously sensitive to visual information for the control of activity. Vision, in fact, can perform not only a teloreceptive but a proprioceptive function as well, as revealed in the elegant experiments of David Lee (see Jones, Chapter 3). To talk then of intermodal co-ordination as a single framework for the acquisition of motor control – as Jones points out – makes little sense. The issue becomes one of specifying *what* information is picked up in the first place as a child explores the environment, and determining the nature of the pick-up process.

1

Herbert Pick and his colleagues' work is, to some extent, continuous with this theme. Unlike Jones, whose arguments focused on the interrelationship between vision and movement, Pick chooses a skill that motor developmentalists — by tradition — have hardly ever considered, namely, the skill of speaking. Like all good research, Pick and his colleagues are motivated by a practical concern: how do we help those people — children and adults — with speech defects? The more global issue of course rests with how people learn to speak, for without some insight into that issue correctional procedures are likely to fall far short of their goal. Given the presumed coupling between hearing and speaking, it seems logical to Pick first to understand how what we hear modulates how we speak. We are thus treated to a clear discussion of a programmatic series of experiments from Pick's laboratory in which auditory information is manipulated and effects on prosodic (mainly vocal intensity) and articulatory processes evaluated. Much remains to be done here — but one interesting though perhaps speculative conclusion is that humans, rather than becoming less sensitive to auditory information with increasing age, actually become *more* sensitive. This is a potentially damaging blow, if true, to the many who have argued that as skill develops, there is a concomitant shift in control processes. Thus the almost universally accepted truism (without much hard data) that individuals become less dependent on monitoring 'feedback' and resort to some intrinsically generated 'programming' mode when the skill is highly learned. But Pick *et al.*'s data are quite suggestive that the perceptual system, even in adult speech, plays a fine-tuning function on the articulatory process.

Of course the latter conclusion is perfectly consonant with one of the themes elaborated upon in the first chapter of this section by Kugler, Kelso, and Turvey. According to these authors the information for a developing animal is not arbitrarily defined; rather it is specific to the design of the animal and the activity that is engaged in. Unlike Jones who pays little homage to the influence of biomechanical constraints (changing dynamics) on development, Kugler, Kelso, and Turvey approach the problem of movement control and co-ordination from the lessons learned in morphogenesis. The facts of growth expressed in the Principle of Similitude as underscored by D'Arcy Thompson are enormous — but oft-ignored — constraints on the activities of the child in relation to the adult, and a solution to the problem of controlling complex living systems (which grow unlike machines!) must be sensitive to that system's dynamics. This dynamic, physical perspective on developing co-ordination contrasts dramatically with more conventional approaches and so requires extensive elaboration of a philosophy of design. The latter is founded on the joining together of the principles emerging from physical biology and the tenets of ecological realism: control and co-ordination in natural systems emerge as an *a posteriori* fact of the synergistic relationship between animal, environment, and activity. They are not – according to Kugler *et al.* – predicated on the *a priori*, animal – arbitrary concept of formal program. This is a long story indeed and we wish the reader good luck and much perseverance.

# CHAPTER 1

# On the Control and Co-ordination of Naturally Developing Systems

P. N. KUGLER, J. A. SCOTT KELSO, AND M. T. TURVEY

## INTRODUCTION

The purpose of this chapter is to present and to discuss certain principles as a backdrop for the thesis that an understanding of the developmental facts of movement control and co-ordination requires a physical (rather than a formal) approach carefully tempered by a realist (rather than a nonrealist) philosophical attitude. Our presentation and discussion are largely in the tutorial mode because the principles are not commonplace departure points for students of the development of movement. The principles are drawn from philosophy, biology, engineering science and, in particular, nonequilibrium thermodynamics and the ecological approach to perception and action. Throughout, our paradigm issue is an aspect of the larger developmental picture, namely, the implications of a scaling-up in the body's magnitudes for the control and co-ordination of movement. And within the scope of this latter issue our concentration is on the notion of information: how can information be conceptualized so that it is continuously co-ordinated with changes in skeletomuscular dynamics that are brought about by changes in skeletomuscular dimensions?

## 1  PRELIMINARY REMARKS: DEGREES OF FREEDOM AND THE PRINCIPLE OF SIMILITUDE

An attractive view of the movements of animals is one that treats movement as form, as an adjacent and successive ordering of the body's skeletal linkages, and which, therefore, aligns the study of movement production and of the changes in movement that accompany growth with the more general study of morphogenesis. Troland (1929, pp. 366–367), some fifty years ago, subscribed to a formational view of movement; for him, movements were 'ordered successions of progressively different postures.' A posture of the skeleton, like the form of any portion of matter, is to be described as due to the action of forces. In D'Arcy Thompson's (1917) terms, the form of an object – here a movement of the body – is a 'diagram of forces' in that one could, in principle, deduce from it the forces currently and previously in action. Skeletal poses progressively transformed are, of course, less analogous to solid objects than they are to fluids; they are varying rather than frozen forms, but they are, all the same, the resultant of a configuration of forces that index the manifestation of various energy kinds.

## 1.1   Movement as a 'Diagram' of Muscular and Nonmuscular Forces Drawn on Many Degrees of Freedom

It was, perhaps, Bernstein (1967) who first gave full emphasis to the totality of forces in interpreting the 'construction' of movements. For Bernstein, to focus on those forces due to muscular contraction was insufficient. A viable account of movement had to include, with equal emphasis, inertia and reactive forces – those that result from motions of the body and those that result from mechanical contact with surfaces and media. (See Gibson's (1979) definitions of these terms and see Hertel's (1966) discussion of flying and swimming.) A movement of the human body, therefore, is a 'diagram' of muscular *and* non-muscular forces and it is, as we will express it below, a diagram drawn over a large number of degrees of freedom.

The human body (in childhood and in maturity) has in the order of 792 muscles that act, rarely singly and almost always in combination, to generate and degenerate kinetic energy in over 100 mobile joints (Wells, 1976). These joints vary in the kinds of anatomical pieces that they link (cartilages, bones) and in the number of axes over which they can change (for example, hinge joints like the elbow are uniaxial whereas ball-and-socket joints like the hip are triaxial). Were we to take a conservative stance on the body's mechanical degrees of freedom, one that assumed the existence of only hinge joints, we would still be facing a system of 100 or so mechanical degrees of freedom (see Turvey, Fitch, and Tuller, in press).

The organizational principles of movement, subsumed by the general (and unevenly interpreted) terms 'control' and 'co-ordination,' realize behaviors of very few degrees of freedom from a skeletal basis of very many degrees of freedom; they define a mapping from a space of multiple fine-grained variables to a space of considerably fewer coarse-grained variables. To put it most bluntly, the organizational principles of movement systematically dissipate degrees of freedom.

One can take a perspective on the largeness of the body's number of mechanical degrees of freedom that regards it as a 'problem' (e.g. Bernstein, 1967; Gelfand *et al.*, 1971; Greene, 1972; Turvey, 1977) and the aforementioned principles as the 'solution'. This perspective identifies the articulation of the 'solution' to the 'problem' as the foremost task of movement science. It will be a central theme of the present chapter that candidate solutions cannot be indifferent to the facts of growth as expressed by the Principle of Similitude.

## 1.2 The Principle of Similitude or Dynamical Similarity

It has long been respected that the limiting condition on the actions and forms of terrestrial creatures is the strength of the earth's gravity: the forms that animals take are proportional to gravity's pull. Imagine a doubling in the magnitude of gravity: the upright posture that marks *homo sapiens* would be rendered inoperative, and the largest inhabitants of the earth would be reduced to short-legged creatures with bodies very close to the ground or to legless, snakelike creatures with bodies in contact with the ground. In contrast, a halving of gravity's strength would yield tall and slender creatures requiring less by way of energy and equipped with metabolic organs – heart, lungs, etc. – of comparatively diminutive size. That form would change proportionately with gravity is one manifestation of the Principle of Similitude or Dynamical Similarity (see Bridgeman, 1922; Thompson, 1917/1941). A further and reciprocal manifestation of the Principle – one that is less demanding of the imagination – is that form changes proportionately with size.

The forces which determine an organism's form vary, some as one power and some as another power of the organism's dimensions such as, for example, its height or its length. That is to say, forces do not configure independently of dimensions: a scale change in the dimensions is accompanied by a change in the relative values of the forces. Necessarily, form as a diagram of forces changes with a change in scale.

To illustrate, suppose that an engineer, after constructing a strong and durable bridge was then confronted by the problem of building a much larger bridge. To save time, the engineer repeated the earlier design by simply applying a scale factor to the bridge's linear dimensions (such as the lengths of its struts and girders). Unfortunately, this new, larger bridge, though geometrically identical to its smaller counterpart, could never match its stability. The resistance of a supporting structure to a crushing stress – its strength, if you wish – varies as the square of a linear dimension (say, its length) whereas the weight of the structure varies as the cube; thus the larger of the two geometrically similar bridges is disproportionately heavier for its strength and is, therefore, more prone to collapse. Though the set of dimensions is the same for the two bridges the difference in scale is accompanied by a difference in the configuration of forces. At the smaller scale the geometric form represents a stable configuration of forces whereas at the larger scale that same form, in terms of forces, is configurationally unstable. Stability of forces at the larger scale necessitates a change in the geometric form.

By these various considerations changes of form, however inappreciable to the eye, will occur as long as growth lasts. This is one lesson to be learned from the Principle of Similitude or Dynamical Similarity. An equally significant lesson for our present purposes follows from considering not the dynamical differences between geometrically similar systems that may accompany a change in scale, but the dynamical *sameness* of geometrically similar systems that may persist over a change in scale. That is, we need to consider the case in which two systems do not distinguish qualitatively though they may distinguish quantitatively.

Suppose that we were investigating a physical process known to depend on an identifiable number of measurable attributes or dimensions. (And in the following we paraphrase Rosen's (1978) development of this topic.) The process can be lawfully described as some functional relation among the dimensions here designated by $x_i$:

$$\phi(x_4 \ldots x_n) = 0 \qquad (1)$$

Assuming that the process is defined on a mechanical system, we can take mass ($M$), length ($L$) and time ($T$) as the fundamental dimensions (identified, for simplicity, with $x_1$, $x_2$, and $x_3$) in terms of which the other dimensions ($x_4$ through $x_n$) of (1) can be described. For example, if frequency, velocity, and force were three of the 'nonfundamental' or derived dimensions then they would be expressed as $T^{-1}$, $L/T$ and $ML/T^2$, respectively (see Stahl, 1962). More generally any derived dimension in (1) (that is, $x_4 \ldots x_n$) would be given by:

$$x_i = M^{\alpha_i} L^{\beta_i} T^{\gamma_i} \qquad (2)$$

If now we rewrite (2) as a ratio:

$$\pi_i = x_i M^{-\alpha_i} L^{-\beta_i} T^{-\gamma_i} \qquad (3)$$

it is readily recognized that $\pi_i$ is *dimensionless* – it is a *pure* number. It follows that (1) can now be rewritten in dimensionless form;

$$\phi(\pi_4 \ldots \pi_n) = 0 \qquad (4)$$

Suppose that we now wish to compare a second process $\phi'$ with $\phi$ where $\phi'$ like $\phi$ is describable by (1) but where $\phi'$ differs from $\phi$ in terms of the values of the observables, $x_i$. Putting each process into the dimensionless form of (4) allows for a determination of their dynamical similarity; precisely, $\phi$ and $\phi'$ are similar if and only if the dimensionless quantities $\pi_i$, $\pi'_i$ are respectively equal. With respect to the two bridges referred to above: their measurable attributes or dimensions are the same but they differ in scale; that they also differ in stability would be interpretable, by the preceding formulation of the Principle of Similitude, as due to the fact that their respective dimensionless numbers are not equal.

We have remarked that in the interests of stability the larger bridge would have to assume a form different from that of the smaller bridge. But it is perhaps intrinsically obvious that there should be a range of magnitudes over which the two bridges could differ yet remain dynamically similar and, therefore, equally stable. That is to say, the dimensionless numbers in their respective equations should remain virtually equal up to some difference in scale. That scale value at which the two bridges can no longer be related by a similarity transformation – that is, the larger must assume a form different from the smaller – is referred to as a *critical value*. The general notion of critical scale values will figure significantly in the discussions that follow. A dimensional analysis of the damped harmonic oscillator will help to clarify the notion; in addition it gives a concrete example of the procedure for arriving at equations in dimensionless form.

The differential equation of a harmonic oscillator with mass $m$, damping $B$, and stiffness $k$ is:

$$m\ddot{x} + B\dot{x} + kx = 0 \tag{5}$$

From the general solution to this equation the frequency $f$ is given by

$$f = \frac{1}{2\pi} \sqrt{\frac{k}{m} - \frac{B^2}{4m^2}} \tag{6}$$

That is to say, there is a basic equation of the form

$$\phi(f, B, m, k) = 0 \tag{7}$$

Taking $m$ and (for simplicity) $k$ as the fundamental dimensions then the derived quantities $f$ and $B$ may be expressed, respectively, as

$$f = k^{1/2} m^{-1/2}, \quad B = m^{1/2} k^{1/2} \tag{8}$$

giving rise to two dimensionless quantities

$$\pi_1 = m^{1/2} K^{-1/2} f, \quad \pi_2 = m^{-1/2} K^{-1/2} B \tag{9}$$

and the dimensionless equation

$$\phi(\pi_1, \pi_2) = 0$$

Let us now see what happens when $B$, described dimensionally, takes on the value $2m^{1/2}k^{1/2}$. This value of $B$ substituted into (6) renders the quantity under the radical equal to zero which is synonymous with driving $f$ to zero. In short, $B = 2m^{1/2}k^{1/2}$ is a critical value associated with a dramatic qualitative change in the behavior of the system described by (5): below this critical value the system oscillates; at and above this critical value it does not.

Let us now relate these remarks on similitude (that two physical processes with common dimensions related by a common function are dynamically *similar* up to some scale value) and 'dissimilitude' (that two physical processes with common dimensions related by a common function are dynamically *dissimilar* beyond some scale value) to the control and co-ordination of movement.

### 1.3 Implications of the Principle of Similitude for the Theory of Co-ordination and Control

The Principle of Similitude is most frequently discussed with reference to biological functions – to goal-directed activities or *effectivities*. A particular bodily form, anatomical structure or physiological arrangement serves as a 'method' for realizing a given effectivity only up to some limiting magnitude of a linear dimension. Beyond that magnitude the 'method' for realizing the same effectivity will have to change. To illustrate, most animals rely on aerobic metabolism and therefore are designed so as to guarantee that their tissues are supplied with adequate amounts of oxygen. The method by which oxygen is transported to tissue is scale-dependent. For the smallest of animals – from protozoa to the flatworm – oxygen transport is solely by diffusion on gradients of partial pressure. However, beyond a tissue thickness of approximately 0.06 cm (Alexander, 1968) this method of transporting oxygen is unworkable and some other method has to be used; for a large number of animals it is the circulation of blood infused with respiratory pigment.

There are two ways in which the magnitudes of a person's bodily dimensions change. They change naturally as an accompaniment of age and they change artificially – for example, as a matter of wielding and carrying objects. By virtue of the Principle of Similitude alone we should expect that as a child grows bigger an effectivity such as walking or throwing will pass through a sequence of qualitatively distinguishable forms, where each form is stable over a limited range of growth in the bodily dimensions. We do not wish to be read here as saying that the simple scaling-up of a linear dimension is responsible for the developmental pattern that is actually observed in walking and throwing (see, respectively, Bernstein, 1967; Roberton, 1978) rather that a scale change is sufficient to induce a sequence of distinguishable stable and unstable movement patterns for the same effectivity. Similarly, by virtue of the Principle of Similitude alone we should necessarily expect that an effectivity supported by skeletomuscular motions will be either subtly or radically modified by 'artificial' magnitude changes in the fundamental dimensions of mass, length, and time wrought by the implements struck with, the missiles thrown, the loads carried, the surfaces walked, run, and stood upon, etc. The child who exhibits a free, natural sidearm swing with a lightweight striking implement transfers to an arm-dominated push at the ball when required to hit with a heavier instrument (Halverson, Roberton, and Harper, 1973).

Whether they be introduced naturally or artificially, increases in the lengths and masses of biokinematic links must be accompanied by changes both in the muscular forces needed to initiate and arrest the motions of the links and in the reactive forces that the links generate in starting, moving, and stopping. This means that a given movement pattern which remains relatively invariant over a period of growth or over an artificial scaling up of dimensions cannot be the result of constant forces generated at fixed times; put differently, the 'diagram of forces' − the form of the movement − remains unchanged although the actual quantities of the forces, muscular and nonmuscular, and their timing do not. Formally speaking, this situation of a constant movement pattern over inconstant magnitudes is analogous to the invariance described above in which two processes defined in the same way over the same set of dimensions are dynamically similar − for nonidentical values of these dimensions − when their respective dimensionless numbers are equal. Physically speaking, this situation of a constant movement pattern over inconstant magnitudes necessitates a principled basis for determining the muscular forces which, together with the circumstantially determined nonmuscular forces, configure to give the constant movement pattern. The related situation − of a qualitative change in a movement pattern at critical magnitudes of one or more dimensions − necessitates a principled basis (i) for determining that at a certain magnitude a given movement pattern, a given diagram of forces, is no longer supportive of a given effectivity; and (ii) for selecting the new movement pattern (or patterns) appropriate conjointly to the dimensional magnitudes and the effectivity. These two cognate desiderata (of accounting in a principled fashion for the scale-associated qualitative invariants and qualitative changes in patterns of movement) identify the restriction on the solution to the problem of degrees of freedom that is imposed by the Principle of Similitude. More generally, they identify a restriction on the solution to the problem of how movements are coordinated and controlled in a system whose dimensions change in magnitude, regardless of whether the changes are abrupt or gradual.

Two frequently promoted conceptions for understanding control and coordination are the motor program (e.g. Keele and Summers, 1976; Keele, 1980) and the schema (e.g. Pew, 1974; Schmidt, 1975; see Shapiro and Schmidt, this volume). These conceptions derive in large part − as we will argue in Section 1.4 − from a particular perspective on biological order. With respect to the task of satisfying the above desiderata of the Principle of Similitude, we ask whether conceptions such as motor program and schema are sufficient and whether they are necessary.

Suppose the ability of a child at age $t$ to strike a ball through a particular movement pattern $m$ was owing to a motor program $p$. And allow that a motor program, roughly speaking, is a detailed set of instructions to contract such and such muscles, to such and such degrees at such and such times (but see Keele, 1980 for a different definition). At some later age, say $t + 1$, the child's muscles are of greater cross-sectional area and the child's bones are of greater length and mass in comparison to their magnitudes at $t$. To produce the same movement pattern at $t + 1$ the child cannot rely on the coded instructions used at $t$ for they are not referential of the current set of skeletomuscular magnitudes. Of course it is generally conceded that motor programs operate with a skeletomuscular context that is not necessarily fixed and therefore programs must be adaptable within reasonable limits. The adjustments to the program's coded instructions are said to be based on feedback, that is, information about the skeletomuscular states of affairs. Under the feedback proviso the program's subgoals or reference signals – roughly of the sentential form 'get this trajectory from this joint at this point in time' – remain the same, just the signals to the musculature change. Though a great deal of unpacking has to be done to make this feedback formulation work, even when relatively few degrees of freedom are involved (Fowler and Turvey 1978; Gelfand and Tsetlin, 1962), we can allow, for sake of argument, that it is tractable. This latter concession is made ungrudgingly because we wish to parlay the double-duty performed by the information about the skeletomuscular states of affairs into a denial of the sufficiency of the program and schema conceptions. What are the two duties?

At age $t + 1$ the child's dimensions had not exceeded a value at which movement pattern $m$ was unreliable. Within the period $t$ to $t + 1$ the aforementioned information is termed 'feedback' and is assimilated to $p$'s referent signals. But now suppose that at $t + 2$ the child's dimensions have magnified critically – $m$ is no longer tenable and a new, qualitatively different movement pattern is required. Within the period $t + 1$ to $t + 2$ the aforementioned information is not just data to be assimilated to $p$ but it is data to be accommodated by $p$ – in short, it is now also 'feedforward' that specifies new subgoals, new referent signals and hence, a new program. What is lacking in the motor program and schema conceptions is any *principled* account of how information about the skeletomuscular states of affairs can do double duty as feedback and feedforward. Without such a principled account these conceptions are insufficient to satisfy the above desiderata. Let us now ask whether they are necessary.

A most obvious response to the double-duty observation is to pursue further the conceptions of program and schema; under some possible elaboration a principled account may be forthcoming. The success of this response cannot be dismissed offhand though we confess to being skeptical and give expression to this skepticism in various sections of the chapter. For present purposes it suffices to note that countenancing an elaboration of the program and schema conceptions with regard to the above desiderata is tantamount to disavowing the continuity of similitude and dissimilitude effects in animal movement and other natural domains. While we should suppose that the worked-through physical account of these effects is most general, the tack of pursuing the program and schema conceptions would have us abandon that generality when animal movements are the object of study and espouse instead explanatory principles of a new and special kind.

The notions of programmed instructions and schemas can have no role in explanations of, say, the forms assumed by water or air as the magnitudes of certain dimensions vary. Nevertheless, one might wish to claim that these notions can have a role in the explanation of scale-associated effects in animal actions. It is doubtful, however, that they can have a *necessary* role in such explanations. The understanding of nature tends to progress through the identifying and gradual extension of very general explanatory principles that accommodate the particular and the novel rather than through the proposing and pursuing of particular and novel explanatory principles *sui generis*. A measure of this latter assertion is to be found in the section that follows. We conclude the present section by noting that if there were some very general physical account of scale-associated invariants of form and changes of form then to that account we should turn for insights into the problem of degrees of freedom in movement and into a conception of the informational basis for movement that is continuously co-ordinate with scale.

## 1.4  Contrasting Perspectives on Order and Regularity

An understanding of the systematic regulation of the body's many degrees of freedom can be sought from two perspectives that are often in opposition where matters of order and regulation in biology are at issue. One perspective (and in many respects the more popular of the two) equates the aforementioned understanding with the resolution of the technical or engineering problem of how, given a multivariable mechanical system, one could effectively control its behavior. In this 'artifactual' perspective: (i) the body's many degrees of freedom are a 'curse' (cf. Bellman, 1961) or a 'problem' (cf. Turvey, 1977); (ii) co-ordination and control are impositions on the skeletomuscular apparatus; and, relatedly, (iii) the central nervous system as the putative source of the co-ordinating and controlling signals is sharply distinguished from the high-powered, energy-converting skeletomuscular system that is the putative recipient of those signals.

Not unexpectedly the artifactual perspective promotes contemporary manmade machines as model sources of ideas for understanding how the degrees of freedom of the body are co-ordinated and controlled. The major candidates are machines in which control is effected through a pre-established arrangement among component parts (here termed 'cybernetic machines') and machines in which control is effected through a pre-established arrangement among specific instructions (here termed 'algorithmic machines').

The artifactual or machine conception (see von Bertalanffy, 1973; Kohler, 1969) has assumed in recent decades an unprecedented status as *the* perspective on order and regulation. This has been owing, in very large part, to the fact that the development of automata theory, information theory, and cybernetics has made secure the concept of machine in ways that appear on *prima facie* grounds to be of special relevance to the 'puzzles' of biology and psychology (see Berlinski, 1976). In automata theory the abstract mathematical notion of a machine was given an explicit reading by tying it to both recursive function theory and the digital computer. By this explicit reading, recalcitrant natural phenomena – such as the cognitive abilities of humans – could be viewed as analogous to machine capabilities and explainable in machine terms (Fodor, 1975; Minsky and Papert, 1972; Pylyshyn, 1980). The formal conception of information, as expressed by Shannon and Weaver (1949), gave a precise and mathematical way of describing communication situations. Moreover, the way in which information theory linked information with probability and with the physical concept of entropy gave it an air of great generality – a theory adaptable, in principle, to many systems and to many phenomena. Thus, in biology the egg-to-organism link could be likened to a communication channel; in principle, the information stored in the egg's nucleus, cytoplasm, and cortex that is eventually transmitted could be estimated (Elsasser, 1958; Raven, 1961). In psychology, stimuli, in principle, could be quantified for their information content and the perceiver's efficacy as a transmission channel, in principle, could be calculated (Attneave, 1959). The fixing of a biologically and psychologically useful conception of machine by automata theory and information theory was abetted by cybernetics which provided an understanding of machine behavior as goal-directed. Thus in biology and psychology the cybernetical closed-loop device that includes a constant reference input (the goal) and negative feedback is a commonplace explanation of conserved values (e.g. Adams, 1971; Powers, 1973, 1978; Riggs, 1970).

Despite the great popularity of the artifactual or machine perspective on order and regularity there are (we believe) good reasons to question its appropriateness. In subsequent sections arguments will be given against the propriety of formal automata theory and classical information theory for understanding motor development. It suffices for the present to question the propriety of the cybernetical closed-loop device for explaining relative stability in biology.

If it is claimed that an output variable of a system is relatively constant – for example, body temperature, respiratory frequency – because of the presence of a constant reference signal then is it not necessary to inquire, further, how it is that the constancy of the reference signal is assured? An infinite regress is enjoined if the latter question is answered – as surely it must be – by an appeal to another negative feedback system which has as its output the previously referred to referent signal and as its input another constant reference signal; for now a further negative feedback machine must be proposed to assure the constancy of this additional, higher order referent. A much better claim – or so we and others (e.g. Yates, 1981; Werner, 1977) would argue – is that any relative constancy in biological systems is an *emergent* and *distributed* property (a steady-state operating point) of physical processes. These processes are sometimes describable by a set of coupled equations whose various parameters, differentially weighted, contribute to achieving the constancy. With regard to temperature regulation Werner (1977) argues that heat flow equations must be calculated for all local co-ordinates; for all parts of the body the characteristic functions are to be found describing (i) metabolism's dependence on heat inflow and (ii) heat outflow's dependence on metabolism. Functions of type (i) are of negative slope while those of type (ii) are of positive slope. For a given body part the only steady-state possible – the only temperature – is that point which is mutual to the two characteristic functions. The gist of Werner's (1977) analysis is shared by Mitchell, Snellen, and Atkins (1970): so-called core temperature is an *a posteriori* fact not an *a priori* prescription.

Zavelishin and Tenenbaum (1968) provide an elegant empirical demonstration that the relative constancy of a given respiratory parameter may best be conceived as an *a posteriori* emergent fact of distributed, paired physical processes with opposite slopes in the relationships between their state variables. Zavelishin and Tenenbaum (1968) first determined the characteristic function relating the duration of inspiration ($D$) to the resistance to inspiration ($R$): $D = f_1(R)$. An artificial feedback relation was then imposed between $D$ and $R$: $R = f_2(D)$. Following the introduction of the artificial feedback link the duration of inspiration underwent variation – driven by the coupled equations – until it achieved a steady state (or steady states) represented by the point (or points) mutual to $D = f_1(R)$ and $R = f_2(D)$.

Further considerations underscore our impression that the negative feedback device with constant reference input has been overvalued. As an example of regulation, the steam escape valve on a common kitchen pressure cooker can be formally analyzed in terms of feedback, referent signal, comparison, etc. Yet to take these terms seriously would be a mistake; they do not stand for anything explicit (Yates, 1980). The regulation band of the pressure cooker is determined by its various parameters (for example, the weight of its stop valve) just as the equilibrium point of a simple mass-spring system is determined by the parameters of mass, stiffness, and friction. To impute to a mass-spring system a reference signal, a feedback loop, a comparator, an error-correcting device and the like would be to impute fictitious entities (Fowler *et al.*, 1980; Kelso *et al.*, 1980; Kugler and Turvey, 1979).

At the heart of these latter considerations is the constrast between order (specifically, an index of stability such as the value of body temperature) as an *a priori* explicit prescription that exists independent of and *causally antecedent* to the dynamical behavior of a system and order as an *a posteriori* fact that arises dependent on and *adjunctively consequent* to (see Shaw and McIntyre, 1974; Turvey and Shaw, 1979) the dynamical behavior of a system. This contrast flags an entry point into the other perspective on order and regulation. In this other perspective, which can be termed 'natural,' the focus is order as a (necessary) *a posteriori* fact. We will make the eccentric claim that the natural perspective is grounded in two necessarily coupled themes: *The proprietary (explanatory) principles of physical theory, with their underscoring of tendencies in dynamics, and the proprietary (ontological and epistemological) tenets of ecological realism.* Because it is the natural (rather than the artifactual) perspective that we take to be proper for the present concerns – viz., moving towards a solution to the problem of degrees of freedom that is consonant with the facts of growth – a large part of what follows is devoted to spelling out in some detail what the two coupled themes of this perspective entail. Initially however, our focus is the artifactual perspective, particularly the concept of information that it inspires.

## 2 INFORMATION AND GROWTH: THE ARTIFACTUAL PERSPECTIVE

The issues raised in Section 1.2 can be reworded as follows: how can the body's degrees of freedom be consistently regulated when the magnitude of the body's dimensions change naturally and artifically? Or, what is the informational base for systematically constraining the body's degrees of freedom and how is that informational base co-ordinated with changes in the body's dimensions?

The artifactual perspective encourages a view of the central nervous system as logically distinct from the skeleton and the musculature. According to this dualism the central nervous system is the source of the signals that inform the skeletomuscular dynamics and it is the site of the information on which such signals are based. If the cybernetical machine is the model then the signals controlling skeletomuscular dynamics derive from reference values or set points; if the algorithmic machine is the model then the signals controlling skeletomuscular dynamics derive from stored rules or programs. In the present section we identify an influential argument for holding information and dynamics distinct; and we consider two generalized conceptions of information that are popular in the artifactual perspective – the linguistic conception and the information theoretic conception – in terms of their relevance to the questions posed above. To anticipate, we express reservations about some steps in the argument and about the general propriety of these two characteristics of information.

### 2.1 The Complementarity of Information and Dynamics

Pattee (1977) provides a view of autonomous complex systems as operating in two complementary modes, the dynamical and the informational or linguistic modes. While there is more than one reading to be given to complementarity there is a potentially significant reading with regard to our present purposes that should be underscored, viz., that the complementarity of information and dynamics is a design requirement of complex systems (Rosen, 1973; Pattee, 1977). This reading is intended to contrast with an interpretation that is commonly ascribed to the complementarity principle in quantum mechanics – that complementarity, continuous as it is with the uncertainty principle, follows from, and gives name to, a technical impossibility. (In standard terms, that of at once precisely locating the position and measuring the velocity of an elementary particle.) The point underscored here is that, with regard to the science of complex systems, the putative complementarity of information and dynamics is seen not as a methodological failing but as an ontological fact.

The reasoning behind the complementarity of informational and dynamical modes is roughly as follows (see Pattee, 1972a, b, 1973, 1977):

1. The microscopic degrees of freedom of all systems, inanimate and animate, abide by the laws of motion and change, that is, dynamical laws.
2. To harness these laws to produce specific and reliable macroscopic functions requires constraints which selectively reduce degrees of freedom.
3. Constraints with relaxation times that are relatively long in comparison to the phenomena of interest may be termed structural: they are said permanently to freeze-out degrees of freedom. Constraints with relaxation times that are relatively short in comparison to the phenomena of interest may be termed functional: they are said effectively to select one trajectory from among the virtual trajectories that a system might exhibit. The latter type of constraint is a control constraint and it is the one of major interest.
4. Unlike the dynamical laws which are expressible as functions of rate, i.e. as derivatives of some variable with respect to time, the constraints that harness these laws are rate-independent. This is the fundamental incompatibility of laws and constraints qua rules.
5. Constraints are unlike dynamical laws in two other ways: they must have a specific material embodiment (laws are incorporeal) and they are local (laws are universal).
6. Because the microscopic degrees of freedom of the physical embodiment of a constraint must abide by the laws of dynamics, the details of their individual motions must be completely determined. Therefore, the only sensible interpretation of a constraint is that it is an alternative description of the behavior of the individual degrees of freedom.
7. Synonymously, a constraint is a classification of the microscopic degrees of freedom; it is a reduced, less detailed description. Being less detailed it is less complex and therein lies its utility: in terms of control a constraint is simple and efficient because it makes the fullest use of the dynamical context without being a description of that context.
8. Constraints are not only extremely simple with respect to the dynamics that they control but the structure of their physical embodiment has no

direct relationship to those dynamics just as the structure of a written injunction (say, STOP) has no direct relationship to the structure of the activities that it might be associated with. Constraints are therefore like symbols – they are arbitrary with respect to that which they signify.

9. Being arbitrary and just symbol vehicles, individual control constraints assume definite meaning only in the context of a system of constraints. This is tantamount to saying that a co-ordination of symbols – a generalized language structure or syntax – defines the informational basis for the control of dynamical processes.

10. There are, therefore, two descriptions of a complex system. One description is of the system's states of affairs as infinite, continuous and rate-dependent (the dynamical description) and the other description is of the system's states of affairs as finite, discrete and rate-independent (the informational or linguistic description). These two descriptions are incompatible but complementary.

## 2.2   The (quasi) Linguistic View of Information

There are two features of the foregoing argument on which we wish to focus: (i) that the proprietary conception of information is (quasi) linguistic; and (ii) that the linguistic mode and the dynamical mode, information and action, are arbitrarily related and logically independent in the significant sense that the structure of either one does not determine (or only weakly determines) the structure of the other.

We may suppose, therefore, from the artifactual perspective that the information base for the control and co-ordination of movement is a language of some kind; and pursuing the questions which introduced this section we can ask whether (given feature (ii) above) the information base so construed can change co-ordinately with changes in skeletomuscular dynamics wrought by changes in the magnitudes of skeletomuscular dimensions. While a definitive answer is not possible, there are strong hints that the answer, when forthcoming, will be negative.

Consider the issue of self-complexing (Apter, 1966): can an information base that is conceived as an internal language become richer in the course of development in the sense that qualitatively distinct predicate types can be added? For the newborn infant to behave any way other than convulsively means that constraints are present at the outset and, as we saw from the argument of 2.1 above, constraints are interpretable as symbols co-ordinated by a grammar. That is, constraints, in the above view, constitute an internal language understood at the very least as a representational medium of predicates and their extensions. If the central nervous system (as the information base and source of controlling signals) and the high-powered, energy-converting skeletomuscular apparatus (as the dynamics to be controlled) are logically independent then some procedure is needed to mediate or co-ordinate the two; the information base must be apprised of the dynamical details of movement. In so far as the dualism of central nervous system and skeletomuscular system is a variant of the dualism of animal and environment (see Turvey and Shaw, 1979 and 4.1 below) then we might expect that procedures logically equivalent to those proposed to mediate an animal's perception of its environment can be proposed to mediate the body's (qua central nervous system) perception of its dynamics (qua activities of the skeletomuscular system). This line of argument suggests that the procedure mediating information base and dynamics is most likely a form of projecting and evaluating hypotheses, for that has been the most popular and the most generally agreed upon contention (e.g. Fodor, 1975; Gregory, 1974; Helmholtz, 1925; Rock, 1975).

It can be ably argued however (e.g. Fodor, 1975) that a hypothesis-testing procedure *cannot give rise to new predicate types*. The general argument, roughly speaking, is that any system whose present competence is defined by a 'logic' of a certain representational power cannot progress, *through the mediary of formal logical operations* (such as forming and evaluating hypotheses), to a higher degree of competence. A hypothesis is a logical formula as is the evidence for its evaluation, and both formulae must be couched in the predicates of the system's internal language. Thus an informational base construed linguistically is closed to complexity; it cannot increase its expressive power, that is, it cannot come to represent more dynamical states of affairs than it can currently represent although it can come to mark off those dynamical states of affairs that do in fact obtain from those that do not.

We see, in short, that information construed linguistically can change co-ordinately with dynamical states of affairs under the condition that the language's power to characterize dynamical states of affairs always encompasses whatever (pragmatically relevant) states of affairs might arise. If it is the case that the set of dynamical states of affairs is open to complexity, unlike the information base, then it will be necessary to include in the information base predicates that are of no use in the present but will be of use in the future. That is, the information base will have to exhibit preadaptive foresight; it will have to include predicates to be used for representing dynamical states of affairs (of a higher order complexity) that are not yet extant.

By way of summary, we have given consideration to the construal of information as language-like and as logically independent from dynamics, and we have looked to the information base and the logical operations that feed upon it as the primary mechanism of development. The upshot of the argument sketched above is that under the foregoing construal of information, the order of complexity a system can achieve is determined by, and identical with the order of complexity with which it began.

## 2.3    The Information-Theoretic View of Information

How fares the classical interpretation of information (Shannon and Weaver, 1949) when extended beyond the narrow problems of communication channels (for which it was designed) to issues of growth and development? A basic result of information theory is that in a closed system in which nothing enters from the surrounding medium – that is, a communication system of source, channel, and receiver that is secured against extraneous signals – the information content of the receiver cannot exceed that of the source. Information (in the information theory sense) cannot be gained. It is true, of course, that information (in the information theory sense) can be changed, as the dots and dashes of the Morse code can be transcribed into the letters of the alphabet. But, importantly, there is change neither in the quantity of the information nor in what it signifies.

Consider a notorious application of the information-theoretic view of information to biology. Raven's (1961) theory of oogenesis addresses the relationship between generations of organisms that are connected by sexual reproduction; to be more precise, it addresses the fact that the ordered structure of the parents is repeated in their offspring. The basic assumption of Raven's theory is that the orderly spatiotemporal patterns, in terms of which the elementary parts and processes are configured from one generation to the next, are based on a transmission of detailed information conventionally measured in *bits*. In such a communication system the sex cells and the fertilized egg cell produced by their union are parts of the communication channel; the parents are the source and the individual arising from the egg is the destination of the information transmitted. Considered in these terms the formation of the egg involves the encoding of information, and development is essentially a process in which this information is decoded. In short, the ordered structure, the encoded pattern of the fertilized egg, faithfully represents specific information concerning the morphology of the organism that develops from the egg. Oogenesis, therefore, advocates a strong preformationist claim that the information content of the mature organism must be wholly contained in the chemical structure of the genes – it is extracted during growth to guide the dynamics of morphogenesis.

This general thesis, that the development of organismic form (the emergence of phenotype from genotype) is *not* a gain of information, seems intuitively nonsensical to most (e.g. Waddington, 1968) and constitutes one good motivation for the abandonment by biology of the information-theoretic view of information (at least its quantitative aspects, see MacKay, 1969). Other reasons for the abandonment of the classical view of information that should be advanced follow from the mathematical and physical origins of the theory. Mathematically speaking, information theory is part of statistics and its concerns are primarily those of quantities and degrees of certainty. With regard to some state of affairs, an information-theoretic analysis reports on what that state of affairs is not, but might have been (cf. Gibson, 1966). Information in the information-theoretic sense reduces uncertainty – it is a metric by which a state of affairs $p$ is distinguished from other possible states of affairs, say, $q$ and $r$; it is not, however, and most importantly, a metric by which a state of affairs $p$ is specified. *In a closed system where the possible states of affairs are fixed and given a priori, the criterion of distinguishing is sufficient for a conception of information. In an open system where new states of affairs arise a criterion of specifying rather than discriminating must be pursued.*

In a similar vein, information theory's physical origins are not those of a potentially successful physical biology. Information theory is based on equilibrium-reversible thermodynamics, a physical theory which is mute on (indeed, without significant qualifications, contrary to) the facts of growth and development (see 3.0 below). Information as classically construed by Shannon and Weaver (1949) is a measure of probability in the terms of 'deviation from the state of entropy'. A system at entropy is assigned an information measure of zero and a thermodynamic probability of one; and deviations from entropy are associated with decreasing thermodynamic probability and increasing information.

## 2.4 Summary

In 2.1 the information mode and the dynamical mode were distinguished as rate-independent and rate-dependent, respectively. We can also add that, under either the (quasi) linguistic or information-theoretic construals, the information mode is further distinguished from the dynamical mode in that it is closed to complexity. The dynamical mode is most obviously open to complexity at the terrestrial scale and how it can be so is the main issue of irreversible non-equilibrium thermodynamics (Section 3.0).

We remarked at the outset of Section 2.0 that the contemporary form of the complementarity argument is agreeable to us in part but not in total. There is agreement with the claim that information (for control) can only be an alternative description of the dynamics; there is disagreement with the claim that this alternative description is symbolic, language-like and arbitrary with reference to the dynamics with which it is associated. To pursue and to abide by a definition of information in which information is closed is to run counter to an understanding of order as an *a posteriori* fact, that is, to run counter to the understanding that a large aggregation of atomistic particulars evolve toward decreasing entropy.

There is a distinction owing to Tomović (1978) that parallels the artifactual–natural distinction drawn above and that similarly expresses the qualms registered here with the direction of the relation between the informational and dynamical modes. Tomović (1978) refers to the conventional view of the relation of the informational mode to the dynamical mode as a direct plant–model relation where the model is derived from the plant by a logical process (of abstraction). The benchmark of a system abiding by this relation is that the products of the system may equal but not exceed the control potential contained in the initial algorithms: computers cannot outperform the control rules that govern their operation. The unconventional view of the relation of the informational mode to the dynamical mode is referred to by Tomovic (1978) as an inverse plant–model relation where the model arises from the plant by a dynamical process. the benchmark of a system abiding by this relation is that the products of the system necessarily exceed its initial control potential.

We are inclined to read these various considerations as follows: (i) a construal of information should be sought such that 'information' can be self-complexing; (ii) for the most general of cases the conception of information cannot be arbitrarily related to dynamics; and, relatedly, (iii) the predicates of information, when properly construed, ought to be dynamical in some sense of that word.

## 3    THE NATURAL PERSPECTIVE: PHYSICAL THEORY AND SYSTEMIC BEHAVIOR AT THE SCALE OF ECOLOGY

The problem of co-ordinating and controlling the body's many degrees of freedom consonant with the Principle of Similitude resides at the ecological scale. It is, therefore, a description of physical theory and systemic behavior at the ecological scale that we seek. The present part of the paper is intended to provide a historical overview of physical perspectives. Our intent will be to highlight the traditional tendency to select as primary a particular scale of physical reality from which to forge an understanding of the nature of 'causal dynamics' at all scales, and to identify the various philosophical attitudes that were deduced from particular physical perspectives. What follows is an identification of the philosophical perspective that we take to be proper for the ecological scale, a perspective that suggests significant constraints on physical theory as it bears on naturally developing systems.

### 3.1    Classical Mechanics

Between the sixteenth and nineteenth centuries physical science made significant advances concerning the laws governing motions of bodies through space at the scale of celestial activity. In particular, Galileo and Newton formulated laws making it possible to determine with precision the past and future states of certain mechanical systems. These laws formed the basis of *classical mechanics*. That these laws might be applicable to scales other than that of celestial activity gave rise to a scientific ideal that received its most celebrated expression in the writings of Laplace in the eighteenth century; namely, that it was possible to regard the behavior of any physical system as determined ultimately and completely by the laws of classical mechanics. Laplace's only requirement was that full knowledge be available, at any instant of time, of the composite forces and positions of the system. Given the composite force configuration, all future and past events could be completely determined merely by applying the laws of mechanics. Laplace's argument was the classical foundation of the so-called mechanistic perspective on natural phenomena (cf. Bohm, 1957). The working hypothesis of mechanism stated that ultimately any set of phenomena could be reduced, completely and unconditionally, to nothing more than the effects of some definite and bounded set of *fixed* laws which *determined* completely and precisely the phenomena. The conclusion drawn from the hypothesis was that systemic behavior on any scale of analysis and under any set of conditions could be determined, requiring only the specification of a set of initial and boundary conditions.

According to the Laplacian philosophy of mechanism, each and every system behaves in a determinate manner indifferent to its complexity. The degree of systemic complexity was not a factor to be considered in applying the philosophy; more importantly, perhaps, the Laplacian mechanistic stance does not refer to any means by which complexity can be fashioned. Laplacian mechanism does not address issues of complexity; rather it addresses issues of state transitions where the successive states are equivalent in complexity. Laplacian mechanism does not provide any means by which the system can change its degree of order and, therefore, the development of new order is outside the purview of a mechanistic philosophy.

### 3.2   Statistical and Quantum Mechanics

During the prior and present century, the view of classical mechanics was profoundly altered by the increasingly apparent confirmation of atomic theory. Whereas representation of macro-physical qualities of classical mechanics was by a *continuous* function of space $x$ and time $t$, $B(x, t)$, kinetic atomistic theory considered matter and energy as collections of a huge number of *discrete* particles moving under the influence of mutual forces and it represented the micro-physical qualities by functions on the phase-space co-ordinates $(q_1, \ldots, q_n, p_1 \ldots, p_n) = (q, p)$ and on the parameters $x$ and $t$: $b(q, p; x, t)$. Moreover, whereas the behavior of systems on the macro scale of classical mechanics could be continuously and *determinately* specified, the behavior of systems on the micro scale of quantum mechanics had a fundamentaly discrete and *statistical* character associated with it. The nature of this statistical character is duly expressed first by mean free path, relaxation time relations in the 19th century and in the Heisenberg uncertainty relations in the 20th century. Even if the maximum possible information about the state of the system is available, only statistical predictions about the values of the observables are possible. According to these discrete formulations of the uncertainty relations, the function defining the phase space $(q_1, \ldots, q_n, p_1, \ldots p_n)$ could have only a statistical distribution associated with it, leading to a probabilistic description of the activity of individual particles.

A statistical description of a dynamical many-body system can be represented as a collection of points in phase space, each point being weighted by a certain number. The total collection of weighted points defines the probability distribution and is termed an *ensemble*. Put simply, an ensemble is a discrete set of atomistic particulars standing in a continuous interrelation, where the interrelation is described by a distribution function. The observed value of a dynamical function, both local and in a more extended sense, is identified with the ensemble average of the microscopic function.

It became apparent by the twentieth century that the laws of quantum mechanics provided a precise description of micro behavior at the atomic or molecular state, and that the laws of classical mechanics provided a sufficiently accurate description of behavior at the macroscopic scale. The strikingly different character of behavior at these two scales, however, underlined the need for an explanation of the laws of continuous macro-physics as a consequence of the microscopic evolution of motion of matter as ensembles of discrete particles. A bridge between the two scales was proposed in the form of statistical mechanics.

Statistical mechanics established a formal link between the microscopic dynamical functions $b(q, p; x, t)$ and the macroscopic dynamical functions $B(x, t)$. It postulated the existence of a unique mapping correspondence between the microscopic phase space and the macroscopic state space:

$$b(q, p; x, t) \to B(x, t)$$

According to the postulate at any point in time the 'state' of a system was determined by a distribution function $F(q, p)$ satisfying

$$\int dq\, dp\, F(q, p) = 1$$

The observable value $B(x, t)$ of a dynamical function $b(q, p; x, t)$ in a system was given by

$$B(x, t) \langle b \rangle = \int dq\, dp\, b\, (q, p; x, t) = F(q, p)$$

By adding the extra condition $F(q, p) \geqslant 0$, $F(q, p)$ could be interpreted as the probability density for finding the system at the point $q, p$ in phase space. Since the probability is postulated to be positive, $F(q, p) \geqslant 0$, the system's state is guaranteed to be somewhere in the phase space. The concept of state of the system is such that at time $t$, every point in the phase space represents a possible configuration of the system where each point is weighted by a value $F(q, p)$ of the distribution function (see Balescu, 1975 for a more complete analysis of statistical mechanics).

Statistical mechanics however proves to be a less than ideal bridge between the two scales. The mapping function from the micro phase space into the macro state space, $b(q, p) \to B$, specifies the existence of a unique correspondence in the direction of the micro-physical to the macro-physical. The mapping states that 'to every $b(q, p)$ there corresponds one and only one $B$.' The reverse of this statement, however, is *not* true. The statement 'to every $B$ there corresponds one and only one $b(q, p)$' is *false*. The reason for this is that not all macroscopic qualities can be expressed in the form of an average of a dynamical function weighted with a distribution function, $F$.

In short, there is a one to many mapping from micro to macro and a many to one from macro to micro. In physical theory it is common that the set of macroscopic qualities is subdivided into two classes: the *mechanical* qualities, of the above form, and the *thermal* qualities, of a different form. The thermal qualities are typical of thermodynamics and are not treated by single particle analysis. It is difficult to assign certain qualities – such as temperature – any microscopic meaning. They generally are conceived of only at the macroscopic scale. For example, one speaks of the energy (that is, a mechanical quality of motion) of a single molecule, but one does not speak of the temperature of a single molecule. With this limitation, one defines these thermal qualities (such as temperature, entropy, etc.) entirely in terms of properties of the ensemble distribution, rather than as averages of single-particle properties. These are examples of *collective* properties whose values are determined by the overall distribution of all the particles in the system. The importance of the relationship between the mechanical and thermal properties will be discussed in the next section (on thermodynamics). Before proceeding, however, let us consider the role played by quantum principles in motivating philosophic attitudes.

The assertion of the statistical nature of quantum mechanics rested on two assumptions: the first one originated in Heisenberg's Uncertainty Principle; the second, following from uncertainty, eliminated the possibility of any precise identification of the initial state of a many-body system. Extending those assumptions, Heisenberg postulated the existence of a formal relationship between quantum mechanics and philosophy. Using the strong form of the law of causality, viz., that 'the exact knowledge of the present allows the future to be calculated,' Heisenberg noted that 'it is not the conclusion that is false but the hypothesis that is false' (cited in Jammer, 1974, p. 75). The uncertainty principle, by ruling out determination of an exact initial condition, eliminates the possibility of exact prediction of future events. Heisenberg concluded that 'since all experiments obey the quantum law and, consequently the indeterminacy relations, the incorrectness of the law of causality is a definitely established consequence of quantum mechanics itself' (p. 75). In short, Heisenberg was promoting a philosophic attitude of *indeterminacy*. Not even a Laplacian superbeing (capable of measuring a system and obtaining information about it without disturbing it) could make precise predictions about a system's future.

A second philosophic attitude arose from the problem of measurement associated with Heisenberg's uncertainty principle: the position and momentum of a particle cannot be determined simultaneously with arbitrary precision. The smaller the error committed in the measurement of momentum, the larger the uncertainty of the position (and vice versa). Most outspoken on this issue was Bohr who in 1927 noted that:

> the definition of the state of a physical system, as ordinarily understood, claims the elimination of all external disturbances. But in that case, according to the quantum postulate, any observation will be impossible, and above all, the concept of space and time lose their immediate sense. On the other hand, if in order to make observation possible we permit certain interactions with suitable agencies of measurement, not belonging to the system, an unambiguous definition of the state of the system is naturally no longer possible, and there can be no question of causality in the ordinary sense of the word. The very nature of the quantum theory thus forces us to regard the space–time co-ordination and the claim of causality, the union of which characterizes the classical theories, as complementary but exclusive features of the description, symbolizing the idealization of observation and definition respectively (cited in Jammer, 1974, p. 87).

According to Bohr, 'space–time co-ordination' and 'causality' are related in a complementary manner on the quantum scale, an interpretation which has come to be known as the 'complementarity interpretation' or 'Copenhagen interpretation' of quantum mechanics (cf. Jammer, 1974, for an excellent account of the entire history of quantum mechanics). We outlined a contemporary version of the Copenhagen interpretation and its bearing on the character of complex systems in 2.1 above.

### 3.3    Classical Equilibrium Reversible Thermodynamics

Within the past hundred years it has become increasingly apparent that at a scale greater than that of the quantum scale and less than that of the celestial scale, certain conditions reveal a dramatically different view of 'causal dynamics.' It is at this scale that variations in thermal flows such as entropy become sufficiently prominent so as to compete with the classically defined mechanical forces such as gravitational (where mass is above a critical level) and electrostatic (where mass is below a critical level). The result of these competing 'flows' and 'forces' is the possibility that the state of the system can systematically 'increase' its order. Thus, the second law of thermodynamics, viz. the principle of increasing entropy, which is prescriptive of *disorder* at the celestial and quantum scale can nevertheless be prescriptive of *order* when certain conditions on the law, such as those found terrestrially, prevail. An understanding of this significant fact rests on an analysis of the conditions that raise and lower thermal flows. The beginning of such an analysis is provided by thermodynamics.

Thermodynamics deals with the transactions of various forms of energy in all of its possible forms. Thermodynamics does so by describing a system in terms of concepts and laws derived from the study of macroscopic phenomena such as pressure, volume, temperature, concentrations, etc. The boundary of such a system is a mathematical surface which separates an exterior or surrounding system from an interior system. Using these guidelines any physical or chemical system can be described as a thermodynamic system.

Thermodynamic system properties are subdivided according to the exchanges of energy (heat and work) and matter through their boundaries. A system can be classified as an *isolated* system when it exchanges neither energy nor matter with its surroundings. An example of an isolated system is a coffee thermos; once the coffee is poured into the thermos and the thermos is sealed no further heat is added. Strictly speaking, however, it is not a real isolated system because it eventually loses (exchanges) heat to its environment (see Figure 1). A second system is classified as *closed* when it exchanges energy but

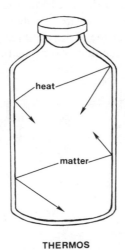

**THERMOS**

FIGURE 1    *Isolated system:* heat and matter cannot leave or
enter the system

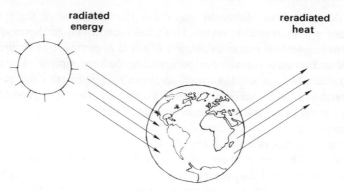

FIGURE 2 *Closed system:* matter cannot cross the boundary but energy can be exchanged across the boundary

not matter with its surroundings. The earth may be viewed as an example of a closed system insofar as it does not receive nor expel significant amounts of matter (the amounts lost into space or gained through meteorite fall, etc. are negligible). It does exchange energy, as heat is both received from and reradiated into outer space (see Figure 2).

Finally, a third system is classified as *open* when it exchanges *both* energy and matter with its surroundings. A biological cell is an example of an open system. Both energy and matter can be exchanged with the cell's surroundings through the cell membrane. The cell's membrane is differentially permeable allowing only certain substances to enter and leave the system (see Figure 3).

Classical thermodynamics originated from a few empirical observations on the behavior of (in principle) isolated systems. These observations were organized and axiomatized in the form of 'three laws.' For our present concerns we need consider only the first two of the three laws. The first law is the

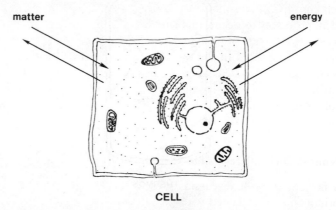

FIGURE 3 *Open system:* both matter and energy pass through the boundaries

law of conservation of energy: in all macroscopic chemical and physical processes, energy is neither created nor destroyed but merely transformed from one form to another. For example, while energy may be transformed (as in the case of a chemical form to a mechanical form in an internal combustion engine) there must exist a *conservative* quantitative correspondence between the different kinds of energy.

The second law of thermodynamics (in one of many equivalent forms) states that: any spontaneous process results in an increase in the disorder of the system plus its surroundings. This law provides a criterion for predicting the temporal *direction* of a given process. First, it recognizes a measure of state or condition of matter and energy called entropy, which can be defined or identified with randomness or disorder. Second, it states that all physical and chemical processes proceed in a direction such that the randomness or entropy of the universe – the system plus its surroundings – increases to a maximum possible; when the local ensemble can no longer undergo any such change, then at this point there is local *equilibrium*. According to the second law no process can occur which results in a decrease in the entropy of the universe. The law predicts destruction of local regions of inhomogeneity of molecular configurations and a tendency to establish uniformity. In short, systems tend to approach equilibrium states in which temperature, pressure, and other measurable parameters of state become locally uniform throughout. Once at equilibrium there is no tendency to spontaneously change back to nonuniform or nonrandom states.

Theoretically the entropy of a system may also remain *constant* during a process, and when it does such a process is defined as being *reversible*. In a reversible process the path described by the process passes through an infinite succession of intermediate states all of which are at equilibrium. While reversible processes are theoretically possible, completely reversible processes in which entropy remains constant are rare physical occurrences. In order for such ideal processes to occur, time would have to approach infinity to provide the necessary slow rate of change. Because of this, time as a variable does not enter into the formalism of the two classical laws. The laws deal strictly with energy changes as a system assumes new equilibrium states. Due to the time independent nature of these laws it has been argued that they should be termed laws of 'thermostatics' rather than thermodynamics (Bridgman, 1941; DeGroot and Mazur, 1962; Iberall, 1978).

### 3.4  Nonequilibrium Irreversible Thermodynamics: The Linear Range

Let us now extend our discussion of thermodynamics beyond the reversible equilibrium states associated with locally isolated systems, and into the nonequilibrium irreversible states associated with open and closed systems. In the previous section we noted that the second law of thermodynamics postulates the existence of a state function – the entropy function – and the tendency of the function to increase monotonically until it reaches its maximum at thermodynamic equilibrium. Using the concept of change in entropy, $dS$, during a time $dt$ we can distinguish between two types of processes: reversible and irreversible. Reversible processes are defined as those processes in which entropy changes are zero. In contrast, irreversible processes are defined as those processes in which entropy changes are always greater than zero. More specifically, irreversible processes are defined on the basis of the properties of the state function, $S$, in terms of the rate of dissipation per unit time, the so-called *entropy production*.

Consider a system *open* to the exchange of energy and matter with its surroundings. The entropy change during a time interval $dt$ may be decomposed as follows (Prigogine, 1947, 1967; Glansdorff and Prigogine, 1971):

$$dS = d_e S + d_i S$$

with

$$d_i S \geqslant 0$$

where $d_e S$ is the flow of entropy due to exchange with the surroundings and $d_i S$ is the entropy production inside the system due to irreversible processes (see Figure 4). According to the second law of thermodynamics $d_i S$ must equal zero for reversible (or equilibrium) processes and be positive for irreversible (or nonequilibrium) processes. For an isolated system, where the flow of entropy between systems is ruled out, the state entropy function reduces to:

$$dS = d_i S \geqslant 0 \quad \text{(isolated system)}$$

The inequality indicates that the entropy production for an isolated system will tend irreversibly to an equilibrium state where $d_i S = d_e S = 0$. The behavior of an isolated system is, therefore, always defined with reference to the second law of thermodynamics, namely, the state entropy function.

Consider, for example, a gas in an initial state where a certain degree of order has been imposed, such as confining it to one half of a container by a partition. And consider further that the system is isolated from the exchange of matter or energy with its surrounds. If the partition is now removed, the gas will rapidly tend to occupy the entire volume and reduce the initial order as

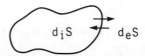

FIGURE 4    Entropy flow ($d_e S$) entropy and entropy production ($d_i S$) in an open system

defined by the second law. In this regard the process irreversibly tends to a state of equilibrium whereby once at equilibrium the inverse process cannot spontaneously occur. Thus once equilibrium is achieved time-dependent reversible processes begin which are stable with respect to disturbances. The behavior of an isolated system may be characterized by a tendency for the state entropy function to increase monotonically until it reaches a maximum at thermodynamic equilibrium. *The spontaneous formation of ordered structures is therefore ruled out for isolated systems.*

Consider next a closed system that is at equilibrium but which can exchange energy (but not matter) with its surroundings. Let the surroundings be at a certain constant temperature. This situation is similar to the isolated condition except that the state function $S$ is not the sole determinant of the resulting behavior, there is an additional state function to be considered, the Helmholtz free energy, $F$, defined by:

$$F = E - TS \quad \text{(closed system)}$$

where $E$ is the energy of the system and $T$ is the absolute temperature (in degrees Kelvin). Whatever configuration an isolated system assumes results from a competition between energy and entropy. At a sufficiently low temperature, energy becomes the dominant factor in the competition with entropy and the isolated system assumes a configuration favoring a minimum of potential energy. In this case the entropy contribution is small compared to that of free energy. At increasing temperatures, however, an isolated system graduates to structures of increasingly higher entropy. Since Boltzmann first identified the shifting outcome of the competition between energy and entropy as a function of temperature in the Boltzmann factor, $\exp(-E/kT)$, an increase in entropy with increasing temperature is termed the *Boltzmann ordering principle* (cf. Nicolis and Prigogine, 1977). The competition at the microscopic scale appears macroscopically in the form of phase transitions, ferromagnetism, etc. The Boltzmann ordering principle prescribes that below a certain critical value of the temperature gradient, microscopic fluctuations due to entropic tendencies are damped and disappear. Thus in equilibrium phase transitions, order arises from the elimination of fluctuation. For example, the gradual elimination of molecular agitation defines the transition from gas (least ordered) to liquid, to ice (most ordered) in the phase changes of water. In sum, Boltzmann's principle provides a primitive means for understanding how order might originate. However, the principle's excessive dependency on (decreased) temperature for the origin of structure strictly curtails its generalizability to biological order.

Classical thermodynamics deals with the equilibrium conditions described above in which the entropy production term goes to zero. We now turn to an analysis of nonequilibrium conditions in which the entropy production term becomes a critical factor. Before extending our analysis to nonequilibrium conditions however, one assumption must be made concerning macroscopic properties such as entropy and thermal flows. It is assumed that the macroscopic properties can be described in terms of a limited number of *local* variables and that these variables continue to relate in the manner that they relate in equilibrium conditions. The validity of the *local equilibrium* description has been investigated extensively starting most notably with Maxwell's kinetic theory of gases. The theory of local equilibrium was advanced historically by way of initial arguments by Boltzmann, with sharp tests provided by Helmholtz and Kirchoff, with codification of the reversible state provided by Gibbs, and the nature of the approach toward equilibrium provided by Boltzmann's H theorem (Chapman and Cowling, 1952; Tolman, 1938). The modern clarification of the *physics* of the linear law operating at local equilibrium was set forth by Onsager (1931). More recently its application has been opened for further discussion, in the theoretical case, by Prigogine and his colleagues (Prigogine, 1947; Nicolis and Prigogine, 1977) and been shown to hold true for conditions near equilibrium. In essence, the validity of the local equilibrium assumption implies that collisional effects are sufficient to *damp* deviations from a steady nonequilibrium state condition (that is to treat the approach toward equilibrium as a linear transport conductance).

Deviations from equilibrium that assume a degree of stability, so-called steady states, are maintained by virtue of *entropy production*. As noted earlier, the total entropy production $dS$ can be decomposed into an entropy flow ($d_eS$) exchanged with the environment and an entropy production ($d_iS$) due to the irreversible processes. The explicit evaluation of the entropy production is described by the following balance equation:

$$P[s] = \frac{d_iS}{dt} = \int dV J_p X_p = \int dV \geqslant 0 \tag{1}$$

where the sign of $d_iS$ is derived from the second law of thermodynamics. The $J_p$s and $X_p$s are, respectively, the conjugate thermodynamic flows and forces of the irreversible processes. It is necessary to understand how the *kinematic* rates of flow ($J_p$), which are in principle unknown quantities, are related to the *dynamic* forces ($X_p$), which are known functions of the composite variables. We begin with the equilibrium condition.

At equilibrium both the flows ($J_p$s) and forces ($X_p$s) vanish

$$\begin{aligned} J_p &= 0 \\ X_p &= 0 \end{aligned} \quad \text{(at equilibrium)}$$

and entropy production goes to zero

$P[s] = 0$ (reversible process connecting two equilibrium states)

$P[s] \geqslant 0$ (irreversible process producing entropy)

For conditions near equilibrium the $J_p$s behave as a *linear* function of the $X_p$s and equation (1) becomes quadratic (Glansdorff and Prigogine, 1971). This argument is based generally on Onsager's reciprocal relationships (1931). In this regard Prigogne (1947, 1967) has shown that when processes do not deviate far from equilibrium and when boundary conditions remain time-independent, *a steady-state condition is specified by the minimum of the entropy production function*. This is known as the *theorem of minimum entropy production*. Under these *nonequilibrium* conditions the entropy production function acts in the same fashion as the state functions of entropy and free energy in the equilibrium conditions. Therefore, when a steady state occurs in near equilibrium conditions the system behaves with reference to the state entropy production function where the steady state is characterized by an extremum principle defining the minimum of the function (Prigogine, 1947; Glansdorff and Prigogine, 1971). Care should be taken not to confuse the steady nonequilibrium state with the equilibrium state that is characterized by a zero entropy production condition.

In terms of stability, the steady nonequilibrium state condition exhibits the same stable properties associated with the equilibrium condition with regard to disturbances. All local perturbations or fluctuations that deviate from the steady state are asymptotically damped back to the steady state by the entropic tendency of irreversible processes. *Because of the asymptotic behavior around a single steady state the development of new and more complex order such as that manifest in biological development must be ruled out within the linear domain of the equilibrium condition*.

Before discussing a nonlinear domain which might potentially exist in far from equilibrium conditions, we summarize systemic behavior in the linear domain: all systems operating at near equilibrium conditions, independent of how complicated the reaction mechanisms are, respond to small deviations from an equilibrium or steady state with a fading or damping behavior which is *linearly* proportional to the magnitude of the deviation.

### 3.5 Nonequilibrium Irreversible Thermodynamics: The Nonlinear Range

A distinction must be made which is commonly passed over. There is a difference in the formal treatment of the mathematical nonlinearities at the macroscopic scale and the mathematical nonlinearities at the scale of local atomistic interactions. Whereas the macroscopic nonlinearities are recognized explicitly in the physical equations, the microscopic nonlinearities cannot be; rather they are captured, in the thermodynamic approximation, by macroscopic *linear* laws. Under the conditions of mathematical nonlinearities the possibility exists for the realization of a threshold beyond which the previous steady state becomes unstable in a mathematical sense and can be replaced by a new class of mathematical regimes having completely different spatial and temporal orderings. Such transformations have been studied in both hydrodynamics and in phase transitions. More recently, Prigogine, motivated by problems in chemically reactive fields, has also made contributions toward understanding these orderings. Prigogine has labeled the orderings *dissipative structures*. In what follows we will briefly describe an extension of thermodynamics to nonlinear ranges that has been advanced by Glansdorff and Prigogine (1971). The approach entails an extension of the theorem of minimum entropy production.

For thermodynamic processes within the linear range, variations in entropy production $dP/dt$ are always less than or equal to zero: $dP/dt \leqslant 0$. The equality refers to a steady-state situation and the inequality refers to irreversible processes tending towards a steady state. When the steady state occurs near equilibrium, the behavior is characterized according to the extremum principle of minimum entropy production. For states far away from equilibrium, the inequality $dP/dt$ may break down such that no extended inequality can be found that would guarantee the stability of a steady state. In fact Glansdorff and Prigogine (1971) have shown that beyond the linear range, $dP/dt$ does not exhibit any inequality which would guarantee the stability of a steady state. While no singular point of stability could be found in the entropy production function, Glansdorff and Prigogine (1971) derived an alternative state function which revealed potential stability points. The new state function was termed *excess entropy production* and was expressed by the following equation:

$$1/2\delta^2 P = \int dV\, \delta J_p\, \delta X_p \geqslant 0 \qquad (2)$$

Here $J_p$, $X_p$ are the *excess* flows and forces resulting from deviations of the system from a stable state. Deviation can result from either random or systematic disturbances acting on the system. For states close to equilibrium $1/2\delta^2 P$ behaves as a quadratic function exhibiting a positive value specifying a stable state. However, for states far from equilibrium this need not be the case. Instead, the excess entropy production can approach zero, creating a marginal state of stability in which a 'sudden' transition occurs moving the system from a previously stable state to an instability. The instability results in the system's *amplification* of its fluctuations which drive the system to a new spatiotemporal ordering. In contrast to equilibrium and steady-state conditions, where fluctuations are asymptotically damped, the above instability results in an amplification of the fluctuations which ultimately reach a macroscopic level and finally stabilize to a new regime. These symmetry-breaking instabilities are of interest since they reveal a means by which the system spontaneously self-organizes in a stable fashion.

It is important to note that the excess entropy production inequality applies not only to the nonlinear range, but also to the linear range, where it becomes equivalent to the theorem of minimum entropy production. Because of the generality, the inequality has been called a *universal evolution criterion* (cf. Glansdorff and Prigogine, 1971). In short, the above inequality provides a thermodynamic criterion for all nonequilibrium states. In regions near equilibrium, the inequality is always satisfied with a positive value. For regions far from equilibrium, the inequality may approach zero, creating an instability, and may ultimately move the system to a new spatiotemporal ordering. In other words, as a system is driven further away from equilibrium, a single solution can 'branch' into several possible solutions, and each of these, in turn, may branch still further from equilibrium. The branches are referred to as *thermodynamic branches* and are similar to the 'bifurcations' or 'catastrophes' described by Thom (1975; and Section 4 below; see also Nicolis and Auchmuty, 1974, for a discussion of how the two concepts differ).

A variety of dynamic regimes may result from the thermodynamic branching surrounding the conditions of a dissipative structure: (i) the systemic behavior may consist of sustained multiple steady states with systematic transitions from one to another; (ii) the systemic behavior may be a rotation on a 'limit' cycle around an unstable singular point, resulting in stable oscillation (several limit cycles are possible); or (iii) the systemic behavior may be a sustained oscillation resulting in waves. Several examples will suffice to demonstrate the manifestation of these instabilities in nature.

The Bénard or convection instability is realized in a situation in which a fluid layer is heated from below and kept at a fixed temperature above so as to create a temperature gradient in opposition to the effects of gravitational force. At small values (within the linear range) of this gradient, heat is transported from lower to upper regions by conduction and macroscopic motion is absent. Random thermal motions of the molecules and a damping of convection currents characterize the state of the fluid. However, when the gradient exceeds a critical value (passes into the nonlinear range) a convective, macroscopic motion occurs generally in the form of rolls or hexagons (for variations see Koschmeider, 1975, 1977). In short, out of an initial state that is completely homogeneous, there arises a well-ordered spatial pattern. Moreover, with further increases in the gradient the spatial pattern becomes oscillatory.

The Taylor instability, similarly a fluid phenomenon, is manifest in a situation in which water is enclosed between two cylinders that can be rotated in opposite directions. At rotation speeds below a critical value (within the linear range) the fluid flow is laminar; above that value (in the nonlinear range) the flow becomes turbulent, progressing toward stable, organized vortices.

The solid-state laser provides a further example. Energy is pumped into a rod of material in which specific atoms are embedded, and at the two endfaces of which mirrors are positioned. At small energy fluxes (within the linear range) the laser operates as a lamp – the atoms emit light wavetracks independently of each other. When the energy flux exceeds a critical value (passes into the non-linear range), all the atoms oscillate in phase emitting a single and very large wave track of light.

In these examples we see that by scaling-up parameters into nonlinear ranges macroscopic structure develops from a homogeneous state of affairs or from a state of affairs of lesser structure. The new stability that develops beyond a critical scale value may in turn give way to a further, different stability at higher scale values. At supercritical values (in both the Bénard and Taylor situations), periodic pulsing characterizes the newer stabilities that replace those that appear at the critical value. The critical scale value may be expressed in terms of dimensionless parameters, such as the Reynolds or Rayleigh numbers.

Let us consider a less familiar philosophic attitude that might be associated with the nonequilibrium-state situations referred to above. We noted that the behavior of dissipative structures is characterized by a tendency not to run down but rather to establish temporary steady-state regimes displaced from global equilibrium. Maintenance of the regimes is through a continual flow of free energy and matter into and out of the operational components of the system (cf. Iberall, 1977, 1978; Morowitz, 1978; Prigogine *et al.*, 1975). Of particular importance is the fact that these systems exhibit: (i) the ability to self-organize and (ii) the phenomenon of autonomy as exhibited by their ability to resist the traditionally dominant effects of initial and boundary conditions. Consider first the phenomenon of self-organization.

Self-organization occurs only under certain *open* conditions, where the amplification of fluctuation leads to an instability resulting in the emergence of a new thermodynamic branch. Symmetry is broken and new structures are formed out of the resulting instability. The new structures may possess new functions that correspond to a higher level of symmetry (interaction) between the system and its environment. The critical event in the symmetry-breaking instability is the realization of a scale change defined over the bifurcation parameters. The scale change is expressible in terms of a dimensionless number (see 1.2 above) such as the generalized Reynolds or Rayleigh numbers. During the scaling-up process there is no explicit *a priori* specification or representation of the new structure, which would remove such a phenomenon from the class of self-organizing systems. Indeed, the new structures arise as an *a posteriori* fact of the system through the act of drawing on a source of high free energy, passing it through the operational component parts of the system and finally dissipating the resulting heat into an external sink. Through amplification of the previously damped nonlinearities on the micro scale, new stabilities may result on the macro scale. Thus dissipative structures are said to exhibit the property of self-organizing or self-complexing: the systemic ability to develop a greater degree of order from a state of affairs of a lesser degree of order.

With respect to the phenomenon of autonomy, we will consider two related properties associated with it. First, dissipative structures exhibit a relative immunity to disturbances in initial and boundary conditions. Small deviations or perturbations in either of these conditions do not change the stable behavioral patterns of these structures. Indeed, the stability of dissipative systems is guaranteed by dimensions *intrinsic* to the system. More commonly this is known as *equifinality*. No longer are the system's dynamics causally linked in a determinate fashion to the system's environment. The system now exhibits a degree of autonomy earmarked by its stability with respect to perturbations.

The second characteristic of autonomy concerns the selection of *particular* stable modes at the bifurcation points. At these points the symmetry-breaking instabilities may reveal multiple stable modes. While the thermodynamic branches are themselves determinately specific, at least in principle, by stability and bifurcation theory, the actual specification of which branch the system enters may ultimately be *nondeterminately* specified by a dimension intrinsic to the system. Only when a system is scaled-up beyond some critical dimension are the nonlinearities sufficiently amplified to lead to these choice points between various solutions (Hanson, 1974). At this point the system achieves additional autonomy with respect to the outside environment. Prior to the scaled-up condition (i.e. within the linear region) the system behaves in a determinate fashion; after the critical condition is reached, the system exhibits stability. In sufficiently complex systems where the thermodynamic branches are multiple, such as those manifest in biological systems, local intrinsic dimensions may specify the particular behavioral mode. This autonomy is ultimately manifest in the macro-structure of the system's behavior.

Nondeterminacy stands in sharp contrast to determinacy, a notion associated with the dynamics of Laplace's celestially scaled system, and to indeterminacy, a notion associated with the dynamics of Heisenberg's quantum system. In contrast to the macro and micro scales associated with determinacy and indeterminacy respectively, nondeterminacy is a phenomenon associated with the dynamics of terrestial activity, activity at the scale of ecology. At this medium-range scale, the micro and macro flows and forces enter into a competing relationship allowing for the possibility of systemic order arising under certain conditions. Only at this scale is there sufficient flexibility and stability to allow for their working relationship to be realized where entropy becomes an active contributor towards order.

If we were to follow the earlier tradition of Laplace and Heisenberg we might now be tempted to postulate that the nondeterminacy revealed in the system's dynamics might be generalized to all scales and to all domains. However, we have seen, in the above analysis of nonequilibrium thermodynamics, that scale factors play a critical role in determining the nature of the causal dynamics associated with any systemic activity. At one scale a system may behave in a causally determinant manner, while at a slightly increased scale the system's behavior may dramatically change such that the previously dominant effects of initial and boundary conditions are now resisted by properties intrinsic to the system.

The upshot of the foregoing for the general conduct of science should be highlighted. The argument given amounts to a strong rejection of the traditional form of reductionism. The advocated strategy for the unity of science was to identify one scale as fundamental and then to identify bridging statements between the (special) predicates of the 'unreduced' scale and the (fundamental) predicates of the 'reducing' scale. This matching of predicates was intended to bring the phenomena at the unreduced scale under the laws governing phenomena at the reducing scale. The assertion that the traditional form of reductionism can succeed even in principle is responded to with well-grounded skepticism (e.g. Bunge, 1977; Fodor, 1975). What the arguments given amount to on the positive side of the ledger is an advocacy of a new strategy for the unity of science – a reductionism (if that word has legitimacy in the new formulation) not to *physical things at some privileged scale* but to *physical principles (or strategies) that are independent of scale.* Iberall (1977), Yates (in press) and Soodak (Soodak and Iberall, 1978) have publicized their pursuit of common principles that can be applied repetitively and with equanimity across scales (and *a fortiori* across disciplines) to embrace the systemic phenomena that characterize them. It is to the version of thermodynamic theory advocated by these theorists – a version termed homeokinetics – that we now turn. Homeokinetic theory is like Dissipative Structure theory in that its principal focus has been the relation of thermodynamics to many complex systems, including living systems. Nevertheless the two theories do distinguish in nontrivial ways and these distinctions are noted.

## 3.6   Homeokinetic Physics

Homeokinetic physics was originally developed by Iberall (Iberall and McCulloch, 1970; Iberall and Soodak, 1978; Soodak and Iberall, 1978; Yates, Marsh, and Iberall, 1972) to provide an integrated account of the dynamics exhibited by biological organisms as a specific form of dynamic regulation (i.e. as an extension of the more static notion of homeostasis). But the notion of homeokinetics proves to be very general and applicable at all scales. *Homeokinetics* is meant to contrast with *homeostasis* (Cannon, 1939; Bernard, 1949). Homeostasis does not explicitly identify the mechanism of biological regulation. What is identified is some quasistatic regulation wherein basic properties and ongoing processes are preserved 'independent of external vicissitudes'. Homeokinetics views the mechanism of biological regulation and of regularity in general as a dynamic process of ongoing engine processes, 'oscillators,' whereby conserved regulated values arise as the consequence of a large spectrum of such autonomous oscillators. A conserved value is an averaged or mean state that emerges as a distributed property defined over the operating parameters of the system. Homeokinetics proposes that the autonomous oscillators are organized in accordance with the design principles of thermodynamic engines that draw on energy from a potential source, reject some to a lower potential sink and have capability to do work in a periodic, limit-cycle fashion (Iberall, 1977). The possible existence of such engine oscillators and their cyclic nature is defined in a theorem by Morowitz (1968, 1978): 'In steady-state systems, the flow of energy through the system from a source to a sink will lead to at least one cycle in the system.' The quality of the cycle is limit-cycle: the source–sink system oscillates between well-defined minimum and maximum values and it does so by virtue of being thermodynamically-open, nonconservative, dissipative and nonlinear.

As anticipated above, in its current and more general form (Iberall and Soodak, 1978; Soodak and Iberall, 1978; Yates, in press), homeokinetic physics argues for a single set of physical principles which are 'scale-independent' (e.g. from the largest to the smallest systems in nature), where scale is meant to define a relative order of magnitude. The principles strategically derive their substance from the domains of statistical mechanics, nonlinear mechanics, irreversible thermodynamics or pure physics in general. While the principles are equally valid for *all* physical systems, it is open systems at the terrestrial scale that we seek as test fields for homeokinetic theory.

### 3.6.1 On the Arbitrariness of the Structure/Function Relationship in Open Thermodynamic Systems

While accepting the observable reality of 'structure,' homeokinetic theory seeks out the dynamical functional basis for both structure and function. Central to the analysis is the identification of the operative thermodynamic engines. These engines are open systems, composed of active, interacting components of very many degrees of freedom. The material composition may vary dramatically from one engine to another, but the set of dynamic events which mark the system as a thermodynamic engine is unvarying. What earmarks thermodynamic engines is the invariant fashion in which these systems do their repetitive 'business' within the source–sink system of available energies. For example, structural properties of a plant, tree, organism or society will differ extensively but not intensively; qualitative dynamic properties (like the cycle) will remain invariant over all of these forms of thermodynamic engines.

In thermodynamic systems 'structure' and 'function' share a common format for their source of order. They differ only in the scale of their relaxation times and their energy levels. Quite generally, structure in the system is associated with a relatively slow relaxation time in comparison to function. In either situation, structure or function, order arises by virtue of cyclical transactions of energy through the source–sink system. In short, functions are not logically distinct from structures but rather partake of the same or related dynamic origins. Significantly, when structural properties are given a dynamic analysis their nonarbitrary relationship to functional properties should ultimately become apparent.

In this regard consider the often cited many-to-one mapping of structure to function. Because many different structural arrangements can be observed supporting the same dynamic event it is generally concluded that the relationship between the material support and its coordinate function is arbitrary. From the homeokinetic view this arbitrariness would be the mistaken consequence of a superficial analysis of the nature of the material composition.

### 3.6.2    The Homeokinetic Methodology: Biospectroscopy

Since the basic element of temporal organization is the cycle, one method of analysis characteristically advocated by homeokinetics is spectroscopy. Spectroscopy is a standard approach to periodic behavior where, for example, time series analysis is used to identify cyclic processes as a precursor to identifying repetitive, possibly invariant and essential, functions of the underlying mechanisms. Broadly speaking, spectroscopic analysis indexes the relationship between the important repetitive business going on within a system, and the process time domains in which it occurs (Iberall, Soodak, and Hassler, 1978).

The physical framework offered by Homeokinetic Theory (Iberall, 1972) for all of nature is an organization of operational components into successive levels of atomisms (A) and continua (c). The use of the term atomism denotes both the unit and the doctrine. It is used in a sense similar to organism. An ensemble of atomisms forms a continuum. The continuum then forms the basis for a new atomism at a larger scale, etc. The . . . A–c–A . . . series may become singular at either end. Each ensemble continuum of atomisms constitutes a collective system of thermodynamic engines with unique distribution functions associated with them. Under the appropriate open conditions thermodynamic engines emerge, where cyclicity will be manifest in accordance with the system's total thermodynamic bookkeeping activities.

At any organizational scale an ensemble of interacting atomistic entities acts in a thermodynamically near-continuous manner, bounded by an appropriate space–time scale (from above and below). While the ensemble may be *far from equilibrium globally, locally the system is thermodynamically near-continuous and in near equilibrium.* Under scale changes this fluid-like continuum may become dynamically unstable locally, whereby a spectrum of patterned functions, or in fact, precipitated structures, of superatomisms may emerge. While a field thermodynamic formulation is appropriate for a continuum condition, it is not appropriate for a discrete atomistic unit. At the atomistic level, more standard kinetic formulations are necessary. Homeokinetics in particular argues that mechanics implies thermodynamics as atomisms transform into continuum (Iberall and Soodak, 1978).

The range of rhythmic cycles exhibited by a system may vary greatly from slow to fast, where each frequency serves as a signature of various autonomous ensembles. From the ensemble perspective the unit of an individual oscillator appears within the thermodynamically complete and relatively autonomous system. However, from the perspective of the individual atomistic units the organization appears 'neighborly,' perhaps even chaotic and random. To capture the dynamics of the large ensemble requires minimally that: (i) the scale of observation be large compared to the mean free path of the atomistic units and (ii) the time of observation be long compared to the relaxation times of the interactions of the atomistic units (Yates, Marsh, and Iberall, 1972; Yates and Iberall, 1973). For example, an organism will exhibit a wide set of signal frequencies which correspond to various organs and tissue systems in the body (for examples see, Iberall and McCulloch, 1970; Iberall, 1969). This range may vary from the order of seconds to years depending on the organ. A set of faster frequencies can also be detected which form the atomistic basis for organs. The range of these frequencies may be on the order of milli- and microseconds. An upper limit may be found in the ecosystem where a single 'relaxation' process is revealed over the entire lifetime spectrum of the individual organism. The general strategy is to select the low frequencies first since they signify the near-static, steady states of the dynamic system. If these are not carefully defined and understood, then the faster frequencies will be less well identifiable (Yates, in press).

Below we present a brief summary of the steps involved in a homeokinetic analysis. We follow closely the steps presented by Yates (in press; see also Iberall and Soodak, 1978; Soodak and Iberall, 1978; Iberall, 1977; Iberall,

Soodak, and Hassler, 1978; Iberall, 1978b, for the complete methodology):

1. Identify the atomisms. Any physical system has atomistic elements that must be identified. These may be extremely simple (i.e. have no internal degrees of freedom), or they may be complex, active elements with many internal degrees of freedom that equipartition energy slowly among these internal degrees of freedom. Examples of the atomism in the neuromuscular system are: muscle fibers, motor units, muscles, co-ordinative structures, and organismic activity (see Bloch and Iberall, 1974). It is important to note that each atomism is an 'ecosystem' on its own scale – it includes a source (of potential energy), a sink and a set of operational components. Moreover, each atomism has its own spectral properties. Significantly, the functional integrity of an atomism – its cyclicity – cannot be attributed to a part; it can only be attributed to the 'ecosystem' as a unit (cf. Turvey, Shaw, and Mace, 1978).

2. Identify the interactions between the atomisms. (Without interaction there is no system. The atomisms exchange energy and are bound together and kept from dissolving into each other by the few physical forces, e.g. electromagnetic and gravitational forces.)

3. Define the ensemble of like-interacting, active atomisms, including the space–time domains in which a continuum view is justified.

4. Define the complexions – the dynamic states in phase space. This constitutes a basis for computing a metric of complexity of the system.

5. Specify the thermostatic description (partitioning of energy, distribution function, thermodynamic potentials, constitutive relations of the equations of state, summational invariants).

6. Specify the field equations of change, in terms of change in average local values of summational invariants. (This is the irreversible thermodynamic account of response to external influence from region to region. This thermodynamic description holds in the response range in which transport coefficients in the equations of change are functions of thermodynamic variables only, but not of time; i.e. are describable by autonomous differential equations. Nonequilibrium, irreversible thermodynamics is limited to conditions that are locally near equilibrium, see below.)

7. Identify the field boundary conditions.

8. Identify the thermodynamic engine processes that are manifest as cyclic processes (limit cycle behavior) at each level.

9. Specify the field mechanics for the whole system, arising out of its various equations of change.

10. Identify the history of the system. This is the trajectory resulting from slow changes in the system parameters. This step is meant to

acknowledge the nonautonomous aspects that arise from outside interactions.

## 3.7 Dissipative Structure Theory and Homeokinetic Theory: Compared and Contrasted

Dissipative Structure theory and Homeokinetics both address questions relative to the design logic for spatiotemporal order in natural systems. Indifferent to the fact that the system is termed a 'dissipative structure' or a 'thermodynamic engine' the following requirements must be satisfied:

1. A source of potential energy from which (generalized) work can arise.
2. A microcosm of operational components with a stochastic fluctuating nature.
3. The presence of nonlinear components.
4. A scale change such that a nonlinear response is critically amplified (in the sense that the system's own dimensions now resist previously dominant initial and boundary conditions).

If these conditions are met, then the possibility exists for the transition from a stochastic steady-state situation to a spatially or temporally structured, steady-state situation (or a time-dependent limit-cycle regime) characterized by homogeneous oscillations or by propagating waves.

According to dissipative structure theory, spatiotemporal orderings are realizable only in the entire field for far from equilibrium conditions. While both theories agree that the 'start-up' phase involving the sudden transition from one ordered state to another requires a far from equilibrium condition, in the entire field, they differ in how they stress their equilibrium requirement. Dissipative Structure theory states that new stability regimes are both 'started-up' and 'maintained' in far from equilibrium conditions. In contrast Homeokinetic theory argues that the local fields before and after start-up are near equilibrium, and thus in the domain of irreversible thermodynamics. After an initial start-up phase, involving some shock waves, a system moves back toward a near-equilibrium state where thermostatic conditions can prevail *locally*. Globally, however, the system is still in a far from equilibrium condition. By maintaining local near equilibrium conditions, a mature biological system does not have to continually transform large energies at high rates as would be required if far from equilibrium conditions also prevailed locally (cf. Morowitz, 1978). Once the spatiotemporal structures are established, maintenance of the structures may be achieved through continuous near-equilibrium transport processes (for more on the transport problem see Iberall, 1977).

A second contrast involves the metholdogy employed by the two theories. For Dissipative Structure theory the methodology entails formulation of a set of nonlinear kinetic equations that correspond to, and form the explanation of, the sudden transition in ordered states. Originally the methodology was applied to test fields involving chemical reactions occurring in series and parallel. Recently the methodology has been extended to ecological and social fields. In these situations sudden transitions in the field reactions are modelled by *kinetic formulation* of 'flow fields,' which are not regarded to be a *thermodynamic formulation* (for examples see Prigogine, Allen, and Herman, 1977). From the perspective of Dissipative Structure theory, kinetic formulations and thermodynamic formulations relate in a *complementary* fashion (Prigogine, 1978; see also, Yates, 1980).

In contrast, Homeokinetic theory employs the methodology of spectroscopy to index the cyclicity generated by thermodynamic engines. The test fields for homeokinetics range from biological cells to societies (cf. Iberall, Soodak, and Arensberg, 1980). Behavior of these systems is modelled by a set of scale independent formulations that relate kinetics/mechanics and thermodynamics in a *continuous*, *not* a *complementary* fashion.

## 4   THE NATURAL PERSPECTIVE: ECOLOGICAL REALISM

Broadly defined, the goal of a theory of perception and action is to explicate the co-ordination of animal and environment. Traditionally, the burden of the animal-environment co-ordination has been carried by a proposed medium of 'between things.' For example, in perception theory the proposed entities mediating animal and environment have been termed ideas, percepts, models, schemas, organizing principles, meanings, sense data, concepts and such like. John Locke's representational realism (Cornman, 1975; Mundle, 1971) formulated in the seventeenth century is the canonical version of perceptual theory in both its past and present forms (see Shaw and Turvey, 1981; Shaw, Turvey, and Mace, in press). Locke assumed that there was an environmental reality that existed independent of the act of perceiving but proposed that the animal was not directly in epistemic contact with that reality but rather with a representation of that reality, precisely, an *idea* that interfaced the animal as perceiver with the environmental object to which the animal's perception referred.

Among the many puzzles to which this view of perception gives rise, there is a particularly notorious puzzle that was a principal focus of Locke's critics, Berkeley and Hume, viz: what guarantees that the ideas (of which the animal is said to be directly aware) represent anything real. Berkeley thought a guarantee was unwarranted, and emphasized the phenomenalism (that there are *only* phenomenal objects such as ideas) implicit in Locke's theory; Hume thought a guarantee unlikely, and emphasized the skepticism (that there may be a real world but of its existence no-one can be sure) implicit in Locke's theory. For reasons that we will not go into here (but see Johnston and Turvey, 1980; Shaw and Turvey, 1981; Shaw, Turvey, and Mace, in press; Turvey and Shaw, 1979) the general argument that an animal is apprised directly not of the animal-environment system of which it is a part, but of phenomenal substitutes for that system (such as ideas) is a dubious starting point for scientific inquiry. For this latter reason and for others, it seems both judicious and prudent to pursue a realist posture, that is, to pursue tenaciously a reformulation of the logical and physical support of perception that deters regression to phenomenalism and skepticism. In short, to commit oneself to a style of inquiry that explicates animal-environment co-ordination without recourse to 'between things' (sometimes originating as analytic or methodologically useful terms but assuming, in the course of time, ontological status) so that science need not feel uncomfortable with the claim that animals perceive the reality that bears on their existence.

The aforementioned commitment to a realist philosophy is most obviously scale-sensitive: the reality that is relevant to animal activity and, therefore, the reality which is to be perceived, is at the scale of ecology and not, for example, at the scale of galaxies or atoms (Gibson, 1966, 1979). It is to an *ecological* realism, therefore, that the commitment is being made. In what follows, we summarize two themes of the ecological-realism program which bear prominently on the physical theory deemed appropriate for the ecological scale of nature: they are the doctrine of mutuality or synergy (with regard to the relation of animal and environment) and the doctrine of necessary specificity (with regard to the nature of information).

### 4.1   The Mutuality or Synergy Doctrine

Ecological realism rejects any variant of the traditional disposition to conduct animal-referential discourse and environment-referential discourse in two distinct and irreducible vocabularies, where matters of perceiving and acting are at issue. That is to say, ecological realism rejects the disposition to describe animal and environment as apart from their joint operation or that each affects the other in the sense of causal interactionism (cf. Dewey and Bentley, 1949). The disposition to treat animal and environment as two parts of a dualism is at the core of the causal-chain theory of perception which attempts to trace a sequence of causes and effects between the environment described in physical terms, and percepts, described in mental terms said to be 'in' the animal. More prominently, for our current concerns, this disposition promotes dichotomies such as that of sensory processes (the consequences of which are described in mental terms) and motor processes (the consequences of which are described in physical terms), the central nervous system (described in a vocabulary appropriate to agents) and the skelotomuscular system (describable in a vocabulary appropriate to instruments), semantics (characterizations in intensional terms identifying what states of affairs *mean*) and syntax (characterizations in extensional terms identifying what states of affairs *are*) and, more generally, information and dynamics. When a system is conceptually severed in two and the consequences of the division held to be irreducible, one to the other, then a third kind of thing must be proposed to bring the separated things together when explanation so demands. Bluntly speaking, animal-environment dualism and its variants mandate 'between things' and repulse (ecological) realism.

Ecological realism starts with the assumption of mutuality or synergy of animal and environment (Gibson, 1979; Shaw, Turvey, and Shaw, in press; Turvey and Shaw, 1979). The animal and its environment are mutually constraining components of a single system (what might be termed an ecosystem) describable by a single vocabulary whose predicates are reflexive and symmetric. The animal is described in terms that reference the environment and the environment is described in terms that reference the animal. To paraphrase Dewey and Bentley (1949), the two terms, animal and environment, cannot be described apart from any joint operation as the two terms, matter and space, cannot be so described in the general theory of relativity. That the two terms, animal and environment, cannot be described in logically independent ways renders inappropriate attempts to co-ordinate them through causal interaction. The formula of causes and effects is, strictly speaking, a formula for binding mutually independent entities. That the two terms are mutually dependent renders unnecessary a third term to mediate them.

In sum, the mutuality of synergy doctrine deters partitioning complex systems (see Yates, 1980, for an informed account of the notion of complexity), of the kind that populate the ecological scale, into components that are described in logically distinct and irreducible vocabularies. A holding apart of information and dynamics, of semantics and syntax, of central nervous system and skeletomuscular system etc., is rejected by the mutuality doctrine, as are the correlated perspectives that any one component overseers any other and that any one component can be adapted to those states of another component that have yet to come into existence. On the positive side the doctrine promotes the idea of systemic components as mutually defined and mutually constraining, related acausally through symmetry principles (Shaw and Turvey, 1981).

## 4.2 The Necessary Specificity Doctrine

Let us turn to the second doctrine of the ecological realist program identified above, namely that of necessary specificity. Following the classical and conventional analysis of vision (which equates the optical support for vision with the inverted, metrically ambiguous and two-dimensional retinal image) it has been held quite generally, that the informational support for animal-environment co-ordination is imprecise, inadequate, and equivocal. The construal given to 'information' has been that of 'evidence,' in the sense of 'clues' or 'hints' about the environment and the animal's relation to it. That is to say, there is a generally accepted doctrine (indifferent to the sensory system of focus) that neither environmental objects and events, nor the perceiver's own movements, structure energy distributions in ways that are specific to their properties. Relatedly, a much-repeated argument has been that the energy distributions are meaningless because they are ambiguous, and because their description is in terms of variables of physics which make no reference to how a given animal can or should relate behaviorally to a given object. In brief, the informational support for animal-environment co-ordination is said to be non-specific to the states of affairs relevant to that co-ordination and, congruently, to be devoid of meaning. It should be underscored that here is encountered once again (2.0) the popular idea of 'information' as arbitrary with respect to the actions that it serves – that 'information' has a syntax but is not intrinsically meaningful; meaning has to be ascribed to the information base by an independent source.

Elsewhere the traditional and conventional conception of the informational support for perception and action has been termed the doctrine of intractable nonspecificity (Shaw, Turvey, and Mace, in press; Turvey and Shaw, 1979). Clearly, because this doctrine mandates 'between things' in the account of animal-environment co-ordination, the doctrine and, therefore, the view of information with which it is associated, must be rejected by ecological realism.

For any activity that an animal performs with respect to an environmental layout, information is needed about the nature of the layout, about the varying relations among the animal's body parts and about the changing relation of the animal to the layout (see Lee, 1976). If these kinds of information are impoverished and equivocal, the animal must embellish and disambiguate them; if they are arbitrary and meaningless the animal must interpret and ascribe meaning to them; and if they are defined over absolute (animal-neutral) dimensions, the animal must redefine them in body-scale terms (its own dimensions). Whenever any one of the above conditionals is accepted, ecological realism is infirmed. Therefore, the definition of 'information' for ecological realism mandates that information be unique and specific to the facts about which it informs, *meaningful* to the control and co-ordination requirements of the activity (what can be done, how it can be done, when it can be done) and *continuously scaled to the dimensions* of the system over which the activity is defined.

## 5    INFORMATION AS THE MORPHOLOGY OF DYNAMICS

Let us now see where the lengthy exegesis of the natural perspective has brought us. The overview of physical theory gives emphasis to the claim that the study of nonequilibrium systems will provide considerable insight into the evolution and functioning of living systems. Dissipative Structure theory and Homeokinetic theory both express the core thesis of such study, namely, that the flow of energy through a system, in the nonequilibrium thermodynamic sense, acts to organize that system; that the flow of energy is a self-organizing, self-complexing principle, and may be so at all physical magnitudes. A generalized energy flow system entails an energy source, an energy sink and an intermediate collection of operational components through which the energy flows. Under an irreversible thermodynamic analysis, the units of action at any scale must be energy flow systems – that is, they must be thermodynamic engines.

The overview of ecological realism denies the legitimacy of separating the animal and environment terms in such a way that a third class of terms has to be introduced to mediate them. Thus, explanation of the co-ordination and control of animal activity cannot be reduced to things which co-ordinate and things which control. Co-ordination and control refer to emergent states of the animal-environment system and not to mediating 'between things' (Fitch and Turvey, 1978; Gibson, 1979; Turvey, 1980). As anticipated in Section 1.3 and as expressed in Section 3.5, co-ordination and control are to be viewed as *a posteriori* facts resulting from distributed physical processes. The latter remark is equivalent to the claim that talk of information and dynamics cannot be conducted in two incompatible vocabularies. To reiterate, ecological realism denies a dualism of information (that controls and co-ordinates) and dynamics (that is controlled and co-ordinated). Fundamentally, ecological realism views information as arising in the dynamics of the animal-environment system, unique and specific to those dynamics and to the system's dimensions.

We can express this conception in another way that is perhaps more useful, given the general concern of the present paper with the problem of degrees of freedom. By the tenets of ecological realism there can be no such notion as an elemental unit of perception or action, from which other, more complex units, are constructed. The contrast of elemental (qua basic) with derived (qua complex) can have no place in explanations of perception and action, for it engenders 'between things' to 'put together' perceptions and actions. The information relevant to activity is not to be construed as elemental information associated with individual degrees of freedom which is somehow concatenated to give complex information associated with an ensemble of multiple degrees of freedom. Ecological realism prescribes that no matter how many degrees of freedom are involved in an action there will be an information base that is unique and specific to the ensemble; it anticipates that there will always be qualitative simplicity in the face of quantitative complexity; it allows that all informational predicates might be termed elementary but disallows that any can be termed elemental. These latter intuitions were prominent in Gibson's (1950, 1966, 1979) attempt to reformulate the optical support for vision through the notion of higher order variables or invariants. Following Gibson's lead, Runeson (1977) and Fowler and Turvey (1978) have remarked on the 'special purpose' nature of both information and a system's sensitivity to it.

Where might we find the confluence of the two themes of (i) energy flow as a self-organizing and self-complexing principle and (ii) information as unique and specific to an act, drawn as they are from the two respective branches of the natural perspective, physical theory and ecological realism? There are hints that the confluence is to be found in the morphology of the dynamics. The particular order exhibited by a thermodynamic engine depends in a very detailed way on the geometric properties that define the source-sink, energy-flow system (Morowitz, 1968). We noted in Section 3.5 that the geometry or form of the excess entropy production indexes points of stability around which the system organizes. The geometric properties are scaled to the dimensions of the thermodynamic system and are specific to its dissipative properties. Qualitative changes in the geometric properties of the excess entropy production function, pursuant to an excessive change in a system dimension, correspond to qualitative changes in the macroscopic properties of the thermodynamic system. We noted, in short, that the particular forms of a system's self-organizing and self-complexing are associated with the geometry of the energy fluxes.

We now move toward the following thesis: when energy is the dependent measure, transformations of a system (in terms of an activity) reveal dramatic gradients and equilibrium points. Sensitivity to the energy variable is synonymous with sensitivity to information specific to properties of the transforming system's dynamics. Furthermore, changes in the system's dimensions, incurred artificially or through growth, will result in a corresponding change in the gradients and equilibrium points revealed under transformation. In other words, *since the biological system of dynamics is functionally self-organizing (as argued in 3.0 above), then the corresponding system of gradients and equilibrium points (as information) is co-ordinately self-organizing.*

Let us consider how it is possible to construe these gradients and equilibrium points as the predicate types in which to characterize an information base. We do this in two steps: first, we consider the important distinction between essential and nonessential variables and second we consider those theoretical perspectives which attempt a qualitative characterization of systems whose quantitative characteristics are poorly known or resist calculation. The review that follows is historical in its organization. It attempts to put into perspective ideas that have been long present in the geometry of modelling and with which the theories of irreversible thermodynamics (Dissipative Structure theory and Homeokinetic theory) are continuous, viz., the emphasis on stability and the qualitative consequences of scale changes.

### 5.1    Essential and Nonessential Variables

The concept of gradients and equilibrium points as an information base stands in sharp contrast to the quasi-linguistic view of information as a finite sequence of letters taken from an alphabet and organized by a syntax; gradients and equilibrium points have their basis in an underlying 'organization' of geometric form. It is difficult to give a complete definition of this notion of organization; for present purposes let us settle on the equating of 'organization' with those characteristic features of a problem that facilitate obtaining a solution (Tsetlin, 1973). We will wish to say that the solution to the problem is achieved by taking advantage of the dynamic morphology of the problem itself. The problems of potential systems are considered 'well-organized' when the function can be partitioned into two classes of variables: essential and nonessential. Essential variables are geometrically defined as being capable of causing abrupt changes and discontinuities in the function's topological qualities (so, to conserve these qualities keep the essential variables fixed). Alternatively nonessential variables produce no qualitative changes in the function's topology but rather are capable of producing scalar changes over the topological qualities (so, to vary the topological qualities without annihilating them, allow the nonessential variables to change). Of significant importance is the fact that: (i) these characteristic features of organization *need not be known in advance* and (ii) *the partitioning of the essential and nonessential variables need not be fixed* (i.e. a continuous change along a dimension of a nonessential variable may cause an abrupt change such that a previously nonessential variable now becomes an essential variable or vice versa). Summing briefly, natural functions are well-organized when the variables may be partitioned into those variables capable of causing qualitative changes (i.e. essential variables) and those capable of causing quantitative changes (i.e. nonessential variables).

The behavior of essential and nonessential variables is distinguished mathematically in the behavior of nonlinear and linear variables respectively. The concept behind the distinction is best appreciated in terms of the operational transformations induced from one vector space to another. In the mapping from one vector space to another, from 'input' to 'ouput,' the behavior of a linear system is characterized by the properties of superposition and proportionality. By superposition is meant that if several inputs are simultaneously applied to the system, their total effect is the same as that resulting from the superposition of individual effects acting on each input separately; in linear theory terms, $L(X_1 + X_2 \ldots + X_n) = L(X_1) + L(X_2) + \ldots + L(X_n)$. And by proportionality is meant that if all the inputs to a system are multiplied by the same factor, then the responses are multiplied by the same factor; in linear theory terms, $L(\alpha X_1, \alpha X_2 \ldots \alpha X_n) = \alpha L(X_1, X_2 \ldots X_n)$. In brief, variations in the 'domain' are precisely captured by variations in the codomain. Put differently, the degrees of freedom specified in the 'input' are identical with the number of degrees of freedom in the 'output.'

In contrast, variations in the domain of a nonlinear system are not associated with linear variations in the codomain. The properties of proportionality and superposition are not preserved in nonlinear systems. Non-linear systems are characterized by inhomogeneities in the codomain where the inhomogeneities identify 'preferred' locations on which the system tends to converge. Variation on the micro scale of 'individual' system parameters (the domain) are not continuously (that is, linearly) associated with changes in the macro scale of systemic parameters (the codomain). Changes in the macro systemic parameters are only realized when critical ratios occur relating individual system parameters on the micro scale. When these ratios are achieved the systemic behavior of the system moves from one stable mode to another (as indexed in the codomain mapping).

One final contrast needs to be drawn. The distinction between nonlinear and linear is a *formal* mathematical distinction; that between essential and non-essential is a *pragmatic* distinction. Within a given range of variation a dimension may continue to meet the formal criteria for nonlinearity but it may not continue to meet the pragmatic criteria for essential. The essential/nonessential contrast owes an obligation to physical realities which the nonlinear/linear contrast does not. We are saying, in short, that the essential/nonessential distinction for a system is system-referential and abides by the resolution power, the self-sensitivity, of the system (Kugler, Kelso and Turvey, 1980).

As a relevant aside, it was to Bernstein's credit that, in his later writings, he gave full recognition to the essential/nonessential distinction as an appropriate way to characterize living systems. Bernstein too was impressed by the fact that many living things embody the features of 'well-organized' functions. Just as the leaves of a tree are never exactly alike in their metrical, nonessential dimensions yet still possess the essential qualitative characteristics of the particular type of tree to which they belong, so the various acts that people perform (e.g. handwriting, gait, piano-playing) retain their essential and individualistic properties over marked variance in nonessential variables (see Kelso, 1981; Kugler, Kelso, and Turvey, 1980) for many examples in the motor system's literature). There are strong hints in Bernstein's later writings of a dissatisfaction with the 'artificial' perspective of cybernetics, with its search for analogs between manmade machines and living systems. In the theory of well-organized functions that applies to the antientropic processes of open systems, Bernstein (1967) foresaw the end of the 'honeymoon' (p. 181) between the sciences of cybernetics and physiology. In short, in the class of natural functions that envelop the behavior of systems with many degrees of freedom, Bernstein envisaged an opportunity to model 'the basic forms of real, not fictitious, life processes' (p. 186).

## 5.2 Qualitative Characterizations of Systems

### 5.2.1 Geometric Similarity

Qualitative characterizations of systems are historically based in Euclid's (300 BC) principle of geometric similarity. Geometric figures were said to be *similar* if they shared the same shape but not necessarily the same size. Preservation of both shape and size meant that the two objects related not only similarly but also congruently. For Euclid similarity was a qualitative measure whereas congruence was a quantitative measure. The principle of similarity formed the basis for one of the earliest theories of modeling.

In general there is a point-to-point correspondence between a model and its prototype. In geometrical terminology, two points that correspond to each other are *homologous*. The concept of homologous points leads immediately to the concept of homologous figures and homologous parts. Figures or parts of the model and the prototype are said to be homologous if they are comprised of homologous points. If transient (i.e. time-variable) phenomena occur in a model, it is necessary to introduce the concept of 'homologous times.' For Euclid, however, geometric similarity was concerned only with the relation between homologous parts. Two systems were said to be *geometrically similar* if homologous parts of the systems were in a constant ratio. Any deviation from the above restriction would annihilate or distort the shared set of geometric qualities.

### 5.2.2 Dynamic Similarity

Extending the principles of similitude from geometric to dynamic systems, Galileo (1564–1642) formulated the first principle of dynamic similarity. Two systems were said to be *dynamically similar* if homologous parts of the system experienced similar net forces. The principle of dynamic similarity was a special case of the general conception of geometrical similarity. If two systems of connected particles and rigid bodies were geometrically similar, additional relationships were required to make them dynamically similar. The two systems were said to be dynamically similar if, in addition to the constant ratio between the linear dimensions, the masses of corresponding portions bore a certain ratio, and the rates of work at corresponding points also bore a certain ratio. It then followed that the forces at corresponding points related as a certain ratio dependent on the other three ratios.

### 5.2.3 Kinematic Similarity

The first principle of kinematic similarity was formulated by Newton (1642–1727). Kinematics is the theory of space-time relationships, consequently kinematic similarity signifies similarity of motions. Two systems are said to be *kinematically similar* if homologous parts of the system lie at homologous points at homologous times. Thus two systems that are kinematically similar have corresponding components of velocity and acceleration that are similar. If kinematically similar systems also share similar mass distributions, they are also dynamically similar.

The above principles of similarity are the basis for modeling methods that allow for the preservation of certain qualities (geometric, kinematic or dynamic) without requiring any exact specification of numerical numbers. Qualitative properties are preserved by virtue of maintaining critical ratios invariant from the prototype to the model. We described this method of modeling in Section 1.2 under its more general label of *dimensional analysis*. Recall that it allows for the specification of similarity between two systems by merely analyzing certain *dimensionless numbers* (like a Reynolds' or Rayleigh number) formed by the required ratios.

### 5.2.4 Qualitative Dynamics

Towards the end of the nineteenth century Poincaré proposed a more abstract characteristic of qualitative properties. By linking calculus and topology, Poincaré conceived of a new qualitative study of differential equations (i.e. $dx/dt = f(x)$), called *qualitative dynamics*. Poincaré found that even if quantitative solutions were impossible, it was still possible to derive qualitative information. For example, qualitative statements such as 'the solution is periodic' were readily revealed, whereas quantitative statements such as 'the solution has a period of 2.5432' were not available without elaborate computational procedures. In fact exact quantitative solutions often defy computation. Using the methods of differential topology, Poincaré could identify the qualitative properties of dynamic systems (e.g. periodicity, equilibrium points, types of stable regions, etc.). Whereas the earlier Principles of Similitude were based in a theory of modeling (preservation of a given set of qualities from a prototype to a model), Poincaré's theory of qualitative dynamics was concerned with a theory of design (understanding the nature and origin of the qualitative properties within a system).

### 5.2.5   Growth and Form

Based on an appreciation of qualitative dynamics and the earlier principles of similitude, Thompson (1917) proposed a unified theory of *growth and form*. With reference to design, Thompson argued that the form an object takes on is intimately linked to the dynamic properties of stability. Moreover, stability was not to be understood merely as the sum total of interacting forces, but rather required a close examination in terms of the qualitative properties inherent in the system's geometry. The exact nature of these stabilities, however, eluded Thompson's mathematics. In terms of modeling, once the qualitative properties were manifest by the system, various transformations (affine, shear, cardiodal, etc.) could be imposed on the system without annihilating them. Growth was explained as a modeling process in which certain qualitative properties were preserved under continuous transformations. This allowed for an explanation of how systems grew and still maintained certain kinematic, geometric, and dynamic similarities. Thompson suggested that the similarity in forms between animate and inanimate systems was the result of the systems sharing similar stable configurations. In short, the fundamental nature of stable configurations is insensitive to material composition. Whether a cloud in the sky or an amoeba in a pond, the qualitative form realized by these dynamic structures is understandable as a stable configuration. Force and material composition can only affect the form in the quantitative fashion of similarity transformations.

### 5.2.6   Relational Biology

A little later, Rashevsky (1938/1950) was to postulate a theory of *relational biology* based on the qualitative properties of functions. Rashevsky's interest was primarily in a theory of design. His insight was the recognition that what biology is directly interested in is primarily dynamic function and behavior and not static structure. On the other hand, it is structure that we can most readily study quantitatively. The two are related, in traditional reductionist terms (as contrasted with the newer version described in 3.6) by the view that 'structure implies function.' As Rashevsky opined, however, even if a reductionistic approach to the study of dynamic systems was in principle correct (which he doubted), that might be the hard way to go about the task. What he attempted to do was to create a mathematical framework in which function, organization, and behavior could be directly characterized and studied apart from any material or structural basis. Through an understanding of qualitative properties of functions, Rashevsky hoped to gain insight into the corresponding organizational constraints manifest in a behaving system. Relational biology was grounded in the realization that the qualitative properties of a function could be expected to place corresponding quantitative constraints on the organization of biological systems.

## 5.2.7   Catastrophe Theory

More recently, Thom's theory of catastrophes (1970, 1975) offered the most formal analysis of qualitative complexity in dynamic systems. Thom's goal in catastrophe theory was to describe the origin of dynamic form, that is, morphogenesis (see Waddington, 1970, for variations on the use of this term in modern biology). Following almost explicitly the arguments of Thompson (1917/1942) Thom used the techniques of Poincaré's differential topology to provide the needed mathematical justification. By giving up quantitative concepts, the topologist gains the ability to analyze certain abstract properties of a function's form. For a problem involving dynamic variables, topological qualities such as equilibrium regions are of crucial importance and may be readily revealed using the techniques of differential topology. The ability to reveal these qualitative properties, however, is only achieved by giving up quantitative concepts such as rate, distance, and magnitude. This allows a topologist to search multidimensional spaces for equilibrium regions with relative indifference to any quantitative measures. The arena of multidimensional spaces with their various equilibrium points constitutes the basic material for Thom's theory of catastrophes.

Essentially, Thom created a mathematical language – catastrophe theory – built on the assumptions of structural stability and qualitative regularity. He proposed that the development of form was completely 'independent of the substrates of form and the nature of forces that create them' (1975, p. 8). Furthermore, 'the only stable singularities are determined solely by the dimensions of the ambient space' (1975, p. 8). In short Thom proposed a theory of form based principally on an appreciation of potential stable points, where these stable points are specified by the dimensionality of the space. The properties of force and material substance are primarily associated with scalar transformations (affine, shear, cardiodal, etc.) on the system's stable dynamic form. Due to the abstract nature of form and stability, the same set of stable points could be manifest by a wide variety of systems. Once again, this commonality could account for the wide similarity in form between many animate and inanimate systems. Because of this fact Thom argued, as Thompson had earlier, that a qualitative study of form should proceed from the mere study of force and substance to the abstract study of form itself. In this regard, Thom moved from the methods of conventional stability theory to the theory of structural stability.

## 5.3    Stability and Catastrophe

Conventional stability theory centers on understanding the dynamical properties associated with certain systems of differential equations. The stability associated with these systems is often represented by the analogy of a marble rolling on a surface (see Figure 5). The system is *stable* if the marble ultimately returns to its initial equilibrium point after a perturbation has been introduced (upper panel of Figure 5). More formally, this stability is referred to as 'point' stability. Conversely, the system is *unstable* if the initial perturbation response does not die away, corresponding to the marble being displaced from the top of the hill (middle panel of Figure 5). Finally, there is *neutral stability* as exemplified by the marble on a flat surface (lower panel of Figure 5). Following initial perturbation the system remains in a new condition dependent on the parameters of the perturbation. This system does not exhibit any tendency systematically to return to or deviate from the initial conditions.

A richer set of building material for dynamical landscapes than the simple hilltops and valley bottoms associated with conventional stability theory is

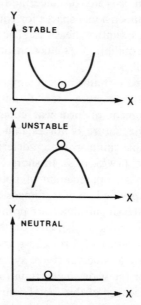

FIGURE 5    Dynamical modes associated with conventional
stability theory (see text for details)

found in the theory of structural stability (cf. Thom, 1975). The theory of structural stability seeks to understand qualitative changes in a system's dynamical character as various independent parameters (which serve to define the dimensions of a system) are changed. Whereas conventional stability theory deals with local response patterns to perturbations, structural stability theory deals with global changes in the dynamical landscapes.

A system of differential equations is referred to as 'structurally stable' if the dynamical landscape remains qualitatively unaltered in the course of changes in the independent parameters. This region of stability may be likened to the similitude region referred to in 1.2, as a *preservation* of qualitative form over a scaling-up in magnitude. At critical scale changes, however, dramatic qualitative changes in the landscape can occur — for example, when a peak and a valley coalesce in mutual annihilation. This region of instability may be likened to the dissimilitude region referred to in 1.2, a *change* in qualitative form over a scaling-up in magnitude. These instabilities are marked by a continuous variation in an independent variable being associated with a discontinuity on a more macro description (such as in the landscape or behavioral descriptions). In these critical regions continuous changes in micro variables which define the system's dimensions may suddenly become associated with dramatic 'jumps' in a system's description on a more macro level. The sudden transition or jump appears to be discontinuous not because there are no intervening states or pathways, but because none of them is stable; the passage from the initial state to the final one is likely to be brief in comparison to the time spent in the stable states. Thom's theorem of 'elementary catastrophes' describes the seven simplest ways for such transitions to occur. According to the theorem, the types of catastrophes which may be associated with a particular system are finitely bounded by the system's dimensionality. In short, each dimensional system has a distinct number of catastrophes associated with it (for example, there are seven distinct catastrophes or bifurcations associated with a system with four dimensions, see Thom, 1975).

The importance of Thom's 1975 discovery was that not only were these patterns of behavior conditioned solely by the system's dimensionality, but they were also limited to a very small number of possibilities. What Thom had formally proven was that as a system increased its organizational complexity the posssibility of increased qualitative complexity was limited. Furthermore, the nature of the qualitative complexity was indifferent to the material substance. In essence Thom was demonstrating the prohibitiveness of multiple solutions to recurring problems in nature. For example, the biological heart and the technological pump are functionally equivalent in terms of pumping fluids; the biological lungs and the blacksmith's bellows are functionally equivalent in terms of pumping of air; and the bacteriophage and the syringe are functionally equivalent in terms of the injecting fluids into and withdrawing fluids from a cavity. Several more general solutions are evident in the problem of locomotion and grooming. Regardless of the species, the solutions to these two problems appear to be fixed. For locomotion, the dynamic relationship between the swing phase and stance phase remains invariant over all locomoting species (Pearson, 1976). Similarly, for grooming, there are strong hints that the temporal relationship among the phases of grooming remains invariant over all grooming species. In short, from Thom's perspective, the functional similarity in the structuring of many natural problems is owing in large part to the limited number of stable possibilities. (And this, we should suppose, is the conceptual backdrop befitting Baerends' (1976) intuition that the phenomenon of convergence — where the same function is seen in largely disparate species — reflects the fact that the solutions to the design problems for living systems extend in age beyond species, families, and even phyla.)

We conclude our brief discussion of stability and catastrophe with a few cautionary notes. Thom's theory of catastrophes provides us with a complete classification of transitions that may occur at points of structural instability. Unfortunately the theory is limited to systems with a finite number of degrees of freedom described by ordinary differential equations. This is a nontrivial restriction because most natural systems involve both spatial and temporal parameters and thus are governed by partial differential equations with an infinite number of degrees of freedom. At present, however, there is no comprehensive theory for the solution of nonlinear partial differential equations (cf. Nicolis and Auchmuty, 1974).

### 5.4    The Principle of 'Order Through Fluctuation' Revisited

From bifurcation and catastrophe theory we learn that scale changes over particular parameters of dynamic systems are sufficient to induce instabilities in the macro structure; ultimately, the instability leads to a higher order of qualitative complexity. What we fail to gain from these theories, however, is an account of the mechanism responsible for inducing the onset of the instabilities. With reference to this issue we re-examine Prigogine's (1976) principle of 'order through fluctuation.'

From our earlier discussions of irreversible thermodynamics we derived the following claim: if systems of any kind are in a sufficiently nonequilibrium state, have many degrees of freedom, have nonlinear components and are open to the inflow of energy and matter, the ensuing instabilities do not lead to random behavior; instead, when critical scale changes are realized the system is suddenly driven to a new stable regime which corresponds to a new state of qualitative complexity. In such transitions the system acquires new margins to produce entropy, new possibilities for activity. We noted above that a closed equilibrium system, with a monotonically increasing entropy function, is

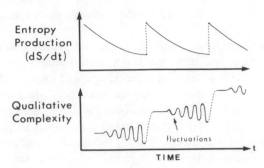

FIGURE 6    Amplified phase of fluctuation

characterized by decreasing activity and entropy production. As it approaches maximum entropy, which corresponds to the lowest state of order, the system asymptotes onto a reversible equilibrium condition. A partially open equilibrium system, in contrast, moves through a sequence of transitions to new regions which, in such cases, generate the conditions of renewed high entropy production within the new regime (see Section 3.5), and thus opens up the possibility for the development and maintenance of new qualitative complexities (see Figure 6).

Prior to realization of a critical scale change, systematic or random fluctuations are asymptotically damped to the previous steady-state condition (see Figure 7). Upon achieving the transition threshold the previously damped fluctuations now amplify and drive the system to new stable regimes. It is also possible for systems close to but below the critical ratio to reach the unstable transition region when certain types of fluctuations are present (cf. Prigogine and Nicolis, 1973). In either case the amplification always occurs in the fluctuation, driving the system to new stabilities. The source of the fluctuations – the spontaneous deviations from some average regime – are a universal

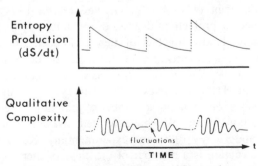

FIGURE 7    Damped phase of fluctuation

phenomenon in systems with large numbers of degrees of freedom (Prigogine, Nicolis, and Babloyantz, 1972).

Let us consider briefly the systematic events associated with the two phases of fluctuation: damped and amplified. Damped fluctuations are associated with thermodynamic systems possessing large numbers of degrees of freedom. The macro behavior of these systems may be said to be determinate since the damping continuously returns the systems to the same steady-state condition. As the thermodynamic system approaches the transition threshold, common fluctuation frequencies emerge allowing for the possibility of entrainment. Previously damped fluctuations are now amplified into a few 'preferred' frequencies. As the operational components are entrained, systematic dissipation of degrees of freedom occurs. Ultimately as the system moves through the critical region, the operational system of many degrees of freedom entrains into an ensemble system exhibiting a single degree of freedom. (This evolutionary sequence is consistent with Iberall's organizational principles for complex physical systems, see Section 3.6.) Prigogine and his colleagues (Prigogine, Nicolis, and Babloyantz, 1972) summarize the above events as follows: 'In the neighborhood of a stable regime, evolution is essentially deterministic in the sense that small fluctuations arising are continuously damped. But near the transition threshold the evolution becomes a stochastic process in the sense that the final state will depend on the probability of creating a fluctuation of a given type. Of course, once this probability is appreciable, the system will eventually reach a unique (apart from small fluctuations) stable state, once the boundary conditions are specified. This state will then be the starting point for further evolution' (p. 27).

### 5.5   Co-ordinative Structures as Dissipative Structures

Let us now draw these arguments to a conclusion by returning to Bernstein's problem concerning the regulation of biomechanical systems possessing multiple degrees of freedom. It has been argued by Bernstein (1967) and those who have pursued his point of view (e.g. Gelfand *et al.*, 1971; Greene, 1972; Turvey, 1977) that the problem of degrees of freedom may be resolved in large part by a systematic linking together of muscles in such a manner that the set of individual muscles is reduced to a much smaller set of muscle collectives. A muscle linkage or a *co-ordinative structure*, as we have come to call it (Kelso *et al.*, 1980; Kugler, Kelso, and Turvey, 1980; Turvey, Shaw, and Mace, 1978) is a group of muscles often spanning a number of joints that is constrained to act as a single functional unit. We have argued elsewhere both theoretically (Kugler, Kelso, and Turvey 1980) and experimentally (Kelso *et al.*, 1980) that a co-ordinative structure is a member of the class of thermodynamic engines qua dissipative structures, and that by virtue of this membership a principled basis is provided for understanding movement co-ordination and control.

A co-ordinative structure as dissipative structure differs from traditional concepts in the motor systems' literature (such as servomechanisms and programs). Instead of pre-established arrangements among components or ordered arrangements of specific instructions, co-ordinative structures constitute a set of organizational constraints which emerge as a function of various energy transactions, and scale changes at multiple levels of organization (ranging from motor units to muscles). Emerging constraints form a dynamic manifold of gradients and equilibrium points. The 'layout' of the manifold *uniquely* and *specifically* indexes biomechanical configurations in terms of *stability* and *energy dissipation*. An important features of the manifold is that it provides an information basis that is continuously scaled to artificially or naturally incurred changes in the systems' dimensions. As an information base the manifold does not 'cause' behavior to occur, but provides continuous information *about* the state of potential dynamic configurations. A manifold is 'structurally-stable' if the topological properties which define the manifold remain unaltered under a range of scale changes in the system's dimensions. Under such conditions the system will continue to exhibit the same set of stable biomechanical configurations. In the event that a scale or dimensional change causes a qualitative change in the manifold's topology – as when a topological property (such as an inflection point) is created or annihilated – then a new set of stable biomechanical configurations may arise. In Thom's terminology, a catastrophe has occurred in the system in the form of a sudden instability in the structure of the dynamic manifold. The catastrophe or bifurcation is always a function of changes in scale or dimensionality.

Let us examine several examples of motor behavior in which a bifurcation occurs in the structural stability of the biomechanical system. Consider the problem of quadruped locomotion. At low velocities, all quadrupeds locomote with a common asymmetry of limbs of the same girdle – they are always half a period out of phase. As the animals scale-up on velocity there is an abrupt transition from an asymmetric gait to a symmetric gait (Shik and Orlovskii, 1965). At higher velocities the stable states of quadruped locomotion are characterized by an in-phase relation of limbs of the same girdle (Grillner, 1975). Sudden changes in biomechanical stabilities wrought by changes in scale and dimensionality are also captured in centipede locomotion. The *Lithobius* normally moves its legs in waves with adjacent legs out of phase by one-seventh of a step. If, however, all but two pairs of the legs are amputated – and regardless of the number of segments separating the pairs – the insects will now display the asymmetrical gaits of quadrupeds. Similarly, *Lithobius* displays the gaits of six-legged insects when all but three pairs of legs are amputated (von Holst, 1973). A final example is drawn from the biomechanics of dolphin locomotion (Brookhart and Stein, 1980). At low velocities the dolphin's swimming pattern can be described as oscillatory. The motion creates a laminar flow of water over the dolphin's body surface allowing a stable form of travel in which energy dissipation is minimally incurred. At higher velocities, however, the laminar flow of water suddenly turns to turbulence. The earlier mode of travel has now become unstable and very expensive in terms of energy dissipation. At this point the dolphin abruptly changes its swimming mode to a more stable form of 'running' in which it periodically leaves the surface. This novel mode of travel now indexes a biomechanically stable solution for the new velocity.

The above examples are meant to emphasize the role of dynamics in the forging of spatiotemporal orderings in biomechanical systems. From this perspective a co-ordinative structure as dissipative structure interprets different locomotory gaits as those stable movement patterns, few in number, that can arise pursuant to the instabilities wrought by scaling-up muscle power (Kugler, Kelso, and Turvey 1980). The general point here is that locomotory patterns are to be explained by an appeal to the concepts and tools of nonequilibrium thermodynamics such as stability theory, bifurcation theory, and fluctuation theory (Haken, 1977; Prigogine et al., 1975; Thom, 1975) rather than an appeal to formal programs of instructions or sets of anatomically fixed constraints.

### 5.6 Co-ordinate Structures as Dissipative Structures: Developmental Comments from the Perspective of Stage Theory

Throughout this chapter our paradigm issue has focused on how it is that the body's many degrees of freedom can be systematically regulated in the face of scalar changes in the body's dimensions. As we have noted earlier, solutions to the degrees of freedom problem cannot be impervious to the Principle of Similitude. Just as a movement's topological qualities remain stable in the face of quantitative changes in scale, so also does scale induce qualitatively different movement patterns. In the previous section – and elsewhere – we have identified these features of movement with co-ordinative structures, and stressed the theoretical and empirical relationship between co-ordinative structures and dissipative structures (cf. Kelso et al., 1980; Kugler, Kelso, and Turvey, 1980). Here we wish to recognize the large body of descriptive data in motor development – as yet unevenly rationalized – and show that it is consistent with the notion of co-ordinative structures as dissipative structures.

There is collective agreement among developmentalists that as a child grows and develops, movement organizations change in a qualitatively step-wise or 'stage-like' fashion (e.g. Roberton, this volume; Smoll, this volume). Although the stage notion is used with varying degrees of sophistication, its universal connotation is one of sudden qualitative changes in the spatiotemporal order-ings of behavior that occur as a consequence of developmental age. With respect to movement development, the categories that constitute 'stages' are derived empirically according to descriptions of movement patterns – usually observed in natural settings. Even though a descriptive analysis may have pre-dictive value – as in the mapping of 'motor milestones' (e.g. Bayley, 1935; McGraw, 1941, 1945) – it lacks explanatory power. Indeed it is crucial for present purposes, to recognize (as so many have, cf. Connolly, 1970) that the descriptive approach is neutral with respect to the question of underlying *process*. We offer here an account of such processes in terms of the theory of co-ordinative structures as dissipative structures.

The data base that we shall consider is provided by the detailed longitudinal descriptions of how movements of an individual change over time (see Halverson and Roberton, 1966; Halverson, Roberton, and Harper, 1973). We refer specifically to the intra-task changes in the overhand throw for force (see Roberton, 1978 and this volume). Figure 8 illustrates the 'staircase' develop-ment of the forearm action in one child from the age of around 2 years to 13 years. The developmental 'steps' correspond to (i) no forearm lag, (ii) partial forearm lag and (iii) full forearm lag (see Roberton, 1978 for details and methods of analysis). This diagram serves to illustrate a stable sequence of spatiotemporal patterns associated with intra-task development as a function of time. The sequence is characterized by a series of qualitatively distinct patterns that are relatively uniform for all subjects despite individual differences in age of occurrence. Note that a relatively short period of time is spent in the transition or unstable period of development, while stable organiza-tion (as reflected in plateaus) is maintained for much longer. In contrast, Figure 9 illustrates a case where the instability – as indicated by the prolonged period of fluctuation – occurs over a longer period of time. How might these qualita-tive changes in movement patterns that develop over time (and take various forms) be interpreted?

The central claim throughout the present paper is that we should construe the development of self-organizing systems as an evolution of a dynamic geometry whose structure is created and maintained by a thermodynamic engine. In addition, we have proposed that information might best be conceived as form. Equilibrium points and gradients emerge from such a proposal as the fundamental building material for a manifold which relates to the evolving system in a unique and specific fashion. Sensitivity to properties of the manifold is synonymous with sensitivity to information *about* the *state* of the system's dynamics. The structural properties of the manifold are created and maintained by a continuous flow of energy into and out of the operational com-ponents of the system. Under certain scale changes the dynamic qualities of the

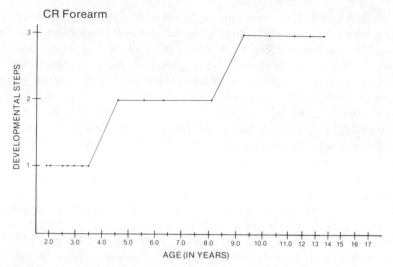

CR Forearm

FIGURE 8 'Staircase' development in overarm throw forearm action in child CR (male) from age 1-10 to 13-2 years. Developmental steps are (i) no forearm lag; (ii) partial forearm lag; and (iii) full forearm lag. (See Roberton, 1978a for complete category descriptions.) Reprinted with permission from Roberton, M. A., and Langendorfer, S., Testing motor development sequences across 9–14 years, In K. Newell, G. Roberts, W. Halliwell, and C. Nadeau (Eds.), *Psychology of motor behavior and sport – 1979*, Champaign, Ill.: Human Kinetics. 1980
(Figures 8 and 9 correspond to Figures 1 and 2 of Roberton (this volume). We are very grateful to Mary Ann Roberton for allowing us to display them here which we do for the sake of completeness.)

system will remain invariant, while under critical scale changes the previously stable organization of the manifold may suddenly break down and be replaced by a new organization. The important feature of this sequence of events is that a *continuous* change in a single variable (or combination of variables) may bring about a sudden *qualitative* change in the macro structure of the manifold associated with the variable(s). The qualitative changes in the manifold reveal themselves in the annihilation or creation of various equilibrium points.

The above explanation of 'stages' of development is obviously conjectural at this point. But let us offer some suggestions as to how these claims might be formalized. The first step in any stage theory of development is to distinguish the various stabilities and instabilities associated with the developmental sequence of interest. Traditionally the descriptive criteria for identifying various stages have suffered from a rather subjective origin. Certain landmark features are selected which purportedly distinguish one stage of development

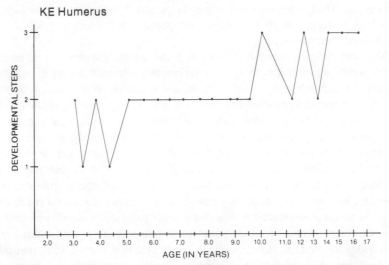

FIGURE 9   Step-to-step development in overarm throw humerus action in child KE (female) from age 3-0 to 16-3 years. Several years of transition occurred before reaching each higher level. Developmental steps are (i) humerus oblique; (ii) humerus aligned but independent; and (iii) humerus lags. (See Roberton, 1978a for complete category descriptions.) Reprinted with permission from Roberton, M. A., and Langendorfer, S., Testing motor development sequences across 9–14 years, in K. Newell, G. Roberts, W. Halliwell, and C. Nadeau (Eds.), *Psychology of motor behavior and sport – 1979*, Champaign, Ill.: Human Kinetics, 1980

from another in an unambiguous way. In general the criteria are motivated by methodological concerns. A more theoretical criterion for selecting different stages might be found in the principles of homeokinetic physics (see Section 3.6). Recall that homeokinetic physics seeks to provide a physical account of the orderly events associated with biological systems. Homeokinetics argues that a thermodynamic engine defines the minimum unit of biological organization. Energy transactions within the thermodynamic engine are always in the form of limit cycle oscillation. The unit of organization may vary in size and order of complexity. A simple unit of organization might constitute a single sink–source, energy-flow system. A more complex system might constitute a collective of sink–source, energy-flow systems which interact in a unified manner so as to exhibit a single collective limit cycle oscillation. An example of a simple system might be a single cell whereas a complex system might be an organ composed of many single cells. In both cases, however, the behavioral unit of organization is an autonomous thermodynamic engine and may be functionally distinguished by the unique spectral properties of the system's limit cycles. Thus, various units of organization may be systematically distinguished in terms of their spectral properties (see Section 3.6.2 for the homeokinetic methodology).

If the limit cycle signature is to be of any use in distinguishing stable patterns of movement organization, then the movement patterns must be chosen with concern for dependent measures which are sensitive to spectral properties. Such movement patterns would require a degree of rhythmicity in their fundamental form (although note that the choice of rhythmical activity is methodologically motivated; elsewhere we have shown how discrete and cyclical movements could emerge from the same limit cycle organization (Kelso *et al.*, 1980; Kugler, Kelso, and Turvey, 1980)). Stable patterns of movement could then be distinguished in terms of their spatiotemporal properties. In short, a methodology based on homeokinetics would entail selection of behavioral sequences which distinguish themselves developmentally in terms of their spectral composition. Such patterns may well share or be elaborations of certain biomechanical configurations that developmentalists have traditionally associated with stages. The point to emphasize however is that the homeokinetic methodology offers a theoretical basis for selecting sequences of stable biomechanical configurations that may constitute developmental stages.

A second methodology for distinguishing various stages of organizational development may be borrowed from Dissipative Structure theory (see Section 3.5). The methodology of dissipative structures entails an identification of the kinetic equations which describe the bifurcations of the biomechanical stabilities associated with scale changes. While homeokinetics focuses on the maintenance of stable organizations, the second methodology – from Dissipative Structure theory – addresses the instabilities associated with transition phenomena. For critical values an instability can arise that causes the biomechanical configuration to change radically and in a discontinuous manner. The beginning of an approach based on dissipative structures starts with an identification of the dimensions which define the system of interest. For the biomechanical system this involves variables such as mass, length, stiffness, etc. Unfortunately even when the dimensions are known, formulation of the appropriate equations can still constitute a formidable task. Such an analysis, we suspect, would allow deep insights into which variables are most critical at which periods in time (see for example, Kugler, Kelso, and Turvey, 1980, Figures 8 and 9).

## 6    A PHYSICAL AND EPISTEMOLOGICAL BASIS FOR DESIGNING AND MODELING NATURAL SYSTEMS: A SUMMARY

The principal goal of this chapter has been to discuss the physical and epistemological basis of order and regularity in natural systems. We have proposed a perspective on the analysis of natural systems that is characterized by a commitment to two coupled themes: first, an explanatory commitment to physical theory, and second, an ontological and epistemological commitment to the tenets of Ecological Realism. The perspective follows the lead of Iberall, Yates, and Soodak in seeking a universal set of design principles that can be applied repetitively and with equanimity across all scales, and across all disciplines that address systematic phenomena in biology.

A major problem confronting theories of biological organization concerns the provision of a principled account of the systematic reduction in a system's potentially large number of degrees of freedom. More formally, the problem focuses on the systematic mapping from a space of multiple fine-grain variables to a space of considerably fewer coarse-grained variables. In terms of movement science the problem is realized in the stable organization of gross movement patterns of a very few degrees of freedom which are derived from a skeletal basis of very many degrees of freedom. The solution outlined in this chapter is derived from many principles that are not commonplace to students of the development of movement. Such principles originate in philosophy, physics, biology, engineering science and, in particular, nonequilibrium thermodynamics and the ecological approach to perception and action. Throughout, our paradigm issue has been the developmental implications of scale changes in the body's dimensions, and the problem of how information can be conceptualized so as to insure continuous control and co-ordination in the face of such scale changes. Below is a summary statement of the physical and epistemological principles implicated in a theory of the control and co-ordination for naturally developing systems. We begin with a summary of physical principles.

## 6.1 Physical Principles That Inform Biological Design

According to classical physical theory (or at least its philosophic view) living systems were viewed as continuously struggling against the laws of physics. The temptation was to ascribe an accidental character to living processes and to imagine their origin as a result of a series of highly improbable events. Indeed, living systems were viewed as the consequence of biological principles that were independent of the laws of physics. The account currently emerging in the field of molecular biology and nonequilibrium thermodynamics supports a different point of view. Far from being outside physical laws, living processes are viewed as following from the laws of physics whenever certain open conditions prevail. The principal results in favor of this conclusion are as follows: systems close to equilibrium always turn toward equilibrium in a linear fashion and evolve to a disordered state corresponding to the steady state of equilibrium. Small deviations, due, say to random perturbations, are continuously damped out by a mechanism ultimately operating on a variational principle of minimum entropy production. The mechanism operates such that for time-independent boundary conditions, the dissipation inside the system (measured by the production of entropy per unit time) attains a minimal value compatible with boundary conditions. If the system is open to the flow of energy and matter, then it is possible to increase its operating distance with respect to global equilibrium. As the distance increases the steady state close to equilibrium continuously shifts up a thermodynamic branch of states, all of which exhibit linear stability of the equilibrium-like behavior. The equilibrium structures which constitute the thermodynamic branch are obtained through a continuous modification of the boundary conditions. As the distance from equilibrium is scaled-up, a critical point is reached where the damping mechanism suddenly breaks down due to nonlinear interactions. No longer does the linear damping mechanism guarantee the global stability of the branch; the disequilibrium state becomes unstable, the amount of dissipation introduced by the fluctuations becomes negative, resulting in amplification rather than damping of the fluctuation. The resulting instability drives the system off the thermodynamic branch (globally but not locally) to a qualitatively new spatiotemporal structure that exhibits the characteristics of nonlinear limit-cycle stability.[1]

An important characteristic of the instabilities is that the relation between order and fluctuation is much more complex than at equilibrium. At equilibrium everything is determined by the strict properties of the thermodynamic potentials and hence the fluctuations are all damped in a characteristically similar manner. This is not the case in the nonlinear range where not only are fluctuations the trigger for the appearance of new structures and processes, but different types of fluctuations may also correspond to different structures. To emphasize the role of fluctuation, Prigogine has termed the new ordering principle *order through fluctuation*.

Two developmental phases may be distinguished. The first phase corresponds to the emergence of a qualitatively new ordering in the macro structure. The second stage entails the stable maintenance of the new structure. The creation phase is associated with *a theory of design*; that is, a theory implicating *change* in various qualitative properties from one system to another. The maintenance phase, on the other hand, is associated with *a theory of modeling*; that is, a theory implicating *preservation* of various qualitative properties from one system to another. The two phases distinguish themselves thermodynamically in the behavior of entropy production: the creation phase operates on the variational principle of excess entropy production, while the maintenance phase operates on the variational principle of minimum entropy production. In addition, the two phases distinguish themselves in the macro structure. Qualitative changes in the spatiotemporal ordering of a system index the establishment of new dissipative structures, while the emergence of a limit-cycle oscillation marks the signature of a stabilized thermodynamic engine. The analysis of the maintenance phase constitutes the chief concern of homeokinetic physics.

Homeokinetics views any relative constancy in biological systems as an emergent and distributed property (a steady-state operating point) of a thermodynamic engine complex. Thermodynamic engines constitute energy-flow systems that draw from a high potential source, reject some to a lower potential sink and do work in a periodic limit-cycle fashion. The amplitude and period of oscillations are determined by the geometric layout of the source–sink, energy-flow system, independent of initial conditions. The limit-cycle periodicity indexes the important energy transactions going on within a thermodynamic system, and the time domains in which it occurs. The limit-cycle, then, is the characteristic signature of an autonomous thermodynamic engine.

The conclusion to be drawn from the theories of Dissipative Structures and Homeokinetics is that there is an inherent possibility for the creation and maintenance of qualitatively new spatiotemporal orderings in thermodynamically-open systems when specific nonlinear interactions are realized. From a more general viewpoint, the principles of nonequilibrium thermodynamics provide a unified framework, as well as an appropriate language for analyzing complex and diverse phenomena in living systems. The core thesis of such an analysis is that the flow of energy and matter through a system, in the nonequilibrium thermodynamic sense, acts to organize and maintain that system. (See p. 43 for a list of general requirements for this organizing principle to manifest itself.)

### 6.1.2 A Commitment to the Tenets of Ecological Realism

*The ecological approach to perception and action incorporates psychology as a companion endeavor to physics and biology for the purpose of studying the epistemological relationship between an animal, as agent and perceiver, and its environment.* The goal of a theory of action and perception is to explicate the organizational principles relating animal and environment on the basis of energy and informational transactions. A commitment to ecological realism starts with the assumptions of (i) a mutuality or synergy of animal and environment as an ecosystem and (ii) information as unique and specific to the dynamics of that ecosystem. Specifically, the ecological perspective denies the legitimacy of approaches that separate animal and environment such that a new and special third class of terms (e.g. set-points, programs, schemas, etc.) must be introduced to mediate the control and co-ordination between them. In addition, the ecological approach denies the introduction of a semantically neutral set of information descriptors (e.g. bits). The concept of information mandated by the ecological approach necessitates that information be defined as *unique, specific* and *meaningful* to the control and co-ordination requirements of activity. Moreover, as we have sought to show in the present chapter, information must be *continuously scaled to the dimensions of the system* over which the activity is defined.

The confluence of the two themes of (1) energy flow as a self-organizing and self-maintaining principle and (2) information as unique and specific to activity may be found in the morphology of a biological system's dynamics. The particular order exhibited by a thermodynamic system depends in a very detailed way on the geometric properties that define the source–sink, energy-flow system. Geometric properties are continuously scaled to the dimensions of the thermodynamic system and unique and specific to its stable and dissipative properties.

### 6.1.3   Information as Form: The Establishment of an Intrinsic Metric

> ... any geometric form whatsoever can be the carrier of information, and in the set of geometric forms carrying information of the same type the topological complexity of the form is the quantitative scalar of the information.
>
> Thom (1975, p. 145)

The concept of information as form has primary application to a class of 'well-organized' functions whose variables may be decomposed into the subdivisions of non-essential and essential. Following Gel'fand and Tsetlin nonessential variables bring about marked changes in the value of the function but leave the topological qualities of the function unaltered, and essential variables determine the function's topological qualities. An important aspect of such functions is that the particular characteristics of the organization need not be known in advance. Transformations over the function are sufficient to reveal the intrinsic properties. When this class of functions is defined over a dynamic system, the qualitative properties of the functions are revealed in the forms of dramatic gradients and equilibrium points. While the division into essential and nonessential may not be possible for all mathematical functions, many of the functions (probably the majority) of living systems capture this decomposition. In formulating the mathematical theory of nonlinear differential equations Poincaré provided the first formal analysis of well-organized functions in dynamic systems. Using the powerful tools of qualitative analytic-topology Poincaré was able to provide a classification of stable temporal periodicities in nonlinear systems. More recently, Thom's somewhat general formulation of morphogenesis in terms of the topological theory of ordinary differential equations has provided a broad classification of situations arising at the bifurcation points or, to use Thom's terminology, at the catastrophe points.

The issue of 'well-organized' functions bears directly on the problems of self-organization and self-maintenance in physical systems. Prior to the establishment of a stable spatiotemporal ordering, the system is at equilibrium and behaves in a linear way. Under sufficient scale changes however, the system shifts from a linear to a nonlinear mode of behavior. Scale changes then create an instability in the system, driving it to a new stable spatiotemporal structure. In the new organization linear and nonlinear variables evolve an organization allowing for the possibility of the creation and maintenance of new stable orderings. This organizational strategy offers a degree of flexibility and precision in the behavior of the system by virtue of the *form* of its linear properties, and a degree of stability in the system's behavior due to the *form* of its nonlinear variables. In short, the organization reveals a functional basis for *control* (precision and flexibility) and *co-ordination* (stability) in the *forms* (as information) of the linear and nonlinear components respectively. (For more details on the concepts of control and co-ordination in terms of functional forms see Kugler, Kelso, and Turvey, 1980.)

In conclusion, in this chapter we have attempted to provide a unified theoretical framework which stands accountable to the developmental problems associated with scale and dimensional changes. A unique aspect of this formulation is its attempt to undercut the classical separation between the high power, energy converting machinery (corresponding to the dynamical aspects of the system) and the low power, communicational signals (corresponding to the linguistic component of the system). In wedding contemporary physical theory to the ecological theory of perception and action, we have taken a first step toward establishing an intrinsic metric for the concept of information. According to this view, information is a *physical* variable that is unique and specific to the changing geometry of a system's dynamics. We suspect rather strongly that only this notion of information places satisfactory and nonarbitrary restrictions on the solution to the degrees of freedom problem in naturally developing systems. That is, without an intrinsic metric for information, we see little chance of an adequate rationale emerging for how movements are co-ordinated and controlled in a system whose dimensions change in magnitude gradually (as in growth) or artificially (as when an organism performs instrumental activity).

## ACKNOWLEDGMENTS

The writing of this chapter was supported by NIH Grants NS 13617, AM 25814 and HD 01994 and Biomedical Research Support Grant RR 05596 to Haskins Laboratories. We are indebted to Arthur Iberall for reviewing an earlier version and Claudia Carello for making the figures.

## NOTE

1. Prigogine has termed the new regime a dissipative structure to emphasize the entropy-producing field processes inside the system which serve to create and maintain the order. Iberall, on the other hand, regards this as the near equilibrium thermodynamic processes – including chemical change – which have been studied by hydrodynamicists since Maxwell, Reynolds, Rayleigh, Helmholtz, Kirchoff, etc. The nonequilibrium of chemistry is only a near equilibrium in thermodynamics. According to the homeokinetic school, what requires novelty of treatment is how to introduce the 'symmetry breaking' of matter condensation.

## REFERENCES

Adams, J. A. (1971). A closed-loop theory of motor learning, *Journal of Motor Behavior*, **3**, 111–150.

Alexander, R. M. (1968). *Animal Mechanics*, University of Washington Press.

Apter, M. J. (1966). *Cybernetics and Development*, London: Pergamon Press.

Attneave, F. (1959). *Applications of Information Theory to Psychology: A summary of basic concepts, methods and results*, New York: Holt.

Baerends, G. P. (1976). The functional organization of behavior, *Animal Behavior*, **24**, 726–738.

Balescu, R. (1975). *Equilibrium and Nonequilibrium Statistical Mechanics*, New York: Wiley.

Bayley, N. (1933). Development of motor abilities during the first three years, *Monograph Society of the Research in Child Development*, **1**.

Bellman, R. E. (1961). *Adaptive Control Processes*, Princeton, NJ: Princeton University Press.

Berlinski, D. (1976). *On Systems*, Boston: MIT Press.

Bernard, C. (1949). *An Introduction to the Study of Experimental Medicine*, New York: Schuman.

Bernstein, N. (1967). *The Coordination and Regulation of Movements*, London: Pergamon Press.

Bertalanffy, L. von. (1973). *General System Theory*, Harmondsworth, England: Penguin.

Bloch, E. and Iberall, A. (1974). The functional unit of mammalian skeletal muscle, *Anatomical Record*, **178**, 312.

Bohm, D. (1957). *Causality and Chance in Modern Physics*, London: Routledge and Kegan Paul.

Bridgeman, P. W. (1922). *Dimensional Analysis*, New Haven, CT: Yale University Press.

Bridgeman, P. W. (1941). *The Nature of Thermodynamics*, Cambridge, Mass.: Harvard University Press.

Brookhart, J. M., and Stein, P. S. G. (1980). *Locomotion*, Quincy, Mass.: Grass Instrument Co.

Bunge, M. (1977). Levels and reductions, *American Journal of Physiology*, **233**, R75–R82.

Cannon, W. (1939). *The Wisdom of the Body*, New York: Norton.

Chapman, S., and Cowling, T. (1952). *The Mathematical Theory of Non-uniform Gases*, Cambridge, England: Cambridge Univ. Press.

Connolly, K. (1970). *Mechanisms of Skill Development*, New York: Academic Press.
Cornman, J. W. (1975). *Perception, Common Sense, and Science*, New Haven: Yale Univ. Press.
DeGroot, S. R., and Mazur, P. (1962). *Non-equilibrium Thermodynamics*, Amsterdam: North-Holland.
Dewey, J., and Bentley, A. F. (1949). *Knowing and the Known*, Boston: Beacon.
Elsasser, W. M. (1958). *The Physical Foundation of Biology*, Oxford: Pergamon Press.
Fitch, H., and Turvey, M. T. (1978). On the control of activity: Some remarks from an ecological point of view, in R. Christina (ed.), *Psychology of Motor Behavior and Sports*, Urbana, Ill.: Human Kinetics.
Fodor, J. A. (1975). *The Language of Thought*, New York: Thomas Y. Crowell.
Fowler, C., Rubin, P., Remez, R., and Turvey, M. T. (1980). Implications for speech production of a general theory of action, in B. Butterworth (ed.), *Language Production*, London: Academic Press.
Fowler, C. A., and Turvey, M. T. (1978). Skill acquisition: An event approach with special reference to searching for the optimum of a function of several variables, in G. Stelmach (ed.), *Information Processing in Motor Control and Learning*, New York: Academic Press.
Gelfand, I. M., Gurfinkel, V. S., Tsetlin, M. L., and Shik, M. L. (1971). Some problems in the analysis of movements, in I. M. Gelfand *et al.* (eds.), *Models of the Structural-functional Organization of Certain Biological Systems*, Cambridge: MIT Press.
Gelfand, I. M., and Tsetlin, M. L. (1962). Some methods of control for complex systems, *Russian Mathematical Surveys*, **17**, 95–116.
Gibson, J. J. (1950). *The Perception of the Visual World*, Boston: Houghton Mifflin.
Gibson, J. J. (1966). *The Senses Considered as Perceptual Systems*, Boston: Houghton Mifflin.
Gibson, J. J. (1979). *The Ecological Approach to Visual Perceptions*, Boston: Houghton Mifflin.
Glansdorff, P., and Prigogine, I. (1971). *Thermodynamic Theory of Structure, Stability and Fluctuations*, New York: Wiley-Interscience.
Greene, P. H. (1972). Problems of organization of motor systems, in R. Rosen and F. Snell (eds.), *Progress in Theoretical Biology* (Vol. 2), New York: Academic Press.
Gregory, R. L. (1974). *Concepts and Mechanisms of Perception*, New York: Scribner.
Grillner, S. (1975). Locomotion in vertebrates. Central mechanisms and reflex interaction, *Physiological Review*, **55**, 247–304.
Haken, H. (1977). *Synergetics*, Heidelberg: Springer-Verlag.
Halverson, L. E., and Roberton, M. A. (1966). A study of motor pattern development in young children, *Abstracts*, Research Section, National Convention, American Association for Health, Physical Education and Recreation.
Halverson, L. E., Roberton, M. A., and Harper, C. J. (1973). Current research in motor development, *Journal of Research and Development in Education*, **6**, 56–70.
Hanson, N. R. (1974). *Patterns of discovery*, Cambridge: Cambridge University Press.
Helmholtz, H. von (1925). In J. P. Southall (ed. and trans.), *Treatise on Psychological Optics*, Rochester, NY: Optical Society of America.
Hertel, H. (1966). *Structure, Form, Movement*, New York: Reinhold.
Holst, F. von (1973). *The Behavioral Physiology of Animals and Man*, Coral Gables, Fla.: University of Miami Press.
Iberall, A. (1969). New thoughts in biocontrol, in C. Waddington (ed.), *Towards a Theoretical Biology* (Vol. 2), Edinburgh: Edinburgh University Press, pp. 166–178.

Iberall, A. S. (1972). *Toward a General Science of Viable Systems*, New York: McGraw-Hill.

Iberall, A. S. (1975). On nature, man and society: A basis for scientific modeling, *Annals of Biomedical Engineering*, **3**, 344–385.

Iberall, A. S. (1977). A field and circuit thermodynamics for integrative physiology: I. Introduction to general notions, *American Journal of Physiology/Regulatory, Integrative, & Comparative Physiology*, **2**, R171–R180.

Iberall, A. S. (1978a). Cybernetics offers a (hydrodynamic) thermodynamic view of brain activities. An alternative to reflexology, in F. Brambilla, P. K. Bridges, E. Endroczi and C. Heusep (eds.), *Perspectives in Endocrine Psychobiology*, New York: Wiley.

Iberall, A. S. (1978b). A field and circuit thermodynamics for integrative physiology: III. Keeping the books – a general experimental method, *American Journal of Physiology/Regulatory, Integrative, & Comparative Physiology*, **3**, R85–R97.

Iberall, A., and McCulloch, W. S. (1970). Homeokinesis – the organization of complex living systems, in A. S. Iberall and J. B. Reswick (eds.), *Technical and Biological Processes of Control: A cybernetic view*, Pittsburgh, Penn.: Instrument Society of America.

Iberall, A. S., and Soodak, H. (1978). Physical basis for complex systems – some propositions relating levels of organization, *Collective Phenomena*, **3**, 9–24.

Iberall, A. S., Soodak, H., and Arensberg, C. (in press). Homeokinetic physics of societies – a new discipline – autonomous groups, cultures, politics, in H. Reul, D. Ghista, and G. Rau (eds.), *Perspectives in Biomechanics*, New York: Harwood Acad.

Iberall, A. S., Soodak, H., and Hassler, F. (1978). A field and circuit thermodynamics for integrative physiology. II. Power communicational spectroscopy in biology, *American Journal of Physiology*, **3**, R3–R19.

Jammer, M. (1974). *The Philosophy of Quantum Mechanics: The interpretations of quantum mechanics in historical perspective*, New York: Wiley-Interscience.

Johnston, T. D., and Turvey, M. T. (1980). An ecological metatheory for theories of learning, in G. H. Bower (ed.), *The Psychology of Learning and Motivation*, New York: Academic Press, pp. 147–205.

Keele, S. W. (1980). A behavioral analysis of motor control, in V. Brooks (ed.), *Handbook of Physiology: Motor control*, Washington DC: American Psychological Society.

Keele, S. W., and Summers, J. (1976). The structure of motor programs, in G. E. Stelmach (ed.), *Motor Control: Issues and trends* New York: Academic Press, pp. 109–142.

Kelso, J. A. S. (1981). Contrasting perspectives on order and regulation in move-of coordinative structures as dissipative structures: II. Empirical lines of con-NJ: Lawrence Erlbaum.

Kelso, J. A. S., Holt, K. G., Kugler, P. N., and Turvey, M. T. (1980). On the concept of coordinative structures in dissipative structures: II. Empirical lines of convergence, in G. E. Stelmach and J. Requin (eds.), *Tutorials in Motor Behavior*, New York: North-Holland.

Kohler, W. (1969). *The Task of Gestalt Psychology*, Princeton, NJ: Princeton University Press.

Koschmeider, E. L. (1975). Stability of supercritical Bénard convection and Taylor vortex flow, in I. Prigogine and S. A. Rice (eds.), *Advances in Chemical Physics*, New York: Wiley.

Koschmeider, E. L. (1977). Instabilities in fluid dynamics, in H. Haken (ed.), *Synergetics*: A workshop, New York: Springer-Verlag.

Kugler, P. N., and Turvey, M. T. (1979). Two metaphors for neural afference and efference, *The Behavioral and Brain Sciences*, **2**.

Kugler, P. N. K., Kelso, J. A. S., and Turvey, M. T. (1980). On the concept of co-ordinative structures as dissipative structures: I. Theoretical lines of convergence, in G. E. Stelmach and J. Requin (eds.), *Tutorials in Motor Behavior*, New York: North-Holland, pp. 1–47.

Lee, D. H. (1976). A theory of visual control of braking based on information about time-to-collision, *Perception*, **5**, 437–459.

MacKay, D. M. (1969). *Information, Mechanism, and Meaning*, Cambridge, Mass.: MIT Press.

Mandle, C. (1971). *Perception: Facts and Theories*. Oxford: Oxford Univ. Press.

McGraw, M. B. (1941). Development of neuro-muscular mechanisms as reflected in the crawling and creeping behavior of the human infant, *Journal of Genetic Psychology*, **58**, 83–111.

McGraw, M. B. (1945). *The Neuro-Muscular Maturation of the Human Infant*, New York: Columbia University Press.

Minsky, M., and Papert, S. (1972). Artificial intelligence, *Artificial Intelligence Memo*, *252*, Cambridge, Mass.: Artificial Intelligence Laboratory, MIT.

Mitchell, D., Snellen, J. W., and Atkins, J. R. (1970). Thermoregulation during fever: Change in setpoint or change in gain, *Pflugers Archives*, **321**, 293.

Morowitz, H. J. (1968). *Energy Flow in Biology; Biological organization as a problem in Thermal Physics*, New York: Academic Press.

Morowitz, H. J. (1978). *Foundations of Bioenergetics*, New York: Academic Press.

Mundle, C. W. K. (1971). *Perception: Facts and theories*, London: Oxford University Press.

Nazarea, A. D. (1974). Critical length of the transport-dominated region for oscillating non-linear reactive processes, *Proceedings of the National Academy of Science* (USA), **71**, 3751–3753.

Nicolis, G., and Prigogine, I. (1971). Fluctuations in nonequilibrium systems, *Proceedings of the National Academy of Science* (USA), **68**, 2102–2107.

Nicolis, G., and Auchmuty, J. F. G. (1974). Dissipative structures, catastrophes, and pattern formation: a bifurcation analysis, *Proceedings of the National Academy of Science* (USA), **71**, 2748–2751.

Nicolis, G., and Prigogine, I. (1977). *Self-organization in Nonequilibrium Systems: From dissipative structures to order through fluctuations*, New York: Wiley-Interscience.

Nicolis, G., Prigogine, I., and Glansdorff, P. (1975). On the mechanism of instabilities in nonlinear systems, in I. Prigogine and S. Rice (eds.), *Proceedings of the Conference on Instability and Dissipative Structures in Hydrodynamics*, New York: Wiley-Interscience.

Onsager, L. (1931). Reciprocal relations in irreversible processes, *Physiological Reviews*, **37**, 405.

Pattee, H. H. (1972a). Physical problems of decision-making constraints, *International Journal of Neuroscience*, **3**, 99–106.

Pattee, H. H. (1972b). Laws and constraints, symbols and language, in C. H. Waddington (ed.), *Towards a Theoretical Biology*, Chicago: Aldine.

Pattee, H. H. (1973). Physical problems of the origin of natural controls, in A. Locker (ed.), *Biogenesis, Evolution, Homeostasis*, Heidelberg: Springer-Verlag, pp. 41–49.

Pattee, H. H. (1977). Dynamic and linguistic modes of complex systems, *International Journal of General Systems*, **3**, 259–266.

Pearson, K. (1976). The control of walking, *Scientific American*, 72–86.

Pew, R. W. (1974). Human perceptual motor-performance, in B. H. Kantowitz (ed.), *Human Information Processing: Tutorials in performance and cognition*, New York: Lawrence Erlbaum.

Powers, W. T. (1973). *Behavior: The control of perception*, Chicago: Aldine.

Powers, W. T. (1978). Quantitative analysis of purposive systems: Some spadework at the foundations of scientific psychology, *Psychological Review*.

Prigogine, I. (1947). *Etude thermodynamique des processus irreversibles*, Desoer, Liege.

Prigogine, I. (1967). *Introduction to Thermodynamics of Irreversible Processes* (3rd edn.) New York: Wiley-Interscience.

Prigogine, I. (1969). Structure, dissipation, and life, in M. Marois (ed.), *Theoretical Physics and Biology*, Amsterdam: North-Holland, pp. 23–52.

Prigogine, I. (1976). Order through fluctuation: self-organization and social systems, in E. Jantsch and C. H. Waddington (eds.), *Evolution and Consciousness: Human systems in transition*, Reading, Mass.: Addison-Wesley.

Prigogine, I. (1978). Time, structure, and fluctuations, *Science*, **201**, 4358.

Prigogine, I., and Nicolis, G. (1971). Biological order, structure and instabilities, *Quarterly Reviews of Biophysics*, **4**, 107–148.

Prigogine, I., and Nicolis, G. (1973). Fluctuations and the mechanism of instabilities, in M. Marois (ed.), *Proceedings of the 3rd International Conference From Theoretical Physics to Biology*, Basel: S. Karger, pp. 89–109.

Prigogine, I., Nicolis, G., and Babloyantz, A. (1972). Thermodynamics of evolution, *Physics Today*, **25**, 11–12.

Prigogine, I., Allen, P., and Herman, R. (1977). The evolution of complexity and the laws of nature, in E. Laszlo and J. Bierman (eds.), *Goals in a Global Community* (Vol. 1), Club of Rowe.

Prigogine, I., Nicolis, G., Herman, R., and Lam, T. (1975). Stability, fluctuations and complexity, *Collective Phenomena*, **2**, 103–109.

Pylyshyn, Z. W. (1980). Computation and cognition: Issues in the foundations of cognitive science, *The Behavioral and Brain Sciences*, **3**, 111–169.

Rashevsky, N. (1938/1950). *Mathematical Biophysics: Mathematical foundations of biology*, New York: Dover Publications.

Raven, C. P. (1961). *Oogenesis: the storage of development information*, London: Pergamon Press.

Riggs, D. S. (1970). *The Mathematical Approach to Physiological Problems: a critical primer*, Cambridge, Mass.: MIT Press.

Roberton, M. A. (1978). Stages in movement development, in M. Ridenour (ed.), *Motor Development: Issues and applications*, Princeton, NJ: Princeton Book Co.

Rock, I. (1975). *An Introduction to Perception*, New York: Macmillan.

Rosen, R. (1973). On the generation of metabolic novelties in evolution. In A. Locker (ed.), *Biogenesis, Evolution, Homeostasis*, Heidelberg: Springer-Verlag.

Rosen, R. (1978). *Fundamentals of Measurement and Representation of Natural Systems*, New York: North-Holland.

Runeson, S. (1977). On the possibility of 'smart' perceptual mechanisms, *Scandinavian Journal of Psychology*, **18**, 172–179.

Schmidt, R. A. (1975). A schema theory of discrete motor skill learning, *Psychological Review*, **82**, 225–260.

Shannon, C. E., and Weaver, W. (1949). *The Mathematical Theory of Communication*, Urbana: University of Illinois Press.

Shaw, R. E., and McIntyre, M. (1974). Algoristic foundations to cognitive psychology, in W. Weimer and D. Palermo (eds.), *Cognition and the Symbolic Processes*, Hillsdale, NJ: Lawrence Erlbaum.

Shaw, R., and Turvey, M. T. (1981). Coalitions as models for ecosystems: A realist's perspective on perceptual organization, in M. Kubouy and J. Pomerantz (eds.), *Perceptual Organization*, Hillsdale, NJ: Lawrence Erlbaum.

Shaw, R. E., Turvey, M. T., and Mace, W. (in press). Ecological psychology: The consequences of a commitment to realism, in W. Weimer and D. Palmero (eds.), *Cognition and the Symbolic Processes* (II), Hillsdale, NJ: Lawrence Erlbaum.

Shik, M. L., and Orlovskii, G. N. (1965). Co-ordination of the limbs during running of the dog, *Biophysics*, **10**, 1148–1159.

Soodak, H., and Iberall, A. S. (1978). Homeokinetics: A physical science for complex systems, *Science*, **201**, 579–582.

Stahl, W. R. (1962). Dimensional analysis in mathematical biology, *Bulletin of Mathematical Biophysics*, **24**, 81–108.

Thom, R. (1970). Topological models in biology, in C. H. Waddington (ed.), *Towards a Theoretical Biology* (3), Chicago, Ill.: Aldine.

Thom, R. (1975). In D. H. Fowler (trans.), *Structural Stability and Morphogenesis*, Reading, Mass.: Benjamin.

Thompson, D. W. (1917/1942). *On Growth and Form*, London: Cambridge University Press.

Tolman, R. (1938). *The Principles of Statistical Mechanics*, London: Oxford Univ. Press.

Tomović, R. (1978). Some central conditions for self-organization – what the control theorist can learn from biology, *American Journal of Physiology: Regulatory, Integrative, & Comparative Physiology*, **3**, R205–R209.

Troland, L. T. (1929). *The Principles of Psychophysiology*, New York: Van Nostrand.

Tsetlin, M. L. (1973). *Automata Theory and Modeling in Biological Systems*, New York: Academic Press.

Turvey, M. T. (1977). Preliminaries to a theory of action with reference to vision, in R. Shaw and J. Bransford (eds.), *Perceiving, Acting and Knowing: Towards an ecological psychology*, Hillsdale, NJ: Lawrence Erlbaum.

Turvey, M. T. (1980). Clues from the organization of motor systems. In U. Bellugi and M. Studdert-Kennedy (eds.), *Signed and Spoken Language: Biological constraints on Linguistic Form*, Dahlem Konferenzen, Weinheim: Verlag Chemie.

Turvey, M. T., Fitch, H. L., and Tuller, B. (in press). The problems of degrees of freedom and context-conditioned variability, in J. A. S. Kelso (ed.), *Human Motor Behavior: An Introduction*, Hillsdale, NJ: Lawrence Erlbaum.

Turvey, M. T., and Shaw, R. E. (1979). The primacy of perceiving: An ecological reformulation of perception for understanding memory, in L-G. Nilsson (ed.), *Perspectives on Memory Research: Essays in honor of Uppsala University's 500th anniversary*, Hillsdale, NJ: Lawrence Erlbaum.

Turvey, M. T., Shaw, R. E., and Mace, W. (1978). Issues in a theory of action: degrees of freedom, coordinative structures and coalitions. In J. Requin (ed.), *Attention and performance VII*, Hillsdale, NJ: Lawrence Erlbaum.

Waddington, C. H. (1969). The basic ideas of biology, in C. H. Waddington (ed.), *Towards a Theoretical Biology*, Chicago: Aldine, pp. 1–32.

Waddington, C. H. (1970). Concepts and theories of growth, development, differentiation, and morphogenesis, in C. H. Waddington (ed.), *Towards a Theoretical Biology*, Chicago: Aldine, p. 177.

Wells, K. F. (1976). *Kinesiology: Scientific Basis of Human Motion*, Philadelphia: W. B. Saunders.

Werner, J. (1977). Mathematical treatment of structure and function of the human thermoregulatory system, *Biological Cybernetics*, 25, 93–101.

Yates, F. E. (in press). Physical biology: A basis for modeling living systems, *Journal of Cybernetics and Information Sciences*.

Yates, F. (in press). Temporal organization of metabolic processes: A biospectroscopic approach, in R. Bergman and C. Cobell (eds.), *Carbohydrate Metabolism; Quantitative physiology and mathematical modeling*, New York: Wiley.

Yates, F. E., and Iberall, A. S. (1973). Temporal and hierarchical organization in biosystems, in J. Urquhart and F. E. Yates (eds.), *Temporal Aspects of Therapeutics*, New York: Plenum.

Yates, F. E., Marsh, D. J., and Iberall, A. S. (1972). Integration of the whole organism: A foundation for a theoretical biology, in J. A. Behnke (ed.), *Challenging Biological Problems: Directions towards their solutions*, New York: Oxford University Press.

Zavalishin, N. V., and Tenenbaum, L. A. (1968). Control processes in the respiratory system, *Automation and Remote Control*, 9, 1456–1470.

The Development of Movement Control and Co-ordination
Edited by J. A. S. Kelso and J. E. Clark
© 1982, John Wiley & Sons, Ltd

CHAPTER 2

# Development of Speech Production as a Perceptual-motor Task[1]

HERBERT L. PICK, JR., GERALD M. SIEGEL, AND SHARON R. GARBER

## INTRODUCTION

In the early seventies around the University of Minnesota the demand by students for relevance in research reached its peak. Up till then, knowledge for knowledge's sake was good enough motivation, but the pressure became too great. Pick caved in and decided to work on a real-life problem: why, when his wife was drying her hair under a hair dryer and he asked her a question, did she shout her answer at him? (No-one said a real-life problem had to be important.) In order to investigate this fundamental problem it was necessary to find other specialists more knowledgeable than he about this research domain. After an exhaustive search of the research community, he identified two speech pathologists, Siegel and Garber, who were used to dealing with such deviant vocal behaviors as his wife had been manifesting under the dryer. They began to collaborate and somehow infected their students with some of their enthusiasm for this endeavor. The work discussed in this chapter is a joint effort of this research group.

In fact, our interests were somewhat more general. Siegel and Garber have been interested in the development of speech production in children. Why do some children have difficulties in acquisition of speech sounds when they can instantaneously monitor their own productions and know when they are correct and incorrect in their articulation? Pick is a perception psychologist who had been interested in feedback processes in visual-motor tasks. Would the same sorts of processes be operating in audio-motor tasks like speaking? Are such feedback processes particularly important in the child developing his speech skills?

The work presented in this chapter focuses mainly on the role of feedback, especially auditory feedback, in the development of speech production. First of all, it seems intuitively obvious that a child would need to have feedback in order to learn to produce the speech of his language – tactual and proprioceptive feedback to help control the actual configurations of the articulatory organs and auditory feedback to know when the speech product approximated the model of the heard external speech. Secondly and probably based on this obvious intuition, some theories of speech pathology suggest that some deviations and pathologies of speech may be based on failures in feedback processes in speech, e.g. Fairbanks (1954). Observations like the following are not at all uncommon: a child is describing the 'Easter wabbit.' A friendly? adult mocks him by saying, 'Tell me more about the Easter wabbit.' The child answers indignantly 'not wabbit – wabbit!' There seems to be a problem with the feedback in this instance in contrast to the apparently accurate perception of the external adult's speech.

Notwithstanding the intuition of the necessity of feedback for speech production, it should be pointed out that feedback is not *logically* required for the development of speech production. One can conceive of an organism programmed to reproduce the speech sounds it hears from outside even though it somehow may be deprived of the opportunity of hearing its own productions. Such a situation seems almost impossible to create experimentally. However, studies of bird-song development have achieved just such an experimental situation (Konishi, 1978). Certain species of birds, e.g. song sparrows and white-crowned sparrows, have a critical period for exposure to their songs which occurs long before they begin to vocalize. Such birds have been experimentally exposed to their species' song during the critical period and have then been deafened. It turns out in this case that our intuition is supported – they develop very abnormal songs in contrast to control birds also exposed during the critical period and not deafened. These control birds develop normal songs in spite of being isolated from further experience with any songs. In regard to our intuition it should also be noted that certain forms of imitation in humans seem to imply production of a motor act without obviously relevant feedback for matching the behavior to the model. Consider, for example, recent evidence for the imitation of tongue protrusion by neonates (Meltzoff and Moore, 1977), and in general the imitation of facial expression by infants.

Nevertheless, let us provisionally accept our intuition about the importance of feedback for humans learning to speak. (We, of course, know for sure that auditory *input* is necessary since deaf children only learn to speak with incredible difficulty, but as suggested above, this does not mean that auditory *feedback* is necessary.) What type of feedback would be useful in learning to speak? Auditory feedback would seem to be the prime candidate since vocal productions must be matched to an external model. While accepting that auditory feedback is necessary in *learning* to speak, it seems clear that auditory feedback is not necessary for speaking once one is a skilled speaker of the language. People can speak quite easily under masking noise so intense that they cannot hear themselves talk. In addition, informal observations of persons who have rather suddenly become profoundly deaf suggest it is possible to go on speaking for years with very little deterioration of speech.[2] It is quite likely that tactual and proprioceptive feedback play an important role in speech production of such persons but there is considerable evidence that speech remains surprisingly intelligible under combined experimental auditory masking and nerve block procedures which drastically reduce, if not eliminate, tactual and perhaps proprioceptive feedback from the oral cavity (Schliesser and Coleman, 1968). In a very careful study of the effects of auditory masking plus oral anesthesia, Borden *et al.* (1979) found that although speech quality was affected by absence of feedback, familiar phonemes were produced within their own boundaries. In short, on intuitive and logical grounds one may argue that auditory feedback must be important for early language learning and on empirical grounds we can assert that it is not necessary for the ongoing speech of the mature speaker. This line of reasoning would suggest that if we examine the role of auditory feedback in children we would find it decreasing in importance as a function of age.

We decided as an initial research strategy to modify the auditory feedback provided to subjects of different ages while speaking and to examine their response to this manipulation. However, before beginning to describe the actual research it is important to note that different characteristics of speech may be differently subject to feedback control. One general distinction in speech can be made between prosodic and articulatory characteristics. Prosodic characteristics are considered to be the intonation patterns and their timing, the intensity and the fundamental frequency of the speech, while the articulatory aspects are those having to do with the phoneme structure. It is again possible to suggest on the basis of logical reasoning that *moment to moment* or on-line control of speech via feedback would more likely function for various prosodic aspects of speech such as fundamental frequency or intensity rather than articulatory characteristics. The prosodic aspects of speech are by definition continuous over time, thus permitting modulation via feedback. Most phonemes on the other hand are short-lived events which are probably completed before they can be modified via feedback or at least the crucial motor act in their production occurs before feedback can tell the speaker it was right or wrong.[3] On the basis of such reasoning it seemed most likely to yield positive results from our research strategy if, to start with, we modified the auditory feedback relevant to prosodic characteristics rather than those of an articulatory nature. Furthermore, the practical technical problems of modifying articulatory aspects of speech in an interesting way seemed immense. For these several reasons we began our research program focusing on a rather easily manipulable prosodic characteristic – that of intensity.

## THE REGULATION OF VOCAL INTENSITY

Our first step in examining the role of auditory feedback in the development of regulation of vocal intensity took advantage of two phenomena well known to speech scientists and speech pathologists, the Lombard sign and the sidetone amplification effect. The Lombard sign refers to the fact that people are almost compelled to raise their voice when speaking in noise – the old hair-dryer effect. The sidetone amplification effect appears to be essentially the opposite effect – people will lower their voices if their auditory feedback is amplified. We were able to produce these phenomena experimentally using the apparatus and setting portrayed in Figure 1. The subject sits at a table in the experimental room wearing earphones. Her speech is picked up by a small microphone similar to that worn by telephone switchboard operators. This microphone is attached to the earphones and thus remains a fixed distance from the lips throughout the experimental session. The signal from the microphone is fed into both channels of a mixer. One channel of the mixer sends its output to a tape recorder on which the subject's speech was recorded for subsequent analysis. The output of the other channel goes to a speech audiometer where

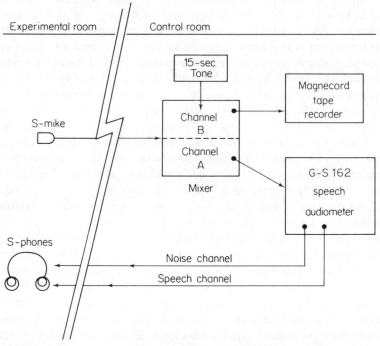

FIGURE 1   Apparatus setting used for research on the role of feedback in regulation of vocal intensity

the signal can be amplified and/or mixed with noise before being transmitted back to the subject's earphones.

In this first experiment (Siegel *et al.*, 1976) three-year-old children, four-year-old children, and adults participated in procedures designed to produce the Lombard sign and sidetone amplification effects. For the Lombard procedure the subjects spoke in quiet, with 60 dB (SPL re 0.0002 dynes/cm$^2$) of noise, and with 80 dB of noise. For the sidetone amplification effect subjects spoke hearing their voice at approximately a normal level (0 dB gain) and with 10 dB (SPL) and 20 dB (SPL) amplification. Subjects spoke for two minutes under each of these conditions. Adults were simply asked to speak extemporaneously. They were given a stack of topic cards to which they could refer if they ran out of ideas. The children were guided through the procedure by an experimenter who was a student teacher in their nursery school. In order to obtain a good sample of speech the children were allowed to select one of several familiar picture books about which they might speak. The experimenter would occasionally prompt them if they ran out of words but generally tried to keep verbal interaction to a minimum.

Vocal intensity measures of the subjects' speech were obtained from the tape-recorded output of one channel of the mixer. Graphic sound level recordings were prepared from these tapes and the intensity peaks on the recordings were averaged for each condition. The results for the Lombard procedure are depicted in Figure 2. All three age groups show a significant Lombard sign, that is, an increase in vocal intensity with increasing noise level. There does not appear to be any difference in magnitude of the Lombard sign among the different age groups, nor is such a difference revealed by statistical analysis. This result provides no support for the hypothesis of decreasing responsivity to auditory feedback as a function of age. (The difference in absolute vocal intensity for the three age groups is reliable but not of particular interest to the present discussion. It may be due to extraneous factors such as differential placement of the microphone on different size subjects or it may be a characteristic of the actual typical speaking intensity of subjects of different ages. The same age trend in absolute intensity occurs in most of our experiments with children.)

The results for the sidetone amplification effect are depicted in Figure 3. Again, all three age groups show a significant sidetone amplification effect, i.e. decreasing vocal intensity as a function of increasing sidetone gain. However, the amount of sidetone amplification effect appears to *increase* with age. The three-year-olds decreased their vocal intensity 3.4 dB over the 20 dB difference in amplification, the four-year-olds 5.2 dB and the adults 7.0 dB. Statistical analysis indicates the difference between the three-year-olds and the other two age groups is significant. This result of greater sidetone amplification effect in the older group is, of course, *opposite* the original hypothesis.

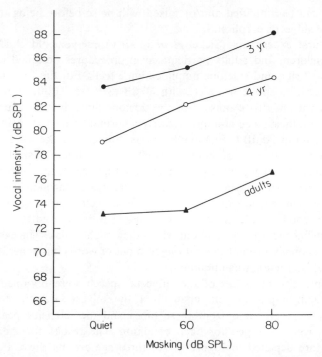

FIGURE 2    Vocal intensity as a function of intensity of masking noise in the study of the Lombard effect in subjects of different ages

It is of some interest to consider whether the Lombard sign and sidetone amplification effects reflect some general sensitivity to auditory feedback of individual subjects. To this end the correlations between the magnitudes of these two effects were examined for each age group. The results proved negative. The correlations were 0.08, 0.52, and 0.10 for the three-year-olds, four-year-olds, and adults respectively. Although that of the four-year-olds reached statistical significance, one can hardly claim these apparently similar phenomena tap a general subject characteristic.

Let us digress for a few moments from research dealing directly with the effect of feedback on speech production and consider a different kind of experiment, but one which we will see does have indirect implications for understanding the role of feedback in production. One aspect of any skill is knowing when and how to use it. In speaking, an important aspect of one's skill is intensity control, i.e. adjusting one's vocal intensity to the needs of the listener. This form of adjustment is especially common as speakers vary their vocal intensity to take into account the distance of the listener. Physically the inverse square

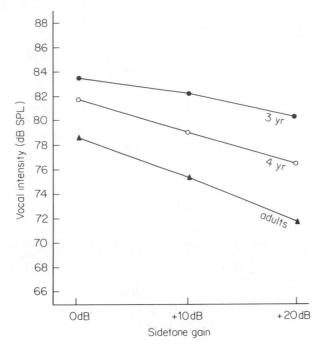

FIGURE 3    Vocal intensity as a function of sidetone gain in
the study of the sidetone amplification effect in subjects of
different ages

law indicates that sound pressure level is inversely proportional to the square of
the distance of the sound source. In acoustic terms this would mean that a
person trying to compensate for a doubling of the distance between herself and
a listener should increase her vocal intensity by about 6 dB (Warren, 1968).
Are children sensitive to this requirement of listeners and do they adjust the
intensity of their voices? A study addressing just this question was conducted
by Johnson *et al.* (in press). Three-year-old children, five-year-old children, and
adults were asked to speak to a listener who stood at different times at
distances of 6, 12, and 24 feet. The subjects wore a microphone of the same
type as described in the previous study through which their speech was
recorded. In order to get good speech samples from the children, the task was
set up as a game in which the subjects told the listener, an artist, what to draw
in a picture. The artist set up his easel at the different distances from the subject
and drew a different picture at each distance.

Vocal intensity was analyzed in the same way as before but now related to
the different distances of the listener. These results are portrayed in Figure 4.
All three age groups show increase of vocal intensity with increasing distance

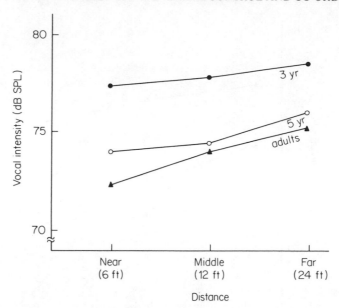

FIGURE 4    Vocal intensity as a function of distance of listener
for subjects of different ages

of the listener. Although Figure 4 suggests the adults might be adjusting to the
distance to a greater degree than the children, analysis of variance did not yield
a significant interaction which would indicate that such a trend was reliable. In
any case, it is clear that the children were *not* adjusting intensity of their voices
to a greater degree than the adults. Indeed, if one analyzes each group
separately (in spite of the nonsignificant interaction), it turns out that the three-
year-olds do not show a significant increase of vocal intensity across distance
while the five-year-olds and adults do. To the degree that the subjects might be
using auditory feedback to help them adjust their vocal intensity for the
different distances, this study again runs counter to the hypothesis that young
children are more sensitive to their auditory feedback. If anything, the results
are just the opposite.

If it is true that the younger subjects are adjusting their voices less than older
subjects, one explanation might be that children perceive changes in intensity in
their own voices as greater than adults perceive comparable changes of
intensity in their voices. In short, the self-perception of loudness of their own
voices by children may be greater than that by adults. As a first step in exploring this hypothesis directly, subjects of different ages were asked to match the
loudness of their own voices to an external sound (Costley, Siegel, and Olsen,
1978). Such a matching procedure hopefully would tell us directly what the

relationship is between the sound of one's own voice and external sound. This relationship has been previously measured for adults by Lane, Catania, and Stevens (1961). Three- to four-year-old children, five- to six-year-old children, and adults participated in the present study. They listened to and tried to repeat exactly a tape recording of the vowel *a*. On different trials it was presented at four different intensities: 60, 70, 80, and 90 dB. To make the task more engaging for the children, the sound was made to appear as if coming from the mouth of a marionette and they were to repeat it exactly as the marionette had said it. In this experiment the recording of the subject's speech was accomplished in the same way as in the previous studies by means of a small microphone attached to a headset and positioned at a fixed distance near the subject's lips. The marionette's vowels were presented through the earphones and the subject received feedback from his own voice at approximately normal levels.

Again, intensity levels were measured from graphic level recordings made from the tape recordings of the subjects' productions. The results are presented in Figure 5. It is evident that subjects of all ages increased, their vocal intensity as a function of the intensity of the externally presented vowels. However, it appears that the change is greater for the adults than for the children in an orderly fashion. That is, the steepest function is that of the adults, the next

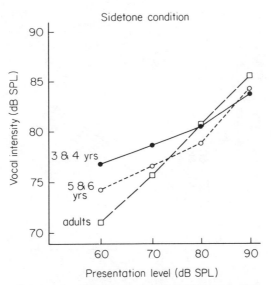

FIGURE 5    Vocal intensity of children and adults under instructions to match sounds of different intensities presented through emphasis

steepest the five-to six-year-olds, and the flattest for the three- to four-year-olds. This appearance is borne out by a significant interaction of an analysis of variance between age and intensity level of the vowels. Similar results were obtained in a second condition in which the subjects did not wear earphones and the vowels were presented over a loudspeaker. These results are presented in Figure 6. Here the five- and six-year-olds are more like the adults than in the previous condition, but the same developmental pattern is evident. The younger children are less responsive to changes in external sounds when their task is specifically to match that sound. If the difference in responsivity is a function of self-perception or feedback, it would seem to mean that the perception of self-produced sound for children is different than that for adults. Specifically, as suggested above, changes in self-produced sounds are relatively greater for children than for adults. Hence, they do not have to change their own productions as much to match a change in externally produced sounds.

It is not surprising that self-produced sounds are perceived differently than externally produced sounds. Self-produced sounds provide bone-conducted auditory stimulation as well as air-conducted auditory stimulation. In addition, self-produced sounds are accompanied by tactual proprioceptive, and efferent cues which are absent in the case of external sounds. These differences presumably account for the fact that, in general, increases in intensity of self-produced sounds are perceived as greater than equivalent changes in the exter-

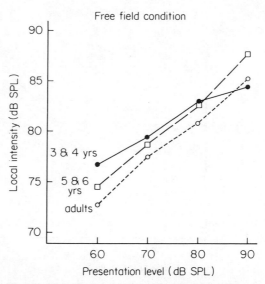

FIGURE 6    Vocal intensity of children and adults under instructions to match sounds of different intensities presented in a free field

nally produced sounds. This is reflected in Figure 6, for example, by the fact that even adults who are most responsive increase their vocal intensity only 13.2 dB to match the 30 dB change in intensity of the external vowel. This result closely replicates that reported by Lane, Catania, and Stevens (1961).

The lower responsivity of children in these self-perception experiments, however, cannot be *unequivocally* attributed to differences in self-perception or sensitivity to feedback. It is possible that it is the external sound which is perceived differently by children and adults. If changes in intensity of external sounds were perceived as smaller by children than by adults, the same pattern of results would be obtained. Still, a third possibility is that both self-produced and external sounds are perceived the same way by children and adults; it is just that children underestimate the change in their matching; that is, they may be less skillful than adults in matching a change. Experiments by Costley are under way in our laboratory to tease these possibilities apart.

## THE REGULATION OF ARTICULATION

In spite of the problems associated with studying the role of feedback in speech articulation, this is still part of our general goal. Indeed, in many ways articulation is a more interesting facet of speech. While the prosodic characteristics of speech help in communication and make speech more or less interesting, it is the phonemic structure which carries the largest amount of information. We can indeed understand computer-generated speech with its very impoverished prosody. However, we get very little information from sound trains which we can judge as having the intonation patterns of speech and even sounding like speech but lacking the phonemic structure. Something like this may be happening when we hear people talking too far away to make out what they are saying at all. One can often tell who is talking, even what language is being spoken; it sounds all right except we cannot understand any words. When beginning this research on articulation, we even had the idea that we might be able to modify the articulatory aspects of auditory feedback in such a way as to induce a person with a particular type of speech defect spontaneously to modify his production in a beneficial direction. We still are far from that goal but we have begun to make some initial steps toward understanding what role auditory feedback does play in children's articulation.

One general strategy has been to generate or take advantage of situations where articulation errors are likely to occur and then to see if the reduction of auditory feedback increases the occurrence of such errors. The first example of this strategy was carried out by Garber, Speidel, and Siegel (1980). They examined the effect of newly fitted dental appliances (palatal plates) inserted into the mouths of five-year-old children. The children's task was simply to name a set of pictures chosen to elicit a variety of phonemes including those considered likely to be affected by the appliance. The children named these pictures with and without the appliance, in quiet and in the presence of 90 dB masking noise. The number of articulation errors increased in the presence of noise and with the appliance in quiet. The combined presence of noise and appliance elicited no greater number of errors than the sum of the two conditions by themselves; that is, there was no interaction. The logic of this experimental design is particularly interesting. Consider what might be expected if proper articulation was very dependent on the presence either of tactual-proprioceptive feedback or auditory feedback but it did not make any difference which. In such a case, a disruption of normal tactual-proprioceptive feedback by itself, such as an appliance might produce, would not be expected to have much of an effect on articulation. Nor would masking noise by itself. However, the combination of the two should have an extreme effect on articulation. Clearly, this pattern did not occur. The pattern obtained is more like what would be expected if the production of some sounds depended on tactual-proprioceptive feedback and others on auditory feedback and still others were perhaps efferent-defined and did not require feedback at all.

Unfortunately, the incidence and distribution of articulation errors did not permit verification of this suggestion with phoneme by phoneme analysis. Some supportive data for this possibility can be derived from an analogous study with adults (Garber et al., 1980). In that study it was found that palatal appliances increase the relative frequency of $s$ and $t_s$ sounds and decrease the relative frequency of $s$ and $z$ sounds. The presence of masking noise did not seem to have any systematically differential effect on the various speech sounds. (It should be kept in mind that the overall increase in errors as a function of noise and/or appliance might not depend on feedback problems but could be a disruptive effect just due to distraction.)

A second example of the articulation error strategy capitalizes on the high likelihood of articulation errors of children who have been undergoing speech therapy. In this study by Yanez et al., (in press) auditory feedback relevant to particular sounds was selectively masked and the subjects' speech was examined for errors in production of these sounds. Two groups of children (ages seven to twelve years) participated in this study. One group of eleven subjects, the $r$-group, had been undergoing therapy for faulty production of $r$ and the other group, of nineteen subjects, the $s$-group, had been receiving therapy for $s$ sounds. The children in both groups were ready to be dismissed from therapy at the time of the experiment. Both groups were given an articulation test (McDonald Deep Test of Articulation) in quiet, in noise specifically selected to mask the $r$ sound (low pass 1250 Hz at 80 dB), and in noise specifically selected to mask the $s$ sound (high pass 2000 at 80 dB). If auditory feedback were especially important for these children's production of the sounds they had been having difficulty with, we would expect an increase in errors for the s-group under s noise but not under r noise and conversely for the r-group, an increase under r noise but not under s noise. The pattern of results was as predicted for the s-group. Errors went from an average of 1.58 under no noise up to 3.89 under s noise but back down to 2.47 under r noise. However, for the r-group both types of noise caused an increase of errors from 1.91 under no noise to 5.0 under the relevant r noise and staying at a high level of 4.64 under the irrelevant s noise. the s-group, as predicted, seemed to be relying on the particularly relevant feedback in the production of that sound. The increase in errors for the r group under both types of noise suggests that the difficulty is not solely dependent on r-relevant feedback. It is possible that their production is more generally feedback-sensitive and any decrease in feedback causes difficulty, or it is possible that the state of their therapy is so fragile that the distracting effect of the masking noise causes the difficulty without regard to feedback. Again, as in the appliance study, the safest conclusion seems to be that speakers exhibit differential sensitivity to control via feedback for different sounds. Thoroughly mapping out this differential sensitivity is a task for the future.

## CONCLUSION

We have reviewed feedback research covering both prosodic and articulatory aspects of speech production. The prosodic aspects (mainly intensity) were investigated rather systematically across a wide developmental range. These results generally indicate that young children are, if anything, less responsive to manipulations eliciting changes in vocal intensity than older children and adults. Such was true for the sidetone amplification, for the effect of a listener at different distances, and in the intensity matching research. Only for the Lombard effect was the developmental pattern different and here there was no change with age. The pattern is clearly counter to an initial hypothesis that there would be decreasing sensitivity to auditory feedback with increasing age. The pattern is consistent with the opposite possibility that there is increasing sensitivity to auditory feedback as a function of age. It is also consistent with a second hypothesis that the loudness of a young child's own voice increases faster with increasing intensity than that of an older child's or adult's own voice. In other words, the autophonic function is steeper for children than for adults (Lane, Catania, and Stevens, 1961). Still a third possibility consistent with the results is that responsivity does not reflect sensitivity. That is, the younger subjects in the various studies may very well detect the experimental differences in feedback but they simply cannot or do not compensate as well as the older subjects. Research currently under way by Costley in our laboratory is aimed at investigating these second and third possibilities directly by a variety of intra and intermodal loudness-matching tasks.

Let us suppose, however, that the pattern of results does reflect the first of the above possibilities, that there is an increasing sensitivity to auditory feedback with increasing age. Let us speculate further. Assume that this age trend could be extrapolated downward and that younger children were even less sensitive to auditory feedback than the children in the research described here. Assume further that such young children were learning the prosodic aspects of their language. It has been suggested, for example, that infants reflect in their speech the fundamental frequency of an adult with whom they are 'conversing' (Lieberman, 1967). The implication of this line of reasoning is that young children may learn the prosodic aspects of their speech production without auditory feedback – perhaps in an imitative manner as was suggested above.

What about articulation? The developmental role of auditory feedback in speech production has not been investigated very systematically. As noted in the introduction, articulation in adults seems to be affected very little by lack of auditory feedback. In a recent fascinating report by Binnie and Daniloff (1979) a five-year-old child who became suddenly profoundly deaf as a consequence of meningitis was described. His articulation deteriorated rapidly after his illness, intelligibility of single words being about 50 percent. Although no systematic pre-illness data were available there were no indications of any speech or auditory problems. If that apparent great dependence on auditory feedback in the five-year-old is indeed generally true it would suggest that the development of articulation might be consistent with our initial hypothesis of decreasing sensitivity to auditory feedback as a function of age. Auditory feedback might well be crucial for learning proper articulation and for its stabilization but once established people could speak without it.

The view expressed here is extremely speculative but it generates the intriguing hypothesis that auditory feedback plays different developmental roles in speech production for different aspects of speech production.

## NOTES

1. The research reported in this paper was supported by Program Project Grant No. HD-03082 from the National Institute of Child Health and Human Development awarded to the Institute of Child Development, University of Minnesota, and by grants awarded to the Center for Research in Human Learning of the University of Minnesota from the National Institute of Child Health and Human Development and the National Science Foundation.
2. Detailed analysis and measurement of the speech of such individuals may indicate subtle changes in the timing of articulatory gestures (Zimmerman and Rettaliata, 1979) but intelligibility remains quite high.
3. Of course 'off-line' feedback or 'knowledge or results' can inform the speaker that she is making frequent articulation errors, e.g. as might happen when one is drunk or feedback can inform a speaker that she is misarticulating a particular phoneme. In such cases one can use feedback by taking extra care, in general, with one's

speech (so as not to let the policeman think one has been drinking) or by attending to the offending phoneme in one's speech. Such knowledge of results may also be important for the very young child in mastering articulatory gestures. It could tell when a gesture resulted in an approximation of a speech sound it was attempting to imitate.

## REFERENCES

Binnie, C. A., and Daniloff, R. G. (1979). Phonetic disintegration in a five-year-old following sudden hearing loss, unpublished manuscript, Department of Audiology and Speech Services, Purdue University.

Borden, G. J., Harris, K. S., Yoshioka, H., and Fitch, H. (1979). Feedback and feedforward mechanisms used by speakers producing familiar and novel speech patterns, International Congress of Phonetic Sciences, Copenhagen.

Costley, M. S., Siegel, G. M., and Olsen, M. G. (1978). Self-perception of loudness in children, paper presented at meeting of American Speech and Hearing Association, San Francisco, CA, 20 November.

Fairbanks, G. (1954). Systematic research in experimental phonetics. 1. A theory of the speech mechanisms as servosystem. *Journal of Speech and Hearing Disorders*, **19**, 133–139.

Garber, S., Speidel, T. M., and Siegel, G. M. (1980). The effects of palatal appliances on the speech of 5-year-old children, *Journal of Speech and Hearing Research*, **23**, 854–863.

Garber, S., Speidel, T. M., Siegel, G. M., Miller, E., and Glass, L. (1980). The effects on speech of alterations in the oral and auditory environment, *Journal of Speech and Hearing Research*, **23**, 838–852.

Johnson, C. J., Pick, H. L., Jr., Gicciarelli, A. W., and Siegel, G. M. and Garber, S. R. (In Press) Effect of interpersonal distance on children's vocal intensity.

Konishi, M. (1978). Auditory environment and vocal development in birds, in R. D. Walk and H. L. Pick Jr. (eds.), *Perception and Experience*, New York: Plenum Press.

Lane, H. L., Catania, A. C., and Stevens, S. S. (1961). Voice level: autophonic scale, perceived loudness, and effects of sidetone, *Journal of the Acoustical Society of America*, **33**, 160–168.

Lieberman, P. (1967). *Intonation, Perception, and Language*, Research Monograph No. 38, Cambridge, Mass.: MIT Press.

Meltzoff, A. N., and Moore, M. K. (1977). Imitation of facial and manual gestures by human neonates, *Science*, **198**, 75–78.

Schliesser, H. F., and Coleman, R. O. (1968). Effectiveness of certain procedures of alterations of auditory and oral tactile sensations for speech, *Perceptual Motor Skills*, **26**, 275–281.

Siegel, G. M., Pick, H. L., Jr., Olsen, M. G., and Sawin, L. (1976). Auditory feedback in the regulation of vocal intensity of preschool children, *Developmental Psychology*, **12**, 255–261.

Warren, R. M. (1968). Vocal compensation for change of distance, paper presented at the 6th International Congress on Acoustics, Tokyo, Japan, August.

Yanez, E. A., Siegel, G. M., Garber, S. R., and Wellin, C. J. (In press) The effects of different masking noises on children with *s* or *r* errors, *Journal of Speech and Hearing Disorders*.

Zimmerman, G., and Rettaliata, P. (1979). Articulatory patterns of an adventitiously deaf speaker: Implications for the role of auditory information in speech production, unpublished manuscript #79–102, Wendell Johnson Speech and Hearing Center, University of Iowa.

The Development of Movement Control and Co-ordination
Edited by J. A. S. Kelso and J. E. Clark
© 1982, John Wiley & Sons, Ltd

CHAPTER 3

# The Development of Intermodal Co-ordination and Motor Control

BILL JONES

## INTRODUCTION: THE SIGNIFICANCE OF DEVELOPMENTAL CHANGES IN MOTOR CONTROL

Theories of intermodal co-ordination have been supposed to provide a 'process' framework for the development of voluntary motor control (e.g. Birch and Lefford, 1963, 1967; Connolly and Jones, 1970). Before examining this idea in particular I shall discuss some general concerns about the development of motor skill in order to focus upon the currently fashionable process-normative distinction (the how?-when? distinction).

Broadly the psychology of motor skill development is concerned with the relationship between the skills of adulthood and those of childhood. In a recent review, Wade (1976) commented on the 'lack of specific theorizing with respect to the development of motor skills in children;' at the same time he noted that there is no lack of normative 'data.' This is a common formulation which is often taken to imply that a process-normative distinction (or more generally a theory-observation distinction) is of some value in categorizing research. Yet at best the formulation is misleading. To dismiss some research as 'merely normative' or 'merely observational' is often to dismiss in a rather *ad hominen* fashion a particular class of theoretical preferences. On the other hand, to regard one's observations as neutral or 'atheoretical' is to refuse to recognize one's own implicit theory.

That said it is not self-evident that we need to theorize specifically about the acquisition of skills *in children* as though children must acquire skills differently than adults. Of course, it is often thought that children and adults differ *qualitatively*. I shall call this the 'developmental' attitude and I want to show that it is altogether odd.

Piaget's claim that the child's thinking proceeds through qualitatively different stages to the final flowering of formal, abstract thought in the adult is, perhaps, the most well-known example of the 'developmental' attitude. Piaget denies in fact that children younger than about seven years of age are capable of deductive logical inference (e.g. Piaget, 1970). I cannot refute Piaget's claim in any detail here. One should simply notice that it is not difficult to demonstrate efficient logical inference on the part of children as young as four years of age (Bryant and Trabasso, 1971). Consider the following syllogism:

(i)   height is equivalent to volume;
(ii)  object $x$ is higher than object $y$;
(iii) therefore object $x$ has the greater volume.

This might be a representation of reasoning by a typical four-, five-, or six-year-old about the so-called conservation of volume problem. As reasoning it is impeccable. An adult or an older child would not always reason in this way, not because they have a qualitatively different ability to reason, but because they do not invariably take height to be equivalent to volume. Like adults, children will reach contingently incorrect conclusions whenever they reason correctly from factually incorrect premises.

Wade (1976) has argued that the child learning a motor skill

> ... is faced with a different matrix of informational uncertainty as compared to the adult ... In informational terms the child is unable to capitalize on any redundancy present in the stream of input and must therefore process more information for the same problem. (p. 377)

This may simply mean that children, by and large, know less than adults, a fact which may be presented without the jargon of information theory.[1] It may also imply that the acquisition of motor skills involves fundamentally different problems for the child and for the adult. Theorizing about motor development often seems to take this latter notion for granted. Wickstrom (1975), for example, writing on the new discipline of 'developmental kinesiology' defines a mature motor skill as 'the basic motor pattern used by skilled *adults*' (p. 167). There is no suggestion that mature patterns may be characteristic of children and Wickstrom simply equates 'unskilled' with 'immature.' Or take Kay's (1970) interesting discussion of a child catching a ball. The fifteen-year-old's performance is described as 'adaptive' and 'complete' while the two-year-old supposedly has no 'general strategy' and no 'timing and co-ordination.' The two-year-old's stance was 'rigid,' her hand movements 'static,' and her eyes were on the thrower, not the ball. But how can the child be said to have had no general strategy when she did look at the thrower and did keep herself still (she did not gaze around aimlessly; her movements were not diffuse or purposeless).

Kay's 'ethological' observational reports are, as they must be, shot through with interpretation, and dubious interpretation at that.

Consider the two-year-old's strategy in comparison to an adult's strategy for receiving a thrown ball. The professional batsman's feet do not move, his hands do not move on the bat and his gaze is often concentrated on the thrower's hand or arm rather than the ball. Of course the adult's timing in catching or hitting a ball is usually smooth and continuous and the child's timing is off. The difference should occasion no surprise. Nor should it suggest the need for some special developmental theory. In the child we are witnessing the beginnings of skill at a specific task so that anything other than poor temporal co-ordination is not to be expected. Comparing a two-year-old catching a ball to a fifteeen-year-old is like comparing a man who has taken his first guitar lesson to Segovia.[2]

I suspect that underlying the 'developmental' attitude to motor skills research is the dogma that one acquires over the course of development not specific skills but general strategies for skill. Thus the fifteen-year-old's ability to catch a ball would reflect general 'skillfulness' rather than some particular ability which the two-year-old has yet to acquire. The dogma is exemplified in current notions of 'schema' control of skilled movements (e.g. Bruner and Bruner, 1968; Pew, 1974; Schmidt, 1975). A quotation from Bruner and Bruner is symptomatic:

> ... skilled action is thus generative in the sense that language is productive, a minimum set of transformation rules serving to produce a large stock of skilled action patterns used in achieving a wide variety of goals. (p. 240)

There is certainly much of interest here; any specific behaviour can be variously achieved. (One can indeed sign one's name in an indefinite number of ways.) A skill is defined by its goal not by the means of its accomplishment. But notice that the Bruners talk about 'a variety of goals' and not about a specific goal accomplished in a variety of ways. They talk as though all skills, all behaviors, have the same common basis. The relationship between transformational rules (what are they in any case?) and the 'stock of skilled action patterns' is not at all clear. Moreover the Bruners' account seems curiously removed from any real skill. One of the virtues of the so-called normative approach was that researchers had to focus on everyday skills. Talk about underlying processes on the other hand is often open to the charge of unreality. The assumption of 'deep' underlying structures of motor control may give rise to little more than superficial discussions of conceptual resemblances between skills.[3]

In practice the process-normative distinction might refer only to a difference between researchers in the kind of skills and in the kind of processes which primarily interest them. It is a mistake to see researchers like McGraw (1935) and Gesell (e.g. Gesell and Amatruda, 1947) who cataloged typical sequences of motor development as innocent of theory. Rather they tended to be concerned with the development of static and dynamic postural control on the theoretical assumption that the sequence of events (neck-righting, head-raising, 'parachute' or 'propping' reaction and body-righting) is under genetic control since it develops in the same way in all normal infants. McGraw (1935) in her 'normative' research distinguished between 'phylogenetic' and 'ontogenetic' skills and talked about corresponding processes of maturation and practice ('learning'). Paillard (1971) who, I suppose, would be regarded as a process-oriented researcher, distinguished heuristically between localizing skills (hand positioning and gross bodily movements) and manipulatory patterns (grasping, consuming, etc.). Yet McGraw's and Paillard's distinctions seem to have essentially the same purpose. Both would distinguish righting and equilibrium reactions ('phylogenetic' or 'localizing' abilities) from patterns of activity which serve to orient objects with respect to the environment ('ontogenetic' and 'manipulatory' skills).

Connolly (1970) attempted to dismiss normative research as 'genetic predeterminism' but this is to say very little. Of course it would be foolish to think that genetic expression is somehow fixed regardless of environmental contingencies. However, there is no conceivable physical environment in which postural anti-gravity reactions would not have significance. In short the maturational process account of early righting responses is inherently plausible,[4] however implausible may be the attempt to generalize from postural control to so-called ontogenetic skills.

I am suggesting here that no single process framework for the acquisition of voluntary motor control can be generally useful. By way of detailed illustration I am going to examine one suggested framework, the development of inter-modal co-ordination (Birch and Lefford, 1963, 1967; Connolly and Jones, 1970). Birch and Lefford (1963, 1967) explicitly assumed that perceptual control of movement must have a different basis in early childhood and adulthood so their account nicely illustrates one version of the developmental attitude.

## INTERMODAL CO-ORDINATION AS A 'PROCESS' FRAMEWORK FOR MOTOR SKILL

### Birch and Lefford's Account

Many theorists have suggested that motor control may be based upon inter-modal organization,[5] though Birch and Lefford (1963, 1967) were undoubtedly the first to propose a detailed developmental account of the possible relationship between intermodal co-ordination and voluntary motor control.

They assumed that the development of cross-modal matching abilities is underpinned by increasing efficiency of neural intersensory organization (Birch and Lefford, 1963, 1967). Cross-modal matching is the ability to make equivalence judgements of forms and so on when information is presented in two modalities. Typically one form will be presented in one modality as a 'standard' and one or more 'comparison' forms are presented either simultaneously or sequentially in a second modality (see Jones, in press).

Birch and Lefford argued that

> ... if visual control of voluntary movement is to be effective, visual information must necessarily be integrated with kinesthetic or other somatosensory information. (1967, p. 8)

Thus the importance of intermodal co-ordination for voluntary control is presented as a logical postulate. Further, they imply that inefficient motor co-ordination in infancy is a function of inefficient intermodal co-ordination. Developmentally they believed that during the first five years of life there is a shift away from reliance upon 'internal' proximal stimulation to reliance upon visual (and auditory) teloreception and

> Simultaneously with the emergence of teloreceptor prominence, a second mechanism of input organization seems to be evolving. It consists of the increasing tendency of the separate sensory modalities to integrate with another and of organization and directed action to be subserved by intersensory or multimodal rather than unimodal patterning. (1967, pp. 5–6)

At the same time they also argued 'that directed and organized action is based upon intrasensory differentiation and definition within each of the sense modalities' (p. 7). In short their position was that efficient voluntary motor control logically requires intersensory, usually visual-somatosensory, integration and that developmentally motor control is associated with a hierarchical shift in sensory dominance from proximal to distant reception, combined with increasing inter and intrasensory efficiency.

Every aspect of this formulation is suspect. Firstly changes with age in the ability to make cross-modal equivalence judgements do not in themselves indicate developmental changes in the nature of intersensory co-ordination. In their 1963 experiment Birch and Lefford had children aged from five to eleven years make same-different judgements of two geometric forms in one of three ways. Either a standard form was presented visually and matched haptically (active manual exploration) or kinesthetically (the subject held a stylus which the experimenter guided around the outline of the form) to a comparison form, or the two forms were presented haptically and kinesthetically. (Just why Birch and Lefford chose these particular comparisons is not at all clear.) They observed a more or less parallel decrease with age in matching errors for all conditions and argued on this basis for developmental gains in efficiency of intermodal organization. However, as Bryant (1968) has noted, improvements with age in accuracy of cross-modal matching do not in themselves show how these improvements occur. He pointed out that cross-modal improvements could arise from the increasing *intra*sensory differentiation which Birch and Lefford themselves regarded as a significant feature of development. In other words developmental gains in their three cross-modal matching conditions may be based upon parallel improvements within one or more modality rather than upon improved intermodal co-ordination.

My own review of cross-modal matching (Jones, in press) has shown that cross-modal efficiency depends largely upon within-modal efficiency. Purely visual matching is very efficient, often asymptotically so, in age groups from about three years on (e.g. Goodnow, 1971). Purely tactual matching often remains far less accurate than visual matching even in adults (e.g. Goodnow, 1971). Indeed tactual matching is sometimes less accurate than matching in the two cross-modal conditions (e.g. Lobb, 1965). I hypothesized that since visual pick-up is more accurate than tactual pick-up it should be easier to match a visual standard to a tactual comparison set than to perform the reverse operation. (I assume that the standard and comparison items are not presented together for then the distinction between visual-tactual and tactual-visual matching is arbitrary.) Examination of fifteen studies confirmed the hypothesis. In short, data from cross-modal matching experiments may be best explained in terms of within-modal performance.

I have also argued in detail elsewhere against the proposition that motor control *necessarily* involves reliance upon somatosensory inputs from proprioceptors in the vestibular system or in the joint-muscle-tendon system (see e.g. Jones, 1978). The proposition is scarcely unique to Birch and Lefford though theorists differ about how vision and proprioception are combined (Legge, 1965, for example, argued that in principle direct integration of visual and proprioceptive is impossible). Birch and Lefford themselves were unclear. Notice that they talked about intersensory *or* multimodal control, by implication two quite different processes. Multimodal control need not be based upon any integration of visual and proprioceptive data; either one assumes that control is somehow delegated from exteroceptors to proprioceptors (Gibbs, 1965) or that proprioception serves to regulate, to 'fine-tune,' exteroceptive control (Gibbs, 1954). A remark in their 1967 paper suggests that Birch and Lefford did not think in terms of integration of information though they consistently use the expression 'intersensory integration:'

... intersensory integration makes it possible for the organism to modify its responsiveness to a given input to the degree that it is accompanied by afferent activity in other modalities, a capacity which permits the modulation of responses in accordance with a broader range of information than is available when the organism is responding separately and independently to stimuli from each of the individual sense systems. (p. 8)

This passage seems to imply that inputs from more than one modality simply provide independent back-up information (redundancy) and not that separate modality inputs are integrated. There are no data which would readily distinguish the independence and integration models and as it stands Birch and Lefford's account may not be different from the usual notion that proprioception can replace vision in initiating and controlling a movement (cf. Gibbs, 1965; Legge, 1965).

What evidence is there that control of movement either demands proprioceptive inputs or is less efficient when such inputs are not available? I have suggested elsewhere that the evidence is slight (e.g. Jones, 1978) and I shall give only one illustration here. Control of movement may require adjustments in velocity, amplitude, or force by means of which terminal position is estimated relative to initial position. Bizzi, Polit, and Morasso (1976) have provided evidence that the terminal position of centrally initiated head movements is not affected by either increased proprioceptive input through stimulation of neck proprioceptors or by abolition of neck proprioception through surgical means. A neat demonstration that somatosensory information is not *necessary* for voluntary control.

Birch and Lefford's developmental sequence is equally dubious. There is little evidence for any hierarchical shift in sensory dominance or that infants primarily process only proximal data (the tradition 'touch teaches vision' notion). We now know, as Berkeley did not, though Birch and Lefford should have, that neonates can make remarkably sophisticated judgements in visual space (e.g. Bower, 1966; Fantz, 1958) and contrary to the traditional line, recent analyses of early righting and equilibrium reactions have demonstrated that control may be achieved through visual rather than vestibular pick-up.

I know of no detailed experimental analyses of neck-righting or head-raising. However, the 'parachute' reaction (e.g. Paine and Oppé, 1966) has been analysed by Peters and Walk (1974). The parachute reaction which appears between six and twelve months in normal development refers to the extension of the hands and arms as though for support which may be observed in an infant lowered toward a visible surface. Presumably, the parachute reaction is an essential factor in the development of basic postural reactions against gravity and it is commonly thought to depend upon vestibular co-ordination (Paine and Oppé, 1966). Analysis by Peters and Walk (1974) suggests alternatively that the response is visually controlled. Infants aged between eight and a half and twelve months were lowered toward the surface of a visual cliff on the 'shallow' or the 'deep' sides. The parachute reaction appeared only given the visual illusion of depth. Consequently the response appears to be solely under visual and not vestibular control.

Similarly Lee and Aronson (1973) following Gibson (1966) argued that standing depends upon visual information rather than activity in the vestibular and in the joint-muscle-tendon systems. They manipulated the optic array for a standing infant (age range thirteen to sixteen months) by moving an experimental room toward or away from the child. If the moving room produces an impression of forward or backward movement of the body then the child should show some compensatory torque about the feet in the direction of movement of the 'room.' Compensatory body-sway was observed on a great majority of trials, strong enough on about one-third of trials for infants to lose their balance. Lee and Aronson suggested that when the child sways forward or backward visual and mechanoreceptors are in conflict. Given that children tend to lose their balance, Lee and Aronson thought that visual data was not only necessary for maintenance of posture while standing but also dominant over mechanoreceptor output.

Butterworth and Hicks (1977) confirmed Lee and Aronson's findings. As well they found that manipulating the optic array affected the sitting posture of infants (average age eleven months) who could sit but not stand unsupported. However, sitting infants were much less likely to lose their balance than standing infants. Butterworth and Hicks argued, therefore, that visual and mechanoreceptive *congruence* is required for maintenance of posture. The standing child is likely to overbalance not because visual is dominant over vestibular and joint-muscle information but because standing is difficult compared to sitting. The standing infant must balance the whole body mass on the relatively small area of the feet. In consequence standing is an inherently unstable posture and we need not argue for visual dominance simply because the standing infant tends to lose his balance. Whatever the case, normal righting and equilibrium responses in infants appear, contrary to the implication of Birch and Lefford's hierarchical shift notion, to be based upon exteroceptive visual control.

Finally the assumption of early proximal specialization is difficult to reconcile with the absolute inefficiency of cutaneous pick-up of form information in infancy. I have already noted that tactual matching seems to be less accurate than visual matching at all ages. In children younger than about five years of age tactual matching seems little better than random (Goodnow, 1971). Preschool children are not in fact likely to explore by hand objects which they can already see (Abravanel, 1972).

Now, I am not arguing here for any version of the visual dominance notion. A number of researchers have indeed suggested, contrary to Birch and Lefford, that infants rely upon a visual map of space (e.g. Warren, 1970) which is only later co-ordinated with proximal (and auditory) space. This account is difficult to sustain and in fact further evidence against both the proximal and telodominance theories can be found in important recent studies of intersensory judgements in infants. Indirectly Bryant *et al.* (1972), and Allen *et al.* (1977), have demonstrated cross-modal equivalence capacities in neonates. Bryant *et al.* (1972) showed that infants aged between six and eleven months were significantly more likely to show visually guided reaching toward an object which they had previously explored manually than toward an object which they had not touched or seen. Visual-auditory cross-modal matching in six-month-old infants has also been demonstrated by Allen *et al.* (1977) using an habituation paradigm.

In sum, Birch and Lefford's (1963, 1967) account is impossible to sustain. The notion that visual information must be combined with somatosensory information for efficient motor control is questionable at best (e.g. Bizzi, Polit, and Morasso, 1976; Jones, 1978). There is no evidence for the traditional view that early development is characterized by relative reliance upon proximal stimulation. On the contrary, visual processing appears to be extremely efficient in infants (e.g. Bower, 1966; Fantz, 1958) and tactual processing is quite inefficient below five years of age (e.g. Goodnow, 1971).

More importantly for understanding processes of motor control, basic righting and equilibrium reactions may depend upon visual exteroceptive control (Butterworth and Hicks, 1977; Lee and Aronson, 1973; Peters and Walk, 1974) though visual-somatosensory congruence is probably well established (Butterworth and Hicks, 1977). In fact some form of intermodal visual-vestibular co-ordination may be present from birth though there is little hard evidence at present.[6] There is, however, no evidence that the sensory modalities are disparately organized in early development; rather, efficient intermodal co-ordination appears to be characteristic of our earliest perceptual judgements and our earliest voluntary movements (e.g. Allen *et al.*, 1977; Bryant *et al.*, 1972; Butterworth and Hicks, 1977; Lee and Aronson, 1973).

### The Connolly and Jones Hypothesis

A basis for voluntary control rather similar to the Birch and Lefford account was assumed by Connolly and Jones (1970). We merely provided a more detailed account of visual-kinesthetic relationships. On our view the development of voluntary control depended on some central translation between peripheral and kinesthetic modalities. We used a reproduction paradigm to study visual (V) and kinesthetic (K) within- and cross-modal judgements of length by schoolchildren and adults. Visual standard and comparison items were presented by mechanically generating a line to a predetermined length (the standard) or until the subject judged it to be equivalent in length to the standard (the comparison). Kinesthetic standards were generated by requiring the subject to draw a line along an unseen path between fixed stops (what I have termed 'constrained' movement – Jones, 1972) and kinesthetic reproduction involved the voluntary production of an unseen line. Hence there were two within- (VV and KK) and two cross-modal (KV and VK) conditions.

We found parallel decline with age in absolute error of matching for all four conditions and the ordering of mean error for the conditions was consistently $VV = KK < KK < VK$. To explain this ordering we assumed that information is translated into the reproduction modality in the cross-modal conditions with noisy translation and unstable kinesthetic memory. Noisy translation increases the error in cross-relative to within-modal conditions and unstable kinesthetic memory produces the relation, $KV < VK$ (cross-modal asymmetry). This inferred process was assumed to be the basis of visual-somatosensory integration and hence, in the traditional way, the basis of voluntary motor control.

Experimental tests have led to the abandonment of our model (e.g. Jones, 1973; Newell, Shapiro, and Carlton, 1979). Newell and his colleagues, for example, informed the subject about the reproduction modality at one of three points, immediately before or after presentation of the standard or immediately prior to reproduction. Assuming that information is stored via the input modality until the reproduction modality is known, delaying translation should on our account have resulted in the relation $VK < KV$ for absolute error. In fact the manipulation had little effect on the ordering of conditions.

However, analysis of our experiment would suggest that each condition involves a quite distinct process (cf. Jones, 1973) so that any general model could at best yield only a spurious fit. Only VV-matching appears to involve a sensory equivalence judgement. KK-matching requires the subject to initiate a voluntary movement on the basis of a constrained movement. The two types of movement are rather different perhaps because the constrained condition does not allow the subject to determine termination of displacement prior to movement (e.g. Jones, 1972, 1974; Stelmach, Kelso, and Wallace, 1975). Conceivably, constrained movement involves some integration of a sequence of voluntary movements via central monitoring of efference (e.g. Jones, 1978). In KV-matching, therefore, efferent output must somehow be compared to afferent visual input. Finally, VK-matching involves the generation of a voluntary movement based on a visual cue (afferent-efferent translation rather than afferent visual-kinesthetic matching). A number of other analyses are possible. They will depend upon one's views on central-peripheral linkages in motor control. In short our experiment and any similar cross-modal comparisons of vision and 'kinesthesis' cannot provide a fruitful model for motor control. Such experiments can only be interpreted if we can take some model of motor control for granted. Were the two cross-modal conditions to be based upon the same process it would make sense to talk about cross-modal asymmetry. As it stands the four conditions may involve quite different (and rather contrived) processes.

## CONCLUSIONS

While developmental changes in intermodal co-ordination, or more precisely in cross-modal matching abilities, have their own interest, they do not provide a framework for understanding the development of voluntary motor control. Neonates are almost certainly capable of efficient intermodal co-ordination (Allen et al., 1977; Bryant et al., 1972) so that the development of motor control need not wait on the maturation of neural intersensory connections. Indeed early postural regulation may depend upon visual-vestibular co-ordination (Butterworth and Hicks, 1977).

In any case the search for a single framework for skilled performance is illusory. 'Skill' is not a unitary concept and no single process can explain how voluntary control is possible in all situations, still less how all skills are acquired in children or in adults. For example, the normative basis for anti-gravity reactions does not provide a model for the acquisition of skill in a ball game though naturally righting and equilibrium reactions are essential for efficient locomotion. 'Phylogenetic' and 'ontogenetic' abilities (McGraw, 1935) do not differ (pace Birch and Lefford, 1963, 1967) in that equilibrium reactions are based upon internal somatosensory control and later manipulative skills upon exteroceptive control. As early as eight or nine months adaptive postural responses seem to be based upon visual control (Peters and Walk, 1974). Early and later abilities do differ in that early control involves a general spatial reaction to a universal gravitational framework. Temporal constraints vis-à-vis the world are relatively unimportant in early development. However, once postural reactions have been established, motor control will often require finely graded spatial responses in a tightly structured environmental time-frame. Consequently the ability to predict events in the world must be acquired.

This is not to say that all skills beyond the level of equilibrium reactions must involve anticipatory timing. It is hard to see how, say, chopping food or sewing on a button involve anticipation at least in the same way as evading a tackle (football games) must involve the preconception and initiation of movement prior to the appropriate environmental contingency. One might argue that sewing on a button is anticipatory in the sense that the sewer has some goal in mind but this would only be to notice the conceptual truth that voluntary actions are always implicitly *intentional*, always defined with reference to a goal.[7]

Too general accounts of processes supposedly underlying skilled performance risk being either obviously wrong or empirically empty. (Practice does after all make perfect, but that is simply how we use the word 'practice.') Inter-modal co-ordination as a basis for skilled performance is far too general. In so far as particular accounts (e.g. Birch and Lefford, 1963, 1967; Connolly and Jones, 1970) are not simply empirically contraverted, they say little more than that motor control is based upon perception since only experimental contrivance can isolate seeing from hearing and touch.

Rather than describing, more or less vaguely, underlying processes of 'skill,' we need to concentrate on particular skills and how they are acquired, whether by children or by adults. There is no particular reason to presume that the processes of skill acquisition in children and in adults are radically different (though there may be a need to remind ourselves from time to time of the obvious: adults know more about the world than do children).

I am not of course suggesting that we abandon theory for normative observation (as though it were possible in any case to make observations without a theory). I am suggesting that we pay much closer attention to how specific skills are acquired without assuming that all skills must necessarily have something in common.

## NOTES

1. In fact the jargon may well be misleading. From the fact that children know less than adults it does not automatically follow that children 'must therefore process more information.' They may work *with* different information.
2. No-one would deny that there are biomechanical differences between children and adults; it may be mechanically easier for a ten-year-old to catch or throw a ball than for a two-year-old. Yet one important consequence of the schema notion (e.g. Schmidt, 1975) is surely that an action can be accomplished in different ways, that biomechanical constraints may have only limited relevance. It is possible that a child may perform actions given a muscular and anatomical apparatus which would be inadequate to their performance in adults.
3. The value of Schmidt's (1975) account seems to me that it goes beyond the conceptual point that a skill is defined by its goal, to ask questions in the traditional transfer-of-training paradigm about how practice of one ability can influence the acquisition of another.
4. A 'maturational' account of the development of early motor control does not do away with the need for fine-grain experimental analyses of performance. See the discussion below of the work of Peters and Walk (1974), Lee and Aronson (1973), and Butterworth and Hicks (1977).
5. E.g. Welford's (1958) off-hand remark that 'It is also obvious that normally we do not perceive with only one sense at a time, but that data from different senses are organized together, and that the resulting perception though it is predominantly, say, visual or auditory, has been partly shaped by stimuli, coming through other sensory channels' (p. 19).
   Birch and Lefford (1963, 1967) claimed historical continuity with the ideas of Baldwin (e.g. 1897) and Sherrington (1951) on intermodal co-ordination and voluntary control. As will be seen they argued that the senses are disparately

organized at birth and that development brings about intersensory liaison. This position they took to be congruent with Sherrington's views on the evolution of the nervous system on the ground that ontogeny repeats phylogeny. Sherrington's exact views on the nature of intersensory liaison are extremely obscure. He spoke of a 'central clearing-house of the senses' which could mean only that he thought of some neural centres (e.g. the motor cortex) as receiving inputs from relatively independent unintegrated sensory channels. Baldwin appears to say, rather like Welford, that we may use several senses which presumably provide correlated information to guide voluntary action.

Incidentally, Baldwin effectively criticized the phylogeny/ontogeny idea, arguing that voluntary control may often require a quite different neural basis in different species.

6. A study by Gregg, Haffner, and Korner (1976) provides some evidence in support. They found that increased vestibular stimulation in infants a few hours to a few days-old improved efficiency of visual tracking.
7. Bruner's work (e.g. 1973) has shown that it makes sense to regard the infant's earliest guided reaching movements as strategic or *intentional*. Hence the infant's movement are *voluntary*.

## REFERENCES

Abravanel, E. (1972). How children combine vision and touch when perceiving the shape of objects, *Perception & Psychophysics*, **12**, 171–175.

Allen, T. W., Walker, K., Symonds, I., and Marcell, M. (1977). Intrasensory perception of temporal sequences during infancy, *Developmental Psychology*, **13**, 225–229.

Baldwin, J. M. (1897). *Mental Development in the Child and the Race*, New York: Macmillan.

Birch, H. G., and Lefford, A. (1963). Intersensory development in children, *Monographs of the Society for Research in Child Development*, **28** (5, Whole No. 89).

Birch, H. G., and Lefford, A. (1967). Visual differentiation, intersensory integration and voluntary motor control, *Monographs of the Society for Research in Child Development*, **32**, (2, Whole No. 110).

Bizzi, E., Polit, A., and Morasso, A. (1976). Mechanisms underlying achievement of final head position, *Journal of Neurophysiology*, **39**, 435–443.

Bower, T. G. R. (1966). The visual world of infants, *Scientific American*, June 80–92.

Bruner, J. S. (1973). Organization of early skilled action, *Child Development*, **44**, 1–11.

Bruner, J. S., and Bruner, B. M. (1968). On voluntary action and its hierarchical structure, *International Journal of Psychology*, **3**, 239–255.

Bryant, P. E. (1968). Comments on the design of developmental studies of cross-modal matching and cross-modal transfer, *Cortex*, **4**, 127–137.

Bryant, P. E., Jones, P., Claxton, V., and Perkins, G. M. (1972). Recognition of shapes across modalities by infants, *Nature*, **240**, 303–304.

Bryant, P. E., and Trabasso, T. (1971). Transitive inferences and memory in young children, *Nature*, **232**, 456–458.

Butterworth, G., and Hicks, L. (1976). Visual proprioception and postural stability in infancy. A developmental study, *Perception*, **6**, 255–262.

Connolly, K. J. (1970). Skill development: Problems and plans, in K. J. Connolly (ed.), *Mechanisms of Motor Skill Development*, New York: Academic Press.

Connolly, K., and Jones B. (1970). A developmental study of afferent-reafferent integration, *British Journal of Psychology*, **61**, 259–266.

Fantz, R. L. (1958). Pattern perception in young infants, *Psychological Record*, **8**, 43–47.

Gesell, A., and Amatruda, C. S. (1947). *Developmental diagnosis*, 2nd edn., London: Harper.

Gibbs, C. B. (1954). The continuous regulation of skilled performance by kinesthetic feedback, *British Journal of Psychology*, **45**, 24–39.

Gibbs, C. B. (1965). Probability learning in step-input tracking, *British Journal of Psychology*, **56**, 233–242.

Gibson, J. J. (1966). *The Senses Considered as Perceptual Systems*, Boston: Houghton Mifflin.

Goodnow, J. (1971). Eye and hand: differential memory and its effect on matching, *Neuropsychologia*, **9**, 89–95.

Gregg, C. L., Haffner, M. E., and Korner, A. F. (1976). The relative efficacy of vestibular-proprioceptive stimulation and the upright position in enhancing visual pursuit in neonates, *Child Development*, **47**, 309–314.

Jones, B. (1972). Outflow and inflow in movement duplication, *Perception & Psychophysics*, **9**, 118–120.

Jones, B. (1973). When are vision and kinaesthesis comparable? *British Journal of Psychology*, **64**, 587–591.

Jones, B. (1974). Role of central monitoring of efference in short-term memory for movement, *Journal of Experimental Psychology*, **103**, 522–529.

Jones, B. (1978). The role of efference in motor control: A centralist emphasis for theories of skilled performance, in D. M. Landers and R. W. Christina (eds.), *Psychology of Motor Behaviour and Sport*, Champaign, Ill: Human Kinetics.

Jones, B. (1981). The developmental significance of cross-modal matching, in R. D. Walk and H. L. Pick (eds.), *Intersensory perception and sensory integration*, New York: Plenum Press.

Kay, H. (1970). Analyzing motor skill performance, in K. J. Connolly (Ed.), *Mechanisms of Motor Skill Development*, New York: Academic Press.

Lee, D. N., and Aronson, E. (1973). Visual proprioceptive control of standing in human infants, *Perception & Psychophysics*, **15**, 529–532.

Legge, D. (1965). Analysis of visual and proprioceptive components of motor skill by means of a drug, *British Journal of Psychology*, **65**, 243–254.

Lobb, H. (1965). Vision versus touch in form discrimination, *Canadian Journal of Psychology*, **19**, 175–187.

McGraw, M. B. (1935). *Growth: A study of Johnny and Jimmy*, New York: Appleton-Crofts.

Newell, K. M., Shapiro, D. C., and Carlton, J. M. (1979). Co-ordinating visual and kinesthetic memory codes, *British Journal of Psychology*, **70**, 87–96.

Paillard, J. (1971). Les déterminants moteurs de l'organisation spatiale, *Cahiers de Psychologie*, **14**, 261–316.

Paine, R. S., and Oppé, T. E. (1966). Neurological examination of children, *Clinics in Developmental Medicine*, (Whole Nos. 20 and 21).

Peters, C. P., and Walk, R. D. (1974). Visual placing by human infants, *Journal of Experimental Child Psychology*, **18**, 34–40.

Pew, R. W. (1974). Human perceptual motor performance, in B. H. Kantowitz (ed.), *Human Information Processing; Tutorials in performance and cognition*, Hillsdale, NJ: Lawrence Erlbaum.

Piaget, J. (1970). *Genetic Epistemology*, New York: Columbia University Press.

Schmidt, R. A. (1975). A schema theory of discrete motor skill learning, *Psychological Review*, **82**, 225–260.

Sherrington, C. (1951). *Man on his Nature*, Cambridge: Cambridge University Press.

Stelmach, G. E., Kelso, J. A. S., and Wallace, S. A. (1975). Pre-selection in short-term motor memory, *Journal of Experimental Psychology: Human Learning and Memory*, **1**, 745–758.

Wade, M. G. (1976). Developmental motor learning, *Exercise and Sports Sciences Reviews*, **4**, 375–394.

Warren, D. M. (1970). Intermodality interactions in spatial localization, *Cognitive Psychology*, **1**, 114–133.

Welford, A. T. (1958). *Ageing and Human Skill*, London: Oxford University Press.

Wickstrom, R. L. (1975). Developmental kinesiology: Maturation of basic motor patterns, *Exercise and Sports Sciences Reviews*, **3**, 163–192.

# PART II

# Development of Schemas, Plans, and Programs

While the papers in the first part of this volume dealt with – in different ways and for different activities – the intrinsic relationship between information, control, and co-ordination in developing systems, more formal approaches were given little air. A contrast is offered in the thorough review by Shapiro and Schmidt of the schema theory of discrete motor learning. Offered initially as a theory to predict the learning of new motor skills in adults, the theory has proven fairly robust, at least with regard to the variability-in-practice prediction, for movement skill acquisition in young children. Fundamental to the schema conceptualization of motor control is the acquisition of rules which structure the relationship between the production of a movement and evaluation of its consequences. The authors make the case that the acquisition of these rules for movement schemata would in all likelihood occur in the early years of life and as such motor skill development might best be viewed as the development of movement schemata.

For Clark the developmental gain in motor control is accomplished by age-related changes in the response selection and programming mechanisms posited in certain theories of information processing. In contrast to the discussion on schema theory, the conceptualizations offered by Clark directly address the issue of response selection, arguing that the developmental evidence on increased error rates and latencies implicates response selection processing as at least one locus of developmental change. Another mechanism considered by Clark is the programming process. Here she forwards the argument that the style of control suggested by Bernstein (1967) and more recently by Greene (1972) and Turvey (1977), might well serve as the proper conceptualization for future investigations of response programming.

These first two chapters provide the reader with the necessary backdrop for the Newell and Barclay paper in which the authors ask the question, 'What can a child know or come to know about his/her action?' They take us through a thorough discussion of knowledge representation systems and leave us with considerable food for thought about what the young child might come to know about his/her own neuromuscular system and the processes that control it. But leave us not to think that this is a simple matter to understand. An example once described by Polanyi (1958) might illustrate the dilemma Newell and Barclay pose. The description is one of a bicyclist attempting to maintain his/her balance on a bicycle. As the cyclist falls to the right he/she turns the handlebars to the right thus bringing the bicycle onto a curving path to the right. This maneuver serves to counteract the gravitational force pulling him/her to the ground by providing a leftward centrifugal force. For a child learning to ride a bicycle this last maneuver might well set up the need for the same action in the opposite direction due to an overzealous correction. Nonetheless, the complexity of the rule governing this action highlights the difficulty identified by Newell and Barclay for understanding the relationship between knowledge and action. For the reader, the rule which governs this balancing act is: 'adjust the curvature of the bicycle's path in proportion to the ratio of unbalance over the square of the speed.' Clearly knowing how to control the system is not necessarily the same as knowing anything about how the system is controlled.

For Griffin and Keogh the problem is much more pragmatic: how to get the child to *try* bike riding? Through all our lengthy discussions and arguments, the practical concern remains: some children choose to and continue to engage in movement situations while others choose not. In the final chapter of this section Griffin and Keogh maintain that the mediator as well as the consequence of movement involvement is a construct called movement confidence. Riding a bike is a very threatening movement situation for some children and the authors have provided a model which may help to predict a child's movement involvement by elucidating those determinants in the development of movement confidence. Indeed the four chapters which comprise this section provide the reader with interesting and hopefully thought-provoking essays on the development of plans, programs, and schemas, their representation and movement consequences.

The Development of Movement Control and Co-ordination
Edited by J. A. S. Kelso and J. E. Clark
© 1982, John Wiley & Sons, Ltd

# CHAPTER 4

# The Schema Theory: Recent Evidence and Developmental Implications

DIANE C. SHAPIRO AND RICHARD A. SCHMIDT

In 1975, Schmidt proposed that a fundamental aspect of the learning of motor skills involved the acquisition of schemata, or rules, that define the relationships among the information involved in the production and evaluation of motor responses. Motivated by the ideas on schema learning generated some forty years earlier (i.e. Bartlett, 1932) and by more recent thinking on abstract rules in pattern recognition (Posner and Keele, 1968, 1970) and motor responses (e.g. Pew, 1974), the idea represented a break in the tradition whereby motor learning was considered to be the establishment of a specific set of commands (e.g. Henry and Rogers, 1960) or references of correctness (Adams, 1971) which defined only a particular movement that was to be acquired in experimental conditions. Rather, the schema theory held that movement programs were generalized, and that complex rules must be formed in order to run them. One such rule was termed the recall schema, which was concerned with the relation between (i) the kinds of commands that the subject sends to the musculature and (ii) the results of those instructions either in terms of the subject's limb movements and/or the effects of those limb movements on the environment. A second rule was termed the recognition schema, and was concerned with (i) the relationship between the nature of the movement produced and (ii) the sensory information that the person received as a result of making that movement. By considering that these two schemata were built up over the course of previously experienced movements, such rules could be generalized to novel movement situations, so that people could produce a movement they had never made previously, or they could evaluate a movement they had never made before.

At this writing, approximately six years have passed since the idea was

113

published, and there has, of course, been a large volume of research done on human motor learning since that time. Some of this work was done in the context of schema-theory predictions. To our knowledge, no comprehensive review of this work has been published, and thus a major goal of this chapter is to bring together the research done on schema theory resulting from published work, conference presentations, and doctoral and masters' theses, in order to provide an examination of how well the various predictions have held up to direct experimental test. As well, there have been many experiments, together with some very important shifts in points of view about the learning and performance of skills, that have not occurred in the context of schema theory; some of this work, nevertheless, has a considerable bearing on the ideas presented in 1975, and we have included what we believe to be the most relevant, if not the most flattering, thinking about motor schemata. These two general bodies of evidence, then, should help us decide whether or not it is still reasonable to consider the learning of motor skills as being based on the acquisition of schemata.

As we shall see, most of this work was conducted with adults and, on the surface at least, would seem to have only limited application for those wishing to understand motor learning in children, or to understand motor development. But a number of us suspected early that the schema theory — even though it was developed using evidence from adult motor-learning experiments — might have considerable applicability for children as well (see, e.g. Schmidt, 1975a, 1977). Therefore, a second major goal of this chapter will be to consider this relationship to motor learning in children, to review the evidence since 1975 in the children's literature, and to provide what we think are reasonable extensions, implications, and future research directions for those interested in motor learning in the early years of life. We have found it convenient to separate the adult and children's work in this review, as the implications for adults and children appear to be different at qualitative levels, with the evidence from children often being far stronger in its statement about schemata than the comparable evidence from adults.

The chapter is divided into essentially five sections. First we provide a brief review of schema theory and some of its predictions. Next, we attempt to provide a review of the work bearing on schema theory since 1975. Third, we treat a separate issue — fundamental to schema theory, but with an importance far beyond it — the concepts of motor programs and generalized motor programs. Next, there are naturally some difficulties with the schema theory, both with respect to its agreement with the evidence, and also with respect to some apparent logical concerns, suggesting that the theory should be modified in certain ways. And, finally, we present what we think are good suggestions for future work in this area, in relation to both the research that could be done and also to the applications that could be made.

## THE THEORY

The schema theory (Schmidt, 1975a) has basically three major components: (i) the generalized motor program; (ii) the recall schema; and (iii) the recognition schema. This section will briefly discuss each of these components within the schema framework in terms of production and evaluation of motor responses. Additionally, since there have been some basic misunderstandings of each of their roles, an attempt has been made to rectify previous confusion. For a more detailed review of the theory, the reader is referred to Schmidt (1975a, 1976a, 1981, in press a, in press b.)

### Generalized Motor Program

At the base of the schema theory lies the notion of a generalized motor program, which is an abstract memory structure that, when activated, causes movement to occur. According to the schema theory, the generalized motor program can be executed in several ways to yield various response outcomes. Thus, not every movement requires a separate motor program for its execution. To attain the various movement outcomes, certain parameters (or 'response specifications') of the program must be determined (e.g. speed or force). Thus, a generalized motor program can be thought of as a program that governs a given class of movements that requires a common motor pattern.

As an example of a generalized motor program, consider an action such as throwing. Given a program for throwing, the speed of the throw can be varied in order to throw an object faster or slower. Additionally, if the subject is presented with objects of different masses, the forces used to propel the objects at constant velocities can also be varied. Therefore, the generalized-motor-program notion implies that by manipulating various parameters, several movement outcomes can be achieved. The specific characteristics of generalized motor programs will be considered in a subsequent section.

A common misunderstanding about schema theory is that the schema selects the appropriate generalized motor program to achieve the required goal. The theory does not concern itself with the selection of a kicking or a throwing program, but instead focuses on the processes that occur after the generalized motor program has been selected (namely, parameter selection) to effectively execute the program. This is where the recall schema is important, since its primary role is parameter selection and not program selection.

### Recall Schema

The recall schema is involved in response production. In order to achieve a desired outcome, the recall schema selects the parameters required to execute the generalized motor program properly. The theory holds that every generalized motor program must have a recall schema, which is a rule based on past attempts at running the program. Three types of information are important to the formation of the recall schema (rule). These are: (i) the initial conditions, which are the limb positions, body positions, and state of the environment prior to the action; (ii) the response-outcome information, which is the actual outcome or knowledge of results (KR), as a result of the action; and (iii) the parameters used when the program was executed.

When selecting a response, a subject receives sensory information about the initial conditions, selects the parameters (response specifications) to generate the movement and then notes the response outcome of his movement. When a number of these responses have been executed, the performer begins to abstract the information about the relationship among the three sources of information. The schema now consists of a rule specifying the relationship among the three pieces of information. The rule (and, of course, the generalized motor program) is stored in memory. Thus we think of schema learning as rule learning, and the strength of the relationship is hypothesized to be a positive function of the number of KR trials and the variability of practice.

The theory suggests that the greater the number of movement experiences (variability) within a response class (for a given generalized motor program) the more effectively the schema is formulated. As the schema becomes more established, the more accurately can the performer select the appropriate

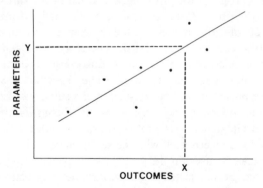

FIGURE 1    Graphical representation of the recall schema demonstrating the relationship between past outcome information and the parameters that have produced them. The points represent individual responses and the 'regression line' represents the rule. In order to produce a novel movement outcome (X) the schema rule selects the appropriate parameter (Y) to achieve the outcome

response specifications to execute a novel movement. Consider Figure 1 as a graphic representation of the recall schema. For this example, assume that the initial conditions are constant, and that the parameters are represented on the ordinate, and the response outcomes are represented on the abscissa. For every movement a performer executes, a point on the graph specifying the response specifications and the actual outcomes for that trial can be displayed. Thus, the more varied the experiences, the more points appear on the graph near the extremes. Consider the rule as analogous to a regression line. The larger the 'spread' of outcomes used to formulate the line, the more accurately the rule is defined. When attempting to produce a novel response, the performer enters his recall schema with the desired outcome. The more well-defined the regression line, the more accurately the performer can estimate the proper response specifications of a novel response. Thus, the recall schema allows the subject effectively to execute a novel response and is strengthened by variability of practice.

## Recognition Schema

The independent memory state responsible for response evaluation is the recognition schema. The recognition schema is composed of initial conditions, past actual outcomes, and past sensory consequences; it is formulated in a way analogous to the recall schema. As a subject practices a task, he formulates a rule specifying the relationship among these sources of information. The strength of the rule is enhanced by increasing the number of trials with KR as well as increasing the variability of practice. The theory predicts that the stronger the recognition schema, the better able is the performer to predict the expected sensory consequences of a novel response. Since it takes a minimal time to process feedback (Keele, 1968), recognition may operate at different times in the response. Evaluation can occur during the response in a slow movement, and only after a response in a rapid movement.

## Summary

In summary, the theory suggests that every movement class is governed by a generalized motor program, although the theory does not specify how the programs are selected. To execute each program to achieve the desired outcome, two independent memory states are required. The first, the recall schema, selects the response specifications that are used to execute the program to achieve the desired goal. The second, the recognition schema, generates the expected sensory consequences necessary to evaluate the correctness of the response. Both schemas are rules whose strengths are positive functions of the number of practice trials and the variability of practice.

Since the conception of the schema theory, there has been evidence generated about it in essentially three areas. The first area — and the issue most extensively examined — has been the variability prediction, tested for both recall and recognition memory. A second group of studies has focused on the independence of recognition and recall schemata. The final issue receiving attention has been that of the generalized motor program. The first two of these issues are examined in this section, while the work on the generalized motor program will be confined to its own section which follows this one.

## Variability of Practice

The schema theory predicts that an increased amount of variability within a schema class will lead to stronger recall and recognition schemata. To test this issue, a variability group experiencing several variations of a task and a constant group experiencing only one instance of that task are used. After an initial practice session under the respective conditions, all groups are transferred to a novel task within the response class. Schema theory predicts that the group receiving variability of practice should perform the novel task more effectively than the group that received constant practice. Given this basic paradigm, the notion of variability has been operationalized in several ways, and other questions concerning variability have been posed (e.g. the amount of variability, the structure of the variability session). Therefore, it will be helpful to review the evidence concerning the variability prediction by grouping the studies according to the experimental design used and the particular issue investigated. Also, an attempt will be made to compare evidence relating to recall and recognition schemata in adults versus children.

### Recall in Adults

Several authors (Hogan, 1977; McCracken and Stelmach, 1977; Zelaznik, 1977) utilized a rapid-timing task where movement time was fixed and movement distance was varied. McCracken and Stelmach used a variable group which practiced at four distances, a constant group which practiced at only one distance, and a third group that practiced at only one distance for less than half the number of trials experienced by the previous groups. When transferred to a novel distance, the variability group performed with significantly less absolute error (but not variable error) than the other groups, supporting the variability prediction for recall memory. Hogan (1977) practiced her subjects at either one, two, or four distances. The absolute error data on the first transfer trial demonstrated that the group receiving variability at four distances performed with significantly less error than the other groups, providing partial support for schema theory.

However, an alternative explanation for Hogan's (1977) results is that the variability group also practiced closer to the criterion transfer task than did the other groups. To control for this problem, Zelaznik (1977) trained a variability group at three distances and a constant group at only one distance; this constant group, however, practiced closer to the transfer target than the variability group did. The transfer data demonstrated that the group receiving variability during practice was not significantly different in absolute error from the constant group on the novel task. In addition, the group means were ordered contrary to the schema prediction, with the variability group demonstrating higher error than a constant group. Zelaznik suggested that the three targets practiced by the variability group may have caused so much response variation that different programs were used for each; the schema-theory prediction involves variations of parameters for a *given* program.

Newell and Shapiro (1976, Experiment 1), using a rapid-timing task with fixed movement distance, allowed subjects to practice at either one movement time (constant) or two movement times (variability) and then to transfer either inside or outside the range of their previous response variations. For absolute error, there were no differences between the constant and variable groups when transferred inside the range; however when transferred outside the range, the group that practiced the rapid response before the slower one had significantly less error on the slower transfer task than the constant group. The results suggest that order of practice may be an important variable in developing schemas. With essentially the same task, Melville's (1976) variability group practiced at two movement times whereas the constant group practiced at only one. The variability group did not perform the transfer trials with significantly less absolute, constant, or variable error, which did not support schema theory.

Using a ballistic positioning task Johnson and McCabe (1977) had subjects slide a ball bushing to rebound off a bumper located at the end of a trackway so that it would stop at a target. Subjects in a variability group experienced six distances and a constant group experienced only one. The variability group did not perform with significantly less absolute error than groups experiencing only one distance, which did not support schema theory.

Wrisberg and Ragsdale (1979) selected a coincident-timing task, where subjects either passively watched (low response requirements) or responded (high response requirements) to a stimulus light moving down a trackway. A constant group only experienced the light moving at one velocity, whereas a variability group experienced the lights moving at four different velocities. During the transfer trials subjects experienced a novel velocity. The high-variability, high-response-requirement group performed the criterion task with significantly less absolute error than the other groups, supporting the variability prediction for an open skill.

Besides using discrete tasks, two studies were performed on continuous tracking tasks (Coleman, 1979; Hawkins, 1977). Hawkins trained variability subjects to track four movement-pattern distortions, while another group tracked only one distortion. Using average integrated error on the transfer trials (prototype pattern), the group means were ordered in a direction predicted by the theory, but no significant differences were present. Coleman (1979) performed a similar study, but the display was extinguished during some of the training trials. This technique was utilized in an attempt to force the subjects to commit the movement patterns to memory. A significant difference in average integrated error was found between the high- and low-variability groups on the first transfer trial. This result partially supported the variability prediction on a continuous task.

Taken together, the results of these studies provide, at best, minimal support for the variability prediction for recall memory for adult subjects. Except for the Zelaznik (1977) experiment, however, the means are ordered in a way predicted by the theory, although the effects were generally not large enough to reach conventional levels of statistical significance.

## Recall in Children

To test the variability prediction on recall memory in children, several authors (Carson and Wiegand, 1979; Pigott, 1979) have trained their subjects to propel objects of varying weights, keeping distance constant, thus changing initial conditions. Carson and Wiegand used a beanbag-tossing task. A variability group trained at four beanbag weights, while a constant group trained at only one weight. When transferred to a novel task, the high-variability group performed with significantly less error than the low-variability group. Also, Pigott (1979) trained seven-year-old children to toss beanbags a fixed distance. Three variability groups and one constant group transferred to a novel location either inside or outside the range of initial variable experience. The absolute error data demonstrated that, on the first transfer block at a novel variation of the task, one of the variability groups performed with significantly less error than the constant group, while another did not. Each of these studies provides support for the variability prediction in children.

Rapid projectile tasks where target distances are varied have also been employed (Dummer, 1978; Hunter, 1977; Kelso and Norman, 1978; Kerr and Booth, 1977, 1978). Kelso and Norman (1978) trained three-year-old children to propel a ball-bushing car down a trackway with sufficient force so that it would coast to a stop at a specified target. The constant group practiced at a single target while a variability group practiced at four randomly assigned targets. During transfer, the groups were divided so that half of the subjects performed a novel task inside the range, and the other half transferred outside the range of previous experience. The variability group performed with less absolute, variable, and constant error than the constant group at both transfer targets. However, Dummer (1978), using the same design on retarded children, found no such support. Hunter (1977), using the same task, had a high-variability group experience eight variations of the task while the constant group only experienced one variation. The variability group performed the novel distance with significantly less absolute error than the constant group. Kerr and Booth (1977) trained seven- and nine-year-old children to toss bean-bags. The variability group practiced at two distances while the constant group practiced at only one. On a novel distance, the group experiencing variability performed with significantly less absolute, constant, and variable error than a constant group. Similar results were found with eight- and ten-year-old children (Kerr and Booth, 1978).

Some authors (Beatty, 1977; Moxley, 1979; Moxley and Fazey, 1977) have changed the initial conditions by varying the subject's position in relation to a fixed target. Moxley (1979) trained six- and eight-year-old children to throw a shuttlecock to an invariant target from a specified initial condition. The variability group threw from three different initial locations and the constant group threw from only one. On transfer, all subjects threw the same object from a novel location. The variability group performed with less absolute and variable error than the constant group, supporting the variability prediction. Moxley and Fazey (1977) and Beatty (1977) used designs similar to Moxley (1979); however, the former had subjects throwing balls and the latter used a modified bowling skill. Both studies demonstrated superior performance by the variability group.

One conclusion that emerges from these experiments is that children's motor skills are apparently more easily affected by variability in practice than are those of adults. From the point of view of schema theory, such results are interpreted to mean that the recall schemata are easily developed in children; adults, on the other hand, may have already developed schemata for the relatively simple tasks employed in the experiments reported here.

## Recognition in Adults

In this section, studies dealing with the learning of recognition tasks in adults are reviewed.[1] Remember that two kinds of performances, according to the schema theory, are involved here. First, slow, positioning responses, although they involve active movement production, are classed as being based on recognition memory, since the schema theory proposes that the subject moves to a position that is *recognized* as correct via ongoing analysis of feedback; this assumption may be incorrect, as we shall see in a later section. Second, in rapid tasks for which the subjects must evaluate their own errors after the movement is completed, the evaluation is based on recognition schemata.

*Positioning tasks.* Magill and Reeve (1978) provided practice at moving a lever to various physical stops for which the subjects knew the distance in advance. Two variability groups, one with a larger standard deviation from one criterion task than the other, and a constant group with but one position, were used. There were differences in favor of the variability group, but only on the second trial where the KR from Trial 1 could be used; the large-variability group performed with significantly less error than the other groups. Thus, there was some support for the notion of a recognition schema.

*Error estimation.* A number of investigators have used the technique where errors are estimated verbally after each performance trial, with the accuracy of the estimate being a measure of the recognition-memory strength (e.g. Hogan, 1977; Newell and Shapiro, 1976; McCracken and Stelmach, 1977). In the Hogan and McCracken–Stelmach studies, there were no significant differences between variability and constant groups on the transfer trials in terms of accuracy of estimations; Newell and Shapiro found effects in favor of the variability conditions, but the effect was limited to only one of the practice orders, and was probably an artifact of the fact that absolute estimated error is spuriously correlated with absolute errors (see Schmidt, 1975a).

Studies such as these, where estimated errors and movement productions are evaluated on the *same* responses, are probably flawed for another reason besides the correlation between estimation and production scores. On any but the first trial, performance (recall) on a given trial will presumably be related to some unknown degree to the strength of the *recognition* mechanisms on the previous trial(s), and vice versa. After a few trials, it could be impossible to separate the recall vs. recognition effects of variables (such as variability in practice) applied earlier, as all differences could be eliminated with but a few trials on transfer-task practice.

There are various ways to eliminate this problem. For example, Amacher (1978) had subjects learn to propel a slide along a trackway through a barrier at a given movement time in a practice session, and then had them estimate (recognize) the movement speed of an *artificially* propelled slide in a transfer session. Thus, estimations of the movement speed on these transfer trials would not be confounded by production of those same responses. However, she failed to find that variable-practice and constant-practice groups were significantly different on these estimation trials. One possible reason for the lack of support here was that subjects, during practice, were not required to estimate their performance times. Hogan and Yanowitz (1978) showed that active estimation produced superior performance on active, no-KR transfer trials relative to a no-estimation control condition; here, performance (recall) was assumed to be improved because of the stronger recognition mechanism being able to provide error information on the no-KR trials, thus allowing subjects to stay closer to the criterion target. Active estimations should probably be used in future investigations of recognition memory.

Another method to separate recognition from recall measures was used by Zelaznik, Shapiro, and Newell (1978). They had subjects listen to tape-recorded sounds of another subject moving a slide, and provided 'KR' about the movement speed on each presentation. Thus, the subjects could presumably associate the sensory consequences of the movements with the outcomes (provided by the 'KR'). Recognition-memory strength was estimated by subjects' *active* performances on a subsequent test session, with no KR being provided on these trials. The reasoning was that on these active performance trials, learning could presumably only occur via the errors evaluated by recognition memory; and performance could be maintained since subjects could evaluate their own errors via recognition memory. In relation to the variability prediction, Zelaznik, Shapiro, and Newell showed that a group that listened to varied responses had less absolute error, and improved performance more, on the no-KR trials than did a group that listened to constant responses. These data provided support for various aspects of the schema theory.

### Criterion versus Varied Practice

This section is concerned with a special contrast among groups found in many of the studies dealing with schema theory. In this contrast, a variable-practice condition is transferred to a novel criterion task; it is compared with another condition in which the same amount of prior practice is provided on the criterion task itself. This contrast is especially interesting, in that many rival theoretical positions (e.g. Adams, 1971), and certainly common sense, would predict that practice on a criterion task itself would be more beneficial for criterion-task performance than practice on variations about the criterion. The authors who have investigated this problem have studied it with respect to both recall and recognition performances; the following sections document this work.

*Recall.* For recall performances in adults, Johnson and McCabe (1977), using a rapid-positioning task, and Melville (1976), using a rapid-timing task, both found no significant differences between their variability conditions and the group that practiced only the criterion task to which both groups were transferred. Hawkins (1977) found similar results for a tracking task.

These studies are difficult to interpret, as the finding of 'no differences' in this contrast does not necessarily mean that the varied practice conditions were as effective as the criterion-task practice. However, in each of these cases, the mean differences were very small, and it seems safe to entertain the possibility that such a conclusion might be correct.

With children, the effects are far more clear-cut. For example, in the Kerr and Booth (1977) study using seven- and nine-year-olds, when the criterion-practice condition was compared to a condition having had prior variability, there was significantly less absolute, constant, and variable error for the variable-practice condition. Similar findings were produced in a later study by the same authors (Kerr and Booth, 1978), and by Carson and Wiegand (1979). Thus, these investigators have shown that not only is varied practice effective in producing novel task performance, it is *more* effective than practicing the constant criterion task itself!

*Recognition.* Using adult subjects with a blindfolded positioning task, Williams and Rodney (1978) had one condition that practiced only the criterion transfer position, while two other groups received experience surrounding this target. Both the group receiving practice at the criterion task and a group having randomly varied experience about the criterion performed the criterion without decrements, and essentially equivalently, for *twenty* trials. Thus, varied practice had produced a response capability that was essentially like that of a group that had practiced the task itself.

In a study cited earlier (Zelaznik, Shapiro, and Newell, 1978), where subjects passively experienced sounds of a slide moving in a rapid-timing task, one of the contrasts was between varied auditory experiences and the actual sound of the criterion task being performed. When subjects were then transferred to the active performance of the rapid-timing task without KR, subjects who had received varied listening experience performed the criterion task as well as subjects who had actually listened to the criterion task. The interpretation is that performance and learning of the criterion task, since it was without KR, must have been based on the subject's receiving self-reports of error based on the prior listening experience and varied experience produced essentially the same capabilities as did actual experience with the sound of the criterion task being performed.

*Theoretical implications.* Taken together, these studies have a number of important theoretical implications. First, they support the idea that schema development occurs much more easily in children than it does in adults. (We found no studies dealing with this contrast for children's recognition performance, however.) Perhaps this is so because adults have already established these schematic representations prior to engaging in the experimental procedures, while the children who have not previously developed them are acquiring them in the experimental settings. Second, and perhaps more important, is the fact that various rival theoretical positions (e.g. Adams, 1971) cannot explain how performance on variations of a task leads to essentially the same transfer performance (in adults) as does practicing the criterion task itself; with children, the varied practice was consistently found to be more effective than practicing the criterion task itself.

At the same time, these findings can easily be handled by schema theory. Here, each trial, whether it be the first one experienced on a novel criterion task or simply one in a long practice series on a constant criterion task, is seen as being novel; that is, subjects presumably prepare the movement on each trial 'afresh,' as Bartlett (1932) put it. With this view, since all responses are, in a sense, novel, then an effective way (the more effective in children) to prepare for the criterion task is with varied practice. This finding, as well, has important practical implications for the structure of practice sessions with children.

## Amount of Variability

Schema theory predicts that the transfer to a novel criterion task will be a function of the amount of variable practice received. The amount of variability can be manipulated by changing the number of trials received (with a fixed standard deviation), by varying the standard deviation of a constant number of trials, or by both. In most of the studies reviewed in this section, the number of trials has been held constant, and the variation of that experience has been altered in the practice session.

*Recall.*    Hogan (1977) used a ballistic-timing task, with one variability group having four different distances and another having only two. The group with the larger variance in prior experience produced more accurate performance on the novel criterion task. This finding should be taken cautiously, however, because it involves the possibility that the four-target condition practiced, on the average, closer to the transfer target than the two-target condition did.

With children, Hunter's second experiment (1977) used a ballistic task in which a slide was propelled down a trackway so that it stopped at a target. She used two versus eight locations for her variable-practice conditions, but arranged them so that the two-location group was actually closer to the criterion transfer target than was the eight-location group. This design effectively eliminated the argument that the more variable condition would have more accurate criterion task performance simply because the prior experience was, on the average, closer to the transfer target. She found that the eight-target condition was more accurate than the two-target condition when transferred to a novel target, but the differences fell just short of statistical significance. As well, Allen (1978), using the same task and design but with distance constant and mass to be pushed variable, found an advantage for an eight-mass condition versus a two-mass condition, with children as subjects; however, the differences were not significant.

Perhaps because both of these investigations used designs in which the low-variability condition was actually closer to the transfer target than the high-variability condition, there may have been an advantage of the close proximity to the transfer target that overshadowed the effects of variability *per se*. Even so, the high-variability condition was more accurate on the transfer task than the low-variability condition was, but these differences were not so large as they were with *constant* versus varied practice discussed earlier. Certainly, both proximity to the transfer target and variability of prior experience seem to be factors that contribute to transfer-task performance.

*Recognition.*    Using adult subjects, Newell and Shapiro (1976, Experiment 2) measured verbal estimations of performance after each trial of a ballistic timing task. Four groups experienced different amounts of variability in prior experience, but there were no significant differences among them in recognition performance on a novel variation of the task. Here, though, the recall and recognition performances were measured on the same trials; we have mentioned the difficulties with this design in a previous section.

Zelaznik, Shapiro, and Newell's (1978) passive-listening study with adults eliminated this problem, as the development of the recognition memory was not associated with active movement performances. They used a high-variable condition with sixty varied listening trials and a low-variability condition with only six such trials. They found that the high-variable condition produced *less* effective performance on the active no-KR transfer task than the low-variable condition, which was contrary to the schema-theory predictions. Similar findings had been produced earlier by Newell (1976). In addition, when the groups in these studies were examined independently on the transfer performance, only the low-variable practice condition maintained performance over the no-KR trials. The authors suggested that a large number of listening trials may have been boring for the subjects, thereby negatively affecting the acquisition of recognition memory, but they offered no evidence in support of this assertion.

## Structure of the Variability Session

*Recall.*    Although the evidence suggests that variability of practice can develop a strong recall schema, perhaps there is an optimal way to structure the variability session in formulating schemata. Some experimenters have examined the structure of the variability session directly by holding constant the amount of variability and the number of practice trials, while varying the structure of the variability. With adults, Newell and Shapiro (1976, Experiment 1) manipulated the order of presenting variable experiences to their subjects in a ballistic timing task. Here, variable practice at a more rapid task before variable practice on a slow one produced more transfer than the reverse order did.

It is certainly not clear as to the reasons for these effects, but the results do suggest that this kind of ordering may be important in the structure of practice sessions. More study is needed.

Pigott (1979) examined the structure of the variability session on seven-year-old children who tossed beanbags of varying weights to a fixed target location. Three variable groups and a constant group transferred to a novel beanbag mass either inside or outside the range of previous experiences. The variability groups received practice at four variations, but the order of experiences was different in each. One group received random presentations, another received the same masses but with fixed mass for blocks of six trials, and a third experienced the varying weights in blocks of three trials. On the transfer task, the three-trial-block condition was more accurate than either of the other two conditions, suggesting that there may be an optimal number of trials for repetition before the child is moved to another variation. Work is only beginning on this problem, but these results suggest that it may be a fruitful direction for future research.

*Recognition.* A study by Williams and Rodney (1978) on adults also demonstrated that the structure of the variability session may be important for producing transfer in recognition memory. Two groups received variability around the criterion target on a positioning task. One received randomly ordered locations around the target, while the other received the same locations but in a systematic order, with repeated over- and undershooting of the criterion target. The performance on the subsequent criterion task was more accurate for the group with unsystematic presentations.

Using the paradigm where the subject was to estimate his or her performance after each trial, Newell and Shapiro (1976, Experiment 1) showed more effective transfer for a fast-to-slow order of variable practice than for the reverse. However, these results are difficult to interpret, as the estimation data appear to be badly confounded with the response-production data (recall). No other studies were found for this issue in recognition memory.

### Across-task Transfer

To this point, we have considered only those investigations that involve transfer to a novel variation of the 'same' task, where the apparatus has remained the same for all variations. While this is the most straightforward kind of test of schema theory, it is possible that variability in practice on one task and apparatus might produce more transfer to another task and apparatus than a constant condition. The only study, to our knowledge, that has investigated this problem is by Carson and Wiegand (1979). Using preschool children, the variable or constant practice was produced with a beanbag toss to a horizontal target on the floor, and the transfer task was with a yarn ball to a vertical target on a wall. Variable beanbag practice was more effective than constant practice in transferring to the yarn-tossing task, suggesting that the variability effects may not be limited to the task on which they were presented.

These results go beyond the schema-theory predictions, as it is difficult to argue that the yarn- and beanbag-tossing tasks involved the same motor program. However, it is certainly possible that there may have been higher-order rules about tossing in general that were formed via variability, and that these rules could then be applied to a new task where a different motor program was required. This investigation has provided a very interesting new direction for the study of rule formation in children's motor behavior.

## Long-term Retention

Schema theory is based on the idea from the perceptual-learning literature (e.g. Posner and Keele, 1970) that a schema or rule is more strongly retained in memory than are the individual experiences upon which the rule was originally based. If so, then we should expect the transfer effects we have seen in the earlier sections to be retained over long periods of no practice, much as Posner and Keele have shown for dot-recognition tasks. As well, for practical reasons, there is a desire to know if the benefits from variable practice might lead to proficiency that would have a more permanent basis than constant practice would, as the relatively permanent capability for responding is a strong goal in most teaching-learning situations, especially with children.

## Recall

For adult subjects, in the study by McCracken and Stelmach (1977) discussed earlier in this section, people were asked to perform the transfer task (knocking down barriers at a novel distance) immediately and then again after a twenty-four-hour retention interval. Although there were immediate differences in absolute timing error between the variable and constant groups, there were no differences found after the one-day layoff. In a study by Coleman (1979) using a tracking task, some subjects experienced a forty-eight-hour retention interval after initial variable or constant practice. A significant difference in average integrated error was observed, but only on the first transfer trial. And no differential variable − versus constant-practice effects were found in a tracking study by Hawkins (1977) after a retention interval of two days.

Using children as subjects, Carson and Wiegand (1979) used a two-week retention interval after an immediate transfer to a novel task. All groups except for the variability condition showed a decrement in performance over the retention interval; this condition continued to display less absolute error than the constant-practice condition. Moxley and Fazey (1977), also using children, showed that between a retention interval of twenty minutes to twenty-four hours, a variability condition maintained performance, with a constant-practice condition losing skill. In a similar design, however, Beatty (1977) did not find improved retention for a variability condition after a retention interval of one week.

## Recognition

The only study we found that examined recognition after a retention interval as a function of previous variability-in-practice conditions was that by McCracken and Stelmach (1977). After a twenty-four-hour retention interval, they failed to find any significant differences (using a within-subject correlation between actual error and estimated error) as a function of variable-practice conditions presented earlier. As mentioned previously, though, these findings were based on recognition and recall performance measures taken from the same trials, and there is a serious risk of masking differences that may have existed with this method. Apparently, no such studies have been done with children as subjects.

## Independence of Recall and Recognition

An additional issue that has been examined, although not to the same extent as the variability prediction, is whether recall and recognition are separate states of memory. The theory posits that, although the two schemata are both comprised of initial conditions and response outcomes, they are different because they involve the relation among these inputs and response specifications (for recall) and sensory consequences (for recognition). This separation of recognition and recall has been thought to be important so that the person can recognize errors; for unless the states responsible for generating the movement and the reference of correctness are postulated to be separate, the motor system would presumably always receive a match between the intended and actual sensory consequences. Also, separating them allows the reference of correctness against which feedback is compared to be based on a correct movement *in the environment* rather than on the movement that was actually produced on a particular trial; the latter movements could, presumably, be different on every trial.

Four studies described earlier (Hogan, 1977; McCracken and Stelmach, 1977; Newell and Shapiro, 1976; Zelaznik, 1977) have all examined recall and recognition schemata in the same experiment. The strength of the recall memory was measured by absolute error, and strength of recognition memory was evaluated using estimated errors. Two of the studies (Newell and Shapiro,

1976; Zelaznik, 1977) demonstrated the same pattern of effects for both mechanisms as a function of variability of practice, while the other two studies (Hogan, 1977; McCracken and Stelmach, 1977) showed no apparent relationship between the measures reflecting each memory state. Based on the inconsistencies in these findings, it is difficult to assess whether recall and recognition were operating independently.

Some incidental findings from Newell (1976) and Zelaznik and Spring (1976) and Zelaznik, Shapiro, and Newell (1978, Experiment 2) also provide some difficulty for the notion that recall and recognition are independent states of memory. In an ingenious technique, these experimenters asked subjects to listen passively to the sound of other subjects producing responses on a rapid ballistic-slide task. Such a procedure should have theoretically strengthened the recognition schema since information about actual movement time was also provided, but it should have had no beneficial effects on the recall schema, since subjects did not *produce* any responses. When the subjects were subsequently transferred to an active condition where they had to produce these movements, there was a reduction of error with successive trials, and without KR. The interpretation was that subjects were using the subjectively generated error information arising from the strengthened recognition schema as a substitute for KR to learn and maintain performance on the novel task.

However, in these studies, the performance on the *first* active trial must be based on previous recall memory, as no trials precede it to provide subjective error information; the schema theory would predict that performance of the groups receiving listening and groups not receiving listening would be equivalent on this trial. Yet listening groups experienced less error on this trial than groups that did not have this experience; and Zelaznik, Shapiro, and Newell (1978, Experiment 2) found that groups with variability in listening were even more effective on this trial than were the constant-listening subjects, all of which appeared contradictory to the notion of separate recall and recognition states.

However, McGhee (1981) hypothesized that the subjects' listening experience may have provided information about the proper speed of the movement that they were to make, so that the movement was initially more rapid (and hence closer to the target movement time) than was the case for the subjects without this listening experience. In a clever experiment, he had one group of subjects listen to others' movements, and then had this listening group instruct yet another group of subjects as to how to move. The instruction, which invariably indicated that the movement was to be extremely rapid, led to first-trial performance equivalent to that for another group having only the listening experience. Thus, McGhee's data suggest that, rather than recognition and recall being functionally dependent, a more proper interpretation of the earlier listening studies is that listening provided information (directions) about what to do on the first trial, leading to more effective first-trial performance.

Wallace and McGhee (1979) also found a first-trial benefit on a *rapid* positioning task that presumably used recall memory; here, experience with passive movements to the criterion position transferred to the active movement production. Thus, having experienced the target location passively (a recognition-memory benefit) transferred to a situation where the same position had to be produced by a rapid action (i.e. by recall memory), contrary to schema theory; analogous results were produced by Williams (1978, Experiment 2). Such findings would, however, be consistent with the recent notion of the mass-spring model (discussed in a later section of this chapter) where the movement *endpoint* is specified as a part of the program; thus, experience at the endpoint in the recognition paradigm may have indicated where the endpoint was so that the person could program it more effectively.

In a more direct test of this issue, Schmidt, Christenson, and Rogers (1975) studied the delay of KR as a variable that might operate differently on recall and recognition memories. One experiment showed that recognition learning (learning to judge lifted weights) was impaired when KR delay was increased, suggesting that KR delay was a variable affecting recognition memory. Their other experiment with a ballistic timing task showed that KR delay had no effect on the development of the recall memory (absolute error), but had negative effects on the development of recognition memory (estimated errors). Together, these findings provided some support for the notion that recall and recognition are separate memory states, since the same independent variable (KR delay) affected measures of them differently. However, these KR-delay effects have not been replicated on a ballistic timing task (Cobb, 1978) and a force-reproduction task (Blair, 1979).

The Schmidt, Christenson, and Rogers (1975) study provides an interesting direction for research in this area. But there are problems. Aside from these failures to replicate, (Blair, 1979; Cobb, 1978) the KR literature (e.g. Bilodeau, 1966) has consistently shown that KR delay has no effect on the learning of positioning responses. This is difficult to reconcile, since Schmidt, Christenson, and Rogers (1975) proposed that KR delay would be a variable that would affect recognition, and the schema theory holds that positioning responses are governed by recognition memory. Therefore, it is surprising to find KR-delay effects in the weight-lifting task, which is also presumably governed by recognition memory. One possibility is that the earlier studies of positioning accuracy have involved *recall* memory, as the authors of these studies (see, e.g. the review by Bilodeau, 1966) have consistently insisted that subjects move 'briskly' to the target, and have not allowed any corrections. If this were the case, then positioning performances might not show KR-delay effects because they were based on recall, not recognition. But subsequently, Schmidt and Shea (1976) failed to show that KR delay was a variable in the learning of slow positioning responses where corrections were allowed (even encouraged), and where the starting positions were shifted on each trial to minimize the possibility that subjects were using a recall memory. The suggestion that KR delay is a variable in recognition memory but not in recall is far from being clear-cut.

A second problem, pointed out to Schmidt, Christenson, and Rogers (1975) by Jahnke (1975), was a logical one. In verbal paired-associates learning, where the recall-recognition distinction was formed, measures of recall consist of the subject's verbal report of the answer based on the stimulus term that is presented. But this is just what we in motor behavior have often used as measures of *recognition* memory; the 'stimulus' is presumably the feedback from the responding limb and apparatus, and the response is the guess about the movement time or other aspect of the response. There does not seem to be an exact parallel to the motor recall measures (i.e. actual performance) in the verbal-learning literature.

To summarize, there seems to be a serious lack of evidence on the question of motor recall versus recognition memory. Logically, it makes sense to postulate that they are separate, or at least capable of being developed separately by different variables (see, e.g. Schmidt, 1975a, for the rationale). But there have been instances where the variables thought to affect recognition have affected recall measures, and the interesting possibility that KR delay may differentially affect recall and recognition has a number of difficulties. We can only conclude that more thinking and research on this issue should be done before any definitive conclusions can be made.


## GENERALIZED MOTOR PROGRAMS

The notion of the motor program, and specifically that the motor program is *generalized*, is critical to the schema theory, as the purpose of the recall schema was to select the parameters (*response specifications*) necessary for the execution of the generalized motor program. As such, the entire theoretical structure rests on the viability of a generalized motor-program notion. Because of its importance, therefore, we treat the idea separately in this section.

The ideas about motor programs and generalized motor programs have been discussed in detail in a number of different places recently, and so only a brief treatment of the fundamental idea and recent evidence will be presented here. We will also attempt to present some problems for the idea that have the most bearing on the schema theory. For a more complete treatment of the notion from a behavioral point of view, see Pew (1974), Schmidt (1976b, 1980, 1981, in press, a); for a treatment in terms of neural-control processes, see Brooks (1979) and Grillner (1975).

## Structure

### Invariant Features

The idea of generalized motor programs emerged from the observation that movements that were slightly different from each other in some ways seemed to be identical to each other in certain other ways. An empirical finding to support this view comes indirectly from a study by Armstrong (1970). He found that when a movement sequence was speeded up accidentally, shortening the movement time, the entire movement sequence was speeded up as a unit; that is, 'relative timing,' or *phasing* as it is usually called, appeared to remain constant in the face of changes in overall movement time. This suggested that phasing was somehow fundamental to a group of responses that might possess different speeds. Pew (1974) and later Schmidt (1975a, 1976a, 1976b) interpreted this finding to mean that phasing was a part of a generalized motor program, that could govern many such response speeds, and that overall movement time was a parameter. Thus, phasing appeared to be an *invariant feature* of this class of movements, while movement time was easily variable from trial to trial.

This kind of thinking led to the idea that the other invariant feature of generalized motor programs was *relative force*, or the relations among the forces called up in the various muscles participating in the action. Thus, an abstract memory structure that defines the relative timing of the contractions (i.e. phasing), and the relative forces that are to be applied was potentially able to account for the production of a set of movements that were quite similar to each other (e.g. overarm throws).

In terms of schema theory, such a generalized motor program defines a *class* of movements; or, if two movements are governed by a certain generalized motor program, then they are said to be members of the same class. Because the generalized motor program, containing phasing and relative force, is capable of defining a *pattern* of activity in the musculature (e.g. one's signature, an overarm throw), even when the details of the pattern (e.g. the speed, the size) are different, a movement class can be thought of as a group of responses that possess the same pattern.

### Parameters

Variations in the movements within a movement class are theoretically produced by changing the parameters used by the generalized motor program during execution. Changing the parameter does not change the basic pattern of action (i.e. the invariant features), but it would be expected to change the 'surface features' of the response. The next section reviews the suggestions for the various parameters.

*Movement time.* As mentioned previously, the overall movement time appears to be a parameter for which there is a great deal of evidence. Using the criterion that the phasing remain constant, various authors have found that the overall speed of the response can be changed without changing the pattern, or phasing of the movement. This has been found in arm movements (Armstrong, 1970), forearm-rotation movements (Shapiro, 1977, 1978), in button-pressing responses (Summers, 1975), in typing and handwriting (Viviani and Terzuolo, 1980), and in the control of walking and running (Shapiro, Zernicke, Gregor, and Diestel, 1981). In fact, Summers (1975) and Shapiro (1977) have shown that, even when the subject was instructed to abandon the phasing that was learned and was to move as quickly as possible throughout the sequence, the original phasing still remained even though movement time decreased.

*Overall force.* Changes in speed of program execution must, according to physical principles, be accompanied by changes in the forces with which the movement is to be made if the movement trajectories are to remain constant. Thus, a second parameter that has been suggested is overall force, where the parameter scales the forces produced by the program so that their relative magnitudes remain invariant. One can think of examples (e.g. Schmidt, 1981, in press, a) where a movement speed parameter would remain fixed, but the overall force parameter would have to be modulated; throwing objects of varying masses a fixed distance would require constant limb speed but varying forces scaled according to the mass.

*Response size.* A third parameter termed 'response size' has been considered. The idea comes from the common observation that we can produce the same signature pattern at various sizes, presumably with the same phasing and relative force (e.g. Merton, 1972). In some situations, however, changes in response size have been argued to be the result of the combinations of two more fundamental parameters – response speed and overall force (e.g. Schmidt, 1980b). This suggestion is in keeping with the finding that increasing the friction applied to a pen in handwriting examples decreases the size of the writing uniformly (Denier van der Gon and Thuring, 1965); here, friction would be expected to scale down the accelerations applied by all aspects of the movement program.

*Muscle selection.* The handwriting examples provide interesting suggestions for a fourth parameter – muscle selection. The fact that small signatures are written with the finger muscles, and larger ones are written with the elbow and shoulder muscles, suggests that the same pattern can be run off with different muscles involved. Thus, a single generalized motor program might not contain information about which muscles are to be involved, with this specification taking the form of parameters that are applied later. Klapp (1977) has provided evidence for this assertion in a reaction-time paradigm, where the pattern could be selected in advance (thereby saving time), without the subject knowing which muscles were going to be used in the response.

## Experimental Tests

Part of the difficulty with the schema theory is the fact that the generalized motor program notion on which it is based has had so little direct experimental examination. As indicated before, much of the evidence, with the exception of the work on the movement-speed parameter, has been based on incidental findings. As we hope to show, more research on the nature of generalized motor programs would give considerable insight into a number of aspects of the schema theory.

### Testing Invariant Features

The fundamental working hypothesis that we have adopted with our work on programming is this: if two movements have the same phasing, then they are governed by the same generalized motor program; if the phasing is different, then the programs governing them are different as well. If such a working assumption can be accepted, this leads the way to a number of experiments to determine some of the characteristics of generalized motor programs.

An example of this is in an experiment by Shapiro et al. (1981), where walking or jogging speed on a treadmill was systematically varied, and various kinematic measures were taken from film records of the movements. One measure of phasing that was used is the proportion of time involved in each of the phases of the Philippson (1905) step cycle, where the stepping action is divided into its four component parts. They found that, during walking, as the treadmill speed was increased, there were nearly no changes in the proportions of time involved in each of the step phases; but when the subject changed from a walk to a jog, the phasing changed to a new pattern which also did not change during the variations in jogging speed. Here, the phasing appeared to be related to a particular gait, with each gait having a distinctly different phasing. Evidence for a program for walking and a program for jogging was produced.

Similar kinds of experiments could be done to determine the extent to which relative force remains invariant across changes in certain parameters; no direct tests of this idea were found in our search of the literature. One prediction would be that the relative force and phasing characteristics of a movement class should be tightly coupled. That is, a given generalized motor program should have a distinct relative force pattern and phasing; and when a different program is employed (e.g. in going from a walk to a jog), *both* relative force and phasing should change to some new (invariant) pattern. This kind of work needs to be done on a variety of movements to test the generality of the idea.

Perhaps the reason that motor behavior researchers have not studied generalized motor programs in this way in the past is that it requires kinematic data that describe what the limbs are doing in an action; heretofore, we have been primarily concerned with movement *outcome* data, where the emphasis was placed on whether the ball went in the basket, the dart hit the target, etc.; we have consistently ignored what the person was doing to produce these skilled actions. Now, with the increased emphasis on biomechanical methods on the part of motor-behavior workers, we should begin to see more and more of this kind of work being done.

### How Large is a Response Class?

With respect to schema theory, an important problem for those who have performed experiments in this context is the definition of a response class. With the orientation provided by the above sections on the generalized motor program, some questions about the size of a response class can be determined empirically. Remembering that the working assumption was that any movements with the same phasing were produced by the same program, we can perform experiments where a certain aspect of the movement is varied systematically (e.g. the weight of a ball to be thrown), and notice the phasing that results from the actions. For example, we might find that throwing a light ball might require one phasing pattern, a medium ball another, and a very heavy ball yet another; e.g. the conclusion might be that throwing, in this context, involves at least three motor programs, each used differentially as a function of the weight of the object to be thrown. Thus, statements of the type 'The response class for throwing a light object has a range of from zero to 5 kg' could result. Thus, as Schmidt (1975a) has discussed, the size of the response class is largely an empirical question, whose answer can be worked out with some assumptions about the invariance of phasing in movements.

### Teaching Implications

Knowing the breadth of a schema class should enable the more effective structuring of variability in teaching situations. For example, if we know that the same motor program for throwing was used for all weights between zero and 5 kg, we could structure a teaching session so that variable practice with this range of responses was experienced. We might also wish to repeat this kind of training for the other motor programs that are discovered for throwing. Even though the schema theory does not address the issue of the selection of different programs, it might be profitable to study the extent to which the forced selection from among *different* programs would enable students to perform novel open skills more effectively; the definitions of the end of one program and the beginnings of the next would aid in the decisions involved in conducting this research.

### The Learning of Generalized Motor Programs

As mentioned before, the theory does not attempt to address the questions about how generalized motor programs are learned. We have the beginnings of a method to do this kind of work now, as we could examine the phasing characteristics of movements on particular tasks to determine changes in the underlying phasing of the responses as a function of practice. An interesting suggestion has been provided by Keele (1976), where a complex movement such as shifting gears in an automobile is initially made up of a group of programs operating in sequence; as practice continues, the same sequence might be governed by a single program. Evidence for such changes should be provided through an examination of the changes in phasing among the movement segments as a function of practice. Initial attempts at this kind of work have been made (Marteniuk, 1978; Shapiro, 1978), but they have not been very successful in coming to a decision about the processes in learning motor programs. But this work represents a good start.

### Importance For Schema Theory

From the point of view that the most important experiments to do are those that are likely to disprove a certain point of view or theory, research on generalized motor programs seems to be very important for schema theory. If the notion of the generalized motor program appears to be incorrect as a result of our critical tests of it, the notion of the schema must be modified.

## SOME CONCERNS FOR SCHEMA THEORY

Aside from some empirical findings, discussed in the previous sections, that do not seem to be in keeping with the predictions from schema theory, there are some other concerns about the theory that should be mentioned. Two of these seem to be of fundamental importance to the theory, and they are discussed in the following sections.

**Initial Conditions**

The theory postulates that one of the kinds of information used by the subject in developing the recall or recognition schemas is the collection of initial conditions that existed when the movement was made. The original notion was that, in making a movement, the system would have to take into account the initial conditions of the limb in order that the parameters to the motor program be specified appropriately. This notion, in turn, was based on our 1975 thinking about the nature of the motor program – a position that we have termed the impulse-timing view of motor programming. This view holds that the program specifies pulses of EMG to the appropriate muscles, in the proper order, and with the proper timing (or phasing, as it is usually called); the net result of these EMG pulses is forces in the muscles that are distributed across time in a way that produces skilled action. In particular, the impulse-timing view holds that if I want to make a 45° flexion movement of the elbow beginning with the elbow at, say, 135°, the program must first apply a force in the direction of flexion, the program turns off this force, and then force in the extension dimension is applied to bring the limb to a stop. According to this kind of idea, the way in which I know how much force to apply, or how long to apply it, is based on 'knowledge' about the limb's initial conditions; it is easy to see that if I produce these forces for too long, or produce too much force in the flexion dimension, the limb will travel too far before it comes to a stop, and I will overshoot my target. Thus, for an impulse-timing view of the program to 'work,' the system must be able to know about the state of the musculature before the move so that the parameters for action (i.e. the overall force parameter, the overall speed parameter, etc.) can be specified properly.

But recently there bas been evidence produced that the impulse-timing view of motor programming might be incorrect, at least for movements such as we have been describing here. The most convincing of this work is by Bizzi and his colleagues (e.g. Bizzi, Dev, Morasso, and Polit, 1978; Bizzi, Polit, and Morasso, 1976; Polit and Bizzi, 1978, 1979), who studied deafferented monkeys trained to make elbow-flexion movements to aim the limb at a target. The arm was not visible to the monkey, and the target light would go off just as the monkey began his move, with the total movement being made in the dark. An important finding was that, when the monkey's arm was moved by the experimenter before the action, either by moving it toward or away from the target, the movement to the target was accomplished accurately. In fact, in some situations the monkeys had the arm displaced *past* the target; the arm in this case achieved the target in a direction *opposite* to the original direction. Thus, the monkeys moved to the target position accurately even when the initial condition was shifted (the monkey, being deafferented, could not sense this shift, of course), implying that 'knowledge' about the initial conditions was clearly not important to making this action.

These findings are in direct contradiction to an impulse-timing view of programming. As we have just argued, without knowledge of where the limb began, there can be no basis for determining the parameters for action. And the monkey could not use feedback-based mechanisms to position the limb, since the animals could do the positioning under conditions of surgical deafferenta-tion, where no feedback was possible.

These results can, however, be explained by a separate hypothesis originally proposed in an obscure paper by Crossman and Goodeve (1963), and (apparently independently) later by Asatryan and Fel'dman (1965) and Fel'dman (1966a, b). This hypothesis, which has come to be known as the 'mass-spring model,' holds that the agonist and antagonist muscles co-contract during the movement, and that the limb is driven by the mechanical spring-like properties of the muscles to achieve a position such that the torques for flexion and extension are equal and opposite. Because of the approximately linear rela-tion between the length of a muscle and the tension it will develop at a given level of innervation, a muscle-joint system can be made to achieve any position by altering the relative innervation levels of the involved muscle groups. Thus, according to this view, the limb achieves the 'equilibrium point' (where the torques are equal and opposite) by purely mechanical means. The output of the motor program in this model consists of appropriate levels of innervation to the opposing muscles, with the temporal aspects (e.g. phasing) being neither involved nor important. For the purposes of the present discussion, it should be emphasized that such a model does not depend on the initial conditions for accurate positioning.

These new findings about the mass-spring model and the independence of the endpoints of (certain) movements from their starting position provide a number of difficulties for the schema theory. First, the motor-program notion on which the schema theory is based appears to be incorrect in at least simple, positioning responses; see Schmidt (1980a, 1980b, 1981) and Schmidt and McGown (1980) for a more complete treatment of this idea. As we have mentioned in a previous section, the schema theory relies heavily on the idea of generalized motor programs and impulse-timing mechanisms, and evidence that such ideas might be incorrect will probably require some modifications in the theory.

As a second problem that these data provide for schema theory, it appears that information about the initial conditions is not always required in order for a movement to be parameterized correctly. The simple arm-positioning responses studied by Bizzi and his colleagues and the work by Kelso (1977) are good examples. If these initial conditions are not important, then the schema theory, which insists that the initial conditions of past movements are elements in recall and recognition schemata, should probably be modified.

A third difficulty is related to the distinction between recognition and recall. The theory specifically states that rapid movements, whose movement time is too short to allow the processing of feedback by the recognition memory, will be handled by recall memory exclusively. Slower movements, which have more within-movement time for feedback analysis and the initiation of corrections, should be handled by recognition memory. The argument here is that the subject moves to that position which is recognized as correct. Thus even though the slow positioning movement is technically active (as opposed to passive), the theory views its control as though it were being moved passively, with the subject stopping when the position is recognized as correct. However, it now appears that at least some positioning responses can be handled by mechanisms that do not require any feedback, and the data from Bizzi and his colleagues, as well as the cuff experiments by Kelso (1977), provide excellent examples. Rather than the system moving to a position that it recognizes as correct, a more reasonable model appears to be the mass-spring view, where the system moves to an equilibrium point defined by the mechanical properties of the muscles. Thus, the schema theory seems to be incorrect in this regard, and the strong stance that slow movements are always controlled by recognition memory may have to be modified (i) because of the mass-spring evidence and (ii) because there is now good reason to suspect that long-duration movements may be programmed using recall memory (e.g. Schmidt, 1980a; Shapiro, 1977, 1978).

It is far from clear as to how these new data should be reflected in modifications to the theory. A major problem is how much generality the mass-spring model has, and modifications of the schema theory should probably wait until this issue can be settled somewhat more completely. For example, there is a suggestion that single-direction movements appear to be controlled via a mass-spring mechanism, whereas multiple-direction and multilimb movements are not (Schmidt, 1980b, 1981; Schmidt and McGown, 1980). And it is still possible that some slow, positioning movements – perhaps of the type used in motor-learning experiments – are controlled by recognition memory, and that only when the feedback channels are degraded does the secondary process of mass-spring control take over (e.g. as in Polit and Bizzi, 1978, 1979; Kelso, 1977). It is clear that some modifications are in order, but we are not sure as to what direction they will take with the state of the evidence as it is. It is too early to tell.

### Learning in Motor-learning Experiments

The second concern we have about the schema theory is related to the theory's internal consistency. It relates to how the theory attempts to explain the learning that typically occurs in the usual motor-learning experiment. In such situations, we usually have a group of subjects practice for a relatively small number of trials (e.g. less than 100). Almost invariably, we observe that the performances – however measured – become more proficient with practice. Such changes in behavior – if they can be shown to be 'relatively permanent' (Schmidt, 1975b) are assumed to be based on motor learning, and it is precisely this learning that the schema theory is attempting to explain.

The explanation is as follows. First, the person selects the program for the action in question. (Remember, the schema does not attempt to explain how *programs* are selected, only how the *parameters* for the program are selected.) Then, estimates of the parameter for the program are selected for the first trial from the subject's recall schema, a rule based on previous experience in running the same program, and the movement is produced. The information from that movement – the response outcome and the parameter – provides additional 'data' for the schema rule, and it is updated, providing a better estimate of the proper parameter for the program on the next trial, and so on. Thus, as a result of practice on the motor-learning task, the schema rule is modified to produce better performance on *that* task.

We find that there are two difficulties with this argument. First, the schema was intended as a construct that represents a very stable dependency between the past response outcomes and the past parameters, with this dependency being established over thousands of trials for which this program was used in the past. If the schema is abstracted from, say, 1000 prior instances, it does not make sense to us to postulate that the schema rule can be severely modified on the basis of only twenty practice trials in the new experimental situation. In fact, the most drastic changes in such experiments typically occur between Trial 1 and Trial 2, and the present version of the schema theory would hold that a schema built up over 1000 trials can be changed drastically in only one trial, essentially negating 1000 trials of previous experience.

The second problem is closely related to this first one. The idea of the recall schema was that a rule could be built up for, say, throwing, which could then be used in a 'new' throwing situation on the first trial. Indeed, some of the strongest evidence that we see for the concept of schemata is that the performance on the *first* trial of a transfer task is more accurate for a variable-practice group than it is for a constant-practice group. The idea that the subject has a stable schema that can be applied to some new situation does not go along logically with the idea that such a schema should be highly modifiable in just a few trials of a motor-learning experiment. If the schema could be modified so quickly, any new motor experience would change the schema rule, and the schema would then be ineffective for the next motor task that came along. We think that it is a mistake to suggest that motor learning *in motor-learning experiments* occurs because of modifications in the schema rule for the motor program in question. Our problem is that we cannot have it both ways: either we argue (i) that the schema changes in a motor-learning experiment, which leaves us with no stable rule to apply to the next use of the motor program in the future; or (ii) that the schema does not change appreciably in a motor-learning experiment, which then fails to explain the large changes in behavior that occur in experiments.

There are a number of ways that we can handle this dilemma. The most simple way is to postulate that the schema does not change appreciably with practice in a motor-learning experiment; this has a very strong advantage theoretically, as it then provides a good explanation of how the person can perform a 'new' motor task (a novel throwing situation, using an 'old' program) so effectively. However, when the individual is confronted with the new throwing task, assume that there are certain aspects of the situation that are not governed by the schema rule, such as the flight characteristics for the object to be thrown, the particular shape of the object, and so on. Thus, one way to view the learning that will occur with repetitions of this new throwing task is to postulate that the learner uses the constant parameters from the recall schema; these are essentially constant from trial to trial since the schema will not change very much, and the task remains objectively constant as well. But, to the constant value for the parameter the subject can add an additional value based on the immediately past performance in the task. For example, if the throw on the first trial is too short, the person uses the same parameter, but adds some force to it so that the next throw is somewhat longer. Thus, the learning in the motor-learning experiment can be regarded as the discovery of the size of the value to be added to the parameters in order to make the program 'work' in this particular situation.

That learning should, however, be situation-specific in contrast to the schema learning which should be general across all the uses of the generalized motor program. This feature should provide a testable means of evaluating whether this modification to schema theory is viable or not. One prediction would be that, if the schema is based on a great deal of prior practice (e.g. as in throwing in adults), practice on four different throwing tasks should not transfer to a fifth throwing task to any greater extent than should an equivalent amount of experience at a single throwing task. On the other hand, if the schema is very poorly developed, as it would be for throwing in infants, then practice at the four different throwing tasks should provide a great deal more transfer to the novel (fifth) throwing task than would the equivalent amount of practice at a single task. This result would be predicted because, in the adults, the schema rule is relatively fixed, so that any learning would be primarily related to the task-specific adjustments to the constant parameter for the program. With children, however, the schema is not well developed, and all practice with the program contributes greatly both to the schema strength and to the selection of the task-specific adjustments. In one sense, this kind of result seems to have been shown previously, as we see very much more effect of variability in practice with children than we do with adults, suggesting that the within-task changes are due to task-specific changes in the adults, and to task-specific changes *plus* changes in the schemata with children. Certainly this issue deserves a great deal more thought and study.

We are not happy about having to make a change in the schema theory in this way, but we see no alternative. The problem we raised earlier in this sub-section needs a solution, and the answer provided here seems to be the simplest one we can discover, while retaining the apparently useful features of the remainder of schema theory. Whether this modification will be a good one will remain to be seen.

## REVIEW, IMPLICATIONS, AND FUTURE DIRECTIONS

Our review of the research in the past six years has revealed about thirty studies that were directly motivated by implications from the schema theory. By far the majority of these studies was concerned with the variability-in-practice prediction in one way or another, with a smaller number being involved with the separation of recognition and recall. The support for the predictions of schema theory is generally quite good. In the variability literature, we nearly always find that a variability condition outperforms a constant condition when transferred to a novel variant of the overall task, but that the differences are not always statistically significant. Only in one study (Zelaznik, 1977) do we find that the direction of the means favors a constant-practice condition. Moreover, the differences appear to be larger and easier to demonstrate with children than with adults, perhaps suggesting that schemata are already developed in adults by the time the experimental tests are given; with children, it is possible that schema-rules are still being formed, and that the varied practice in the experiments provides substantial increases in schema strength.

But there are some troubling findings for the theory as well. Probably the most important of these is the concern that the underlying motor-program representations may not be as the theory has assumed. For example, recent evidence about the mass-spring model suggests that the conceptualization of initial conditions might be incorrect for at least some movements, that the separation of recognition for slow movements and recall for fast movements is in doubt, and that movements may not be parameterized in the way suggested by the theory. Also, there is concern with the independence of recall and recognition memories, as some studies have shown that practice on a purely recognition task (e.g. listening) provides transfer to actual movement situations (i.e. recall) on the first trial; something about the recall mechanisms was strengthened during recognition practice, and the theory cannot explain how these effects occur. And the theory does not seem capable of explaining how motor *learning* occurs in motor-learning experiments. So, clearly, in spite of the weight of evidence that we have reviewed here that seems to support the theory, most of the work is related to variability in practice where solid support is usually found; but when we look to other issues and kinds of evidence, the theory seems to be in need of some revision.

As can be seen from the previous paragraph, the revision will require many different aspects of the theory to be reconsidered in the light of this new evidence. It is possible that small modifications, along the lines suggested in the section on learning in experiments, will remedy the situation, leaving the essential structure intact. But, on the other hand, it is possible that small revisions cannot be made in such a way that they are all consistent with each other, and the fundamental framework of schema theory may have to be abandoned for some different set of assumptions about human performance and learning. Of course, for any replacement of this framework to be adopted, it will have to be demonstrated that it can account for the existing data on motor-performance phenomena *more* effectively than schema theory can.

There are many future directions that experimental and theoretical work might take, and we offer a few of them here. First, there is still not very much work − related to schema or to any theory of motor learning − on motor learning in children. The preliminary evidence suggests that much of rule-learning might occur in these ages, and certainly much more could be done to understand motor learning in children. There could be work on how movement programs are selected, and how abstract rule-learning for this selection process might take place, both in children and in adults. (Recall that the schema theory is silent on these issues.) And we should consider other aspects of motor performances than simply accuracy tasks. Zelaznik and Schmidt (1978) reasoned that increased variability in practice should lead to more *rapid* selection of movement parameters than constant practice would, but the experiment was very preliminary and we cannot say very much about this kind of criterion. Nevertheless, we still believe that it is a good idea to consider tasks that have speed, as well as maximum force, maximum height, etc. as criterion behaviors. Finally, more work should be done on recognition. We seldom practice our own motor learning tasks (in recreational sports, etc.) within the sight of a teacher who can provide effective KR. We therefore provide our own KR, perhaps as the schema theory has it in terms of subjective reinforcement. Understanding the variables that will lead to maximizing the strength of our recognition-memories (or schemata, if you will) should have pay-offs in terms of the learning that occurs in self-practice situations; the study by Hogan and Yanowitz (1978) provides a good example of how such studies could be done; it is easy to see how it might apply to learning away from a purely instructional setting.

But probably the most pressing future direction involves the structure of the motor program. First, understanding when, and under what conditions or tasks, feedback versus motor programs is used will be a large step forward. Within the realm of motor programs, though, there is beginning to be great controversy over their structure. Much of this debate concerns what can be considered as part of the program itself, and what kinds of parameters need to be added to execute it. Some (e.g. Schmidt, 1976a) have suggested that phasing and relative force are integral parts of the movement program, while others (e.g. Polit and Bizzi, 1978, 1979) have provided evidence leading to the idea that movement *endpoints* are represented in the program. How much variation in behavior can be governed by a single motor program? What parameters does the performer have under his or her control? These questions are fundamental to a theory like schema theory, since the postulations about how movements are learned must be based on our understanding of how movements are controlled. The next large step in learning theory will probably occur when a better understanding of motor programs is obtained, so that the theory will be more able to specify its constructs and postulates in ways that are in keeping with motor control.

As well, our ability to apply the theory is restricted by our limitation in understanding motor control. If we know, for example, what control processes changed when we provided variation in a movement – i.e. whether the variation resulted in the selection of a new program, or simply in the selection of a new set of parameters for a given program – we would be in a far better position to design learning environments for children (e.g. in movement education). Such knowledge seems essential to understanding how to structure the variability in practice to maximize learning of schemata for later use.

Finally, we need to understand how motor programs themselves are learned. Recently, there have been a number of such attempts (e.g. Marteniuk, 1978; Shapiro, 1978) to study how the structure of a movement sequence is changed as a result of practice. These studies were quite preliminary, though, and it is not possible to say very much from them. Almost nothing is known about how a complex series of muscle contractions, such as are involved in playing a piano or in the execution of a pole vault, come to be associated so effectively and efficiently into a single unit. Schema theory cleverly sidesteps this issue by assuming that the programs are already there and are selectable by the subject; but the theory is largely silent on the program's genesis. We all recognize that a motor-learning theory that does not explain how programs are learned will fall considerably short of providing an understanding of the motor-learning process.

Our position, after having reviewed the literature cited here, is that the theory still provides a great deal of structure to the evidence about motor learning and performance. It has some strong features, such as the account of the performance of novel tasks and the learning without KR, that set it apart from other theories of learning. But it has problems that we have tried to bring forth here and the theory is somewhat limited in terms of the kinds of learning phenomena it tries to explain. Hopefully, our readers will be able to evaluate this evidence for themselves, with such thinking and new experimentation leading to a modification or replacement of the schema theory with one that explains more of the data. We are taught that such is a theory's lot in life.

## ACKNOWLEDGEMENT

This paper has been supported in part by a UCLA Biomedical Research Support Grant and also by the Bureau of Education for the Handicapped (No. G007700997) to the first author. Also, this paper was supported in part by the National Science Foundation Grant No. BNS-7910672, to the second author.

## NOTE

1. To our knowledge, there have been no studies performed on children's recognition memory within the context of schema theory. This section is limited to adults.

## REFERENCES

Adams, J. A. (1971). A closed loop theory of motor learning, *Journal of Motor Behavior*, **3**, 111–150.

Allen, L. (1978). Variability in practice and schema development in children, unpublished master's thesis, University of Southern California.

Amacher, J. E. (1978). Variability of practice and recognition schema development, unpublished master's thesis, University of Southern California.

Armstrong, T. R. (1970). Training for the Production of Memorized Movement Patterns, Technical Report No. 26, Human Performance Center, University of Michigan.

Asatryan, D. G., and Fel'dman, A. G. (1965). Functional tuning of the nervous system with control of movement or maintenance of a steady posture. I. Mechanographic analysis of the work on the joint on execution of a postural task, *Biophysics*, **10**, 925–935.

Bartlett, F. C. (1932). *Remembering*, Cambridge, England: Cambridge University Press.

Beatty, J. A. (1977). Play, schema development and motor skill acquisition, unpublished master's thesis. Dalhousie University.

Bilodeau, I. M. (1966). Information feedback, in E. A. Bilodeau (ed.), *Acquisition of Skill*, New York: Academic Press.

Bizzi, E., Dev, P., Morasso, P., and Polit, A. (1978). Effect of load disturbances during centrally initiated movements, *Journal of Neurophyisology*, **41**, 542–556.

Bizzi, E., Polit, A., and Morasso, P. (1976). Mechanisms underlying achievement of final head position, *Journal of Neurophysiology*, **39**, 435–444.

Blair, W. O. (1979). A force reproduction test of the schema theory, paper presented at the International Congress in Physical Education, Trois-Rivières, Quebec.

Brooks, V. B. (1979). Motor programs revisited, in R. E. Talbott and D. R. Humphrey (eds.), *Posture and Movement: Perspective for integrating sensory and motor research on the mammalian nervous system*, New York: Raven Press.

Carson, L., and Wiegand, R. L. (1979). Motor schema formation and retention in young children: A test of Schmidt's schema theory, *Journal of Motor Behavior*, 11, 247–251.

Cobb, R. B. (1978). A test of the independence of the recall and recognition states of motor memory, paper presented at the National Convention of the American Alliance for Health, Physical Education and Recreation, Kansas City, MO.

Coleman, C. (1979). The variability of practice prediction and schema theory, unpublished master's thesis, Dalhousie University, April.

Crossman, E. R. F. W., and Goodeve, P. J. (1963). Feedback control of hand-movement and Fitt's law, in the *Proceedings of the Experimental Society*, Oxford.

Denier van der Gon, J. J., and Thuring, J. Ph. (1965). The guiding of human writing movement, *Kybernetik*, 2, 145–148.

Dummer, G. M. (1978). *Information processing in the acquisition of motor skills by mentally retarded children*, unpublished Ph.D. Dissertation, University of California, Berkeley.

Fel'dman, A. G. (1966a). Functional tuning of the nervous system with control of movement or maintenance of a steady posture. II. Controllable parameters of the muscles, *Biophysics*, 11, 565–578.

Fel'dman, A. G. (1966b). Functional tuning of the nervous system with control of movement or maintenance of a steady posture. III. Mechanographic analysis of the execution by man of the simplest motor tasks, *Biophysics*, 11, 766–775.

Grillner, S. (1975). Locomotion in vertebrates: Central mechanisms and reflex interaction, *Physiological Reviews*, 55, 247–304.

Hawkins, B. (1977). Variability of practice in a pursuit tracking task: A test of schema theory, unpublished Master's thesis, Dalhousie University, September.

Henry, F. M., and Rogers, D. E. (1960). Increased response latency for complicated movements and a memory drum theory of neuromotor reaction, *Research Quarterly*, 31, 448–458.

Hogan, J. C. (1977). The effect of varied practice on the accuracy of ballistic movements: A test of Schmidt's schema theory, unpublished manuscript.

Hogan, J. C., and Yanowitz, B. A. (1978). The role of verbal estimates of movement error in ballistic skill acquisition, *Journal of Motor Behavior*, 10, 133–138.

Hunter, M. D. (1977). Unpublished experiments, University of Southern California.

Jahnke, J. C. (1975). Personal communication to R. A. Schmidt.

Johnson, R. W., and McCabe, J. F. (1977). Variability of practice on a ballistic task: A test of schema theory, unpublished manuscript.

Keele, S. W. (1968). Movement control in skilled motor performance, *Psychological Bulletin*, 70, 387–403.

Keele, S. W. (1976). Paper presented at the University of Waterloo, June.

Keele, S. W., and Posner, M. E. (1968). Processing of feedback in rapid movements, *Journal of Experimental Psychology*, 77, 353–363.

Kelso, J. A. S. (1977). Motor control mechanisms underlying human movement reproduction, *Journal of Experimental Psychology: Human Perception and Performance*, 3, 529–543.

Kelso, J. A. S., and Norman, P. E. (1978). Motor schema formation in children, *Developmental Psychology*, 14, 153–156.

Kerr, R., and Booth, B. (1977). Skill acquisition in elementary school children and schema theory, in D. M. Landers and R. W. Christina (eds.), *Psychology of Motor Behavior and Sport* (Vol. 2), Champaign, Ill.: Human Kinetics, pp. 243–247.

Kerr, R., and Booth, B. (1978). Specific and varied practice of motor skill, *Perceptual and Motor Skills*, **46**, 395–401.

Klapp, S. T. (1977). Response programming, as assessed by reaction time, does not establish the commands for particular muscles, *Journal of Motor Behavior*, **9**, 301–312.

Magill, R. A., and Reeve, T. G. (1978). Variability of prior practice in learning and retention of a novel motor response, *Perceptual and Motor Skills*, **46**, 107–110.

Marteniuk, R. G. (1978). Personal communication, June.

McCracken, H. D., and Stelmach, G. E. (1977). A test of the schema theory of discrete motor learning, *Journal of Motor Behavior*, **9**, 193–201.

McGhee, R. C. (1981). The contribution of sensory feedback to response production ability. Paper presented at NASPSPA, Asilomar, CA, June.

Melville, D. S. (1976). Test of motor schema theory: Performance of a rapid movement task in absence of knowledge of results, unpublished doctoral dissertation, University of Iowa.

Merton, P. A. (1972). How we control the contraction of our muscles, *Scientific American*, **226**, 30–37.

Moxley, S. E. (1979). Schema: the variability of practice hypothesis, *Journal of Motor Behavior*, **11**, 65–70.

Moxley, S. E. and Fazey, J. A. (1977). Schema: The variability of practice hypothesis, paper presented at North American Society for Psychology of Sport and Physical Activity, Ithaca, New York, May.

Newell, K. M. (1976). Motor learning without knowledge of results through the development of a response recognition mechanism, *Journal of Motor Behavior*, **8**, 209–217.

Newell, K. M., and Shapiro, D. C. (1976). Variability of practice and transfer of training: Some evidence toward a schema view of motor learning, *Journal of Motor Behavior*, **8**, 233–243.

Pew, R. W. (1974). Human perceptual-motor performance, in B. H. Kantowitz (ed.), *Human Information Processing: Tutorials in Performance and Cognition*, New York: Lawrence Erlbaum.

Philippson, M. (1905). L'autonomie et la centralisation dans le systeme nerveux des animaux, *Trav. Lab. Physiology Institute solvay (Bruxelles)*, **7**, 1–208.

Pigott, R. E. (1979). Motor schema formation in children: An examination of the structure of variability in practice, unpublished master's thesis, University of California, Los Angeles.

Polit, A., and Bizzi, E. (1978). Processes controlling arm movements in monkeys, *Science*, **201**, 1235–1237.

Polit, A., and Bizzi, E. (1979). Characteristics of motor programs underlying arm movements in monkeys, *Journal of Neurophysiology*, **42**, 183–194.

Posner, M. I. and Keele, S. W. (1968). On the genesis of abstract ideas, *Journal of Experimental Psychology*, **77**, 353–363.

Posner, M. I., and Keele, S. W. (1970). Retention of abstract ideas, *Journal of Experimental Psychology*, **83**, 304–308.

Schmidt, R. A. (1975a). A schema theory of discrete motor skill learning, *Psychological Review*, **82**, 225–260.

Schmidt, R. A. (1975b). *Motor Skills*, New York: Harper & Row.

Schmidt, R. A. (1976a). The schema as a solution to some persistent problems in motor learning theory, in G. E. Stelmach (ed.), *Motor Control: Issues and trends*, New York: Academic Press.

Schmidt, R. A. (1976b). Control processes in motor skills, *Exercise and Sport Sciences Reviews*, **4**, 229–261.

Schmidt, R. A. (1977). Schema theory: Implications for movement education, *Motor Skills: Theory into Practice*, **2**, 30–38.

Schmidt, R. A. (1980a). Past and future issues in motor programming, *Research Quarterly for Exercise and Sport*, **51**, 122–140.

Schmidt, R. A. (1980b). On the theoretical status of time in motor program representations, in G. E. Stelmach and J. Requin (eds.), *Tutorials in motor behavior*, Amsterdam: North-Holland.

Schmidt, R. A. (1981). *Motor Control and Learning: A behavioral emphasis*, Champaign, Ill.: Human Kinetics Press.

Schmidt, R. A. (in press, a). More on motor programs, in J. A. S. Kelso (ed.), *Human Motor Behavior: An Introduction*, Hillsdale, NJ: Lawrence Erlbaum.

Schmidt, R. A. (in press, b). The schema concept, in J. A. S. Kelso (ed.), *Human Motor Behavior: An Introduction*, Hillsdale, NJ: Lawrence Erlbaum.

Schmidt, R. A. Christenson, R., and Rogers, P. (1975). Some evidence for the independence of recall and recognition in motor behavior, in D. M. Landers, D. V. Harris and R. W. Christina (eds.), *Psychology of Sport and Motor Behavior II*, Pennsylvania: Penn State HPER Series.

Schmidt, R. A., and McGown, C. (1980). Terminal accuracy of unexpectedly loaded rapid movements: Evidence for a mass-spring mechanism in programming. *Journal of Motor Behavior*, **12**, 149–161.

Schmidt, R. A., and Shea, J. B. (1976). A note on delay of knowledge of results in positioning responses, *Journal of Motor Behavior*, **8**, 129–131.

Shapiro, D. C. (1977). A preliminary attempt to determine the duration of a motor program, in D. M. Landers and R. W. Christina (eds.), *Psychology of Motor Behavior and Sport* (Vol. I), Champaign, Ill.: Human Kinetics, (17–24).

Shapiro, D. C. (1978). The learning of generalized motor programs, unpublished Ph.D. Dissertation, University of Southern California.

Shapiro, D. C., Zernicke, R. F., Gregor, R. J., and Diestal, J. D. (1981). Evidence for generalized motor programs using gait pattern analysis, *Journal of Motor Behavior*, **13**, 33–47.

Summers, J. J. (1975). The role of timing in motor program representation, *Journal of Motor Behavior*, **7**, 229–242.

Viviani, P., and Terzuolo, C. (1980). Space–time invariance in learned motor skills, in G. E. Stelmach and J. Requin (eds.), *Tutorials in Motor Behaviour*, Amsterdam: North-Holland.

Wallace, S. A., and McGhee, R. C. (1979). The independence of recall and recognition in motor learning, *Journal of Motor Behavior*, **11**, 141–151.

Williams, I. D. (1978). Evidence for recognition and recall schemata, *Journal of Motor Behavior*, **10**, 45–52.

Williams, I. D., and Rodney, M. (1978). Intrinsic feedback, interpolation, and closed-loop theory, *Journal of Motor Behavior*, **10**, 25–36.

Wrisberg, C. A., and Ragsdale, M. R. (1979). Further tests of Schmidt's schema theory: Development of a schema rule for a coincident timing task, *Journal of Motor Behavior*, **11**, 159–166.

Zelaznik, H. N. (1977). Transfer in rapid timing tasks: An examination of the role of variability in practice, in D. M. Landers and R. W. Christina (eds.), *Psychology of*

*Motor Behavior and Sport* (Vol. I), Champaign, Ill.: Human Kinetics (36–43).

Zelaznik, H. N., Shapiro, D. C., and Newell, K. M. (1978). On the structure of motor recognition memory, *Journal of Motor Behavior*, **10**, 313–323.

Zelaznik, H. N., and Schmidt, R. A. (1978). Unpublished experiment, University of Southern California.

Zelaznik, H. N. and Spring, J. (1976). Feedback in response recognition and production, *Journal of Motor Behavior*, **8**, 309–312.

The Development of Movement Control and Co-ordination
Edited by J. A. S. Kelso and J. E Clark
© 1982, John Wiley & Sons, Ltd

# CHAPTER 5

---

# The Role of Response Mechanisms in Motor Skill Development[1]

JANE E. CLARK

A motor skill may be viewed as the harmonious co-ordination of component movement elements organized in time and space to achieve a desired goal. As expressed in its mature form, motor skill behavior is graceful, adaptive, and seemingly effortless. As expressed in the developmentally young, motor behavior is clearly less than skillful. The newborn infant has but a limited repertoire of movement actions and those actions are awkward and diffuse. Yet as we watch an individual grow, as we watch the newborn stand, walk, and finally run, we are witness to the evolution of motor skill behavior. How the amazing degree of adult virtuosity displayed by an Olga Korbut is attained after such crude and awkward beginnings is the unique focus of motor skill development theorizing. Indeed, it is the study of motor development which describes the lawful changes in motor skill behavior across the lifespan and attempts to explain the relationship between antecedent and subsequent movement skill behaviors.

One approach to the study of motor skill development is to identify underlying mechanisms which either change or control the change observed in the antecedent-consequent relationships of the overt movement behavior. In the present chapter, I have attempted to describe such a set of underlying mechanisms. Couched in the theory of information processing, the mechanisms to be examined are those postulated to control the musculoskeletal apparatus as it performs a movement. These mechanisms, referred to as response-processing mechanisms, select, structure, and regulate the neuromuscular interactions required to accomplish a motor skill. Clearly, moving the multisegmented body in a smooth, precisely timed manner requires a control system which must not only signal the appropriate time for the muscular contraction but also the precise duration for that contraction. How this control system changes over an individual's lifespan is certainly an important issue to those studying motor development. Focusing on the response-processing mechanisms provides a framework not only within which to understand the central nervous system and its control over the multisegmented body, but also and of equal importance to the present discussion, one in which to understand how such control develops from infancy to adulthood.

Although the chapter focuses on the response of output mechanisms, it should not be interpreted that little or no importance is ascribed to the sensory perceptual mechanisms in the development of motor control. Rather it is the thesis here that very little attention has been focused on the response mechanisms required in motor skill development and that they, like the perceptual mechanisms, may contribute to the developmental changes observed. It remains, therefore, the purpose of the present review to examine the response-processing mechanisms and to discuss their possible role in the development of motor skills.

## DEFINITIONAL CONSTRAINT

Prior to a review of response mechanisms, a definition and clarification of motor development will be considered. This is not a superfluous discussion, but rather one essential to understanding the perspective on motor development from which the focus on underlying mechanisms derives. The discussion revolves around a definitional constraint to motor development; namely, that the study of motor development is, in fact, the study of motor *skill* development.

All living biological systems are characterized by their capacity to move. From inception, movement is a defining characteristic of the human being. But for movement to be skillful, it must be more than a spatial and temporal displacement, it must be purposeful, efficient, and adaptable. For example, motor skill has been defined as the solution of a movement problem constrained with a spatial, temporal and/or force requirement (Bernstein, 1967). Others have defined motor skill as the organization of actions into a purposeful plan to achieve some goal (Elliott and Connolly, 1974). Clearly, motor skill is *not* synonymous with the term movement behavior. And yet definitions of motor development have failed to appreciate this distinction. For example, Seefeldt (1974) describes the study of motor development as:

... the study of progressive modifications in motor performance which occur as a biologically changing organism interacts with its environment. (p. 39)

The definition offered by Halverson and her colleagues (Halverson, Roberton, and Harper, 1973) is similarly unconstrained; they define motor development as '. . . the study of ontogenetic change in human movement' (p. 56). These and similar definitions seem too broad and inclusive. A theory of motor development must start with a clear and constrained definition of the phenomenon unique to its study. Assuming the definitional constraint offered here, we are asked to focus our attention not on motor behavior *per se*, but on the proper subset of motor behavior, skillful motor acts.

This definitional constraint serves two purposes. First, it establishes the end goal for motor skill development. By defining our focus as motor skill, the teleological determination of motor development is defined. The end state for the developmental process is now skillful movement. Theoretical questions are focused then on the process by which the developing person achieves this end goal or the degree to which it is achieved.[2] Second, it directs our attention to the acquisition (i.e. development) of motor skill. By focusing on motor skill development, there is a subtle shift in the questions asked by the theorist. Telling questions revolve around the underlying mechanisms which control motor skill and its changes across the lifespan. Now, as we watch the developing child progressively change in his/her throwing or kicking behavior, we are compelled to describe and explain the gradual acquisition of these skills not merely by a one-to-one isomorphism, but with higher inferential statements necessary for any developmental theory (Zigler, 1963). To do so, however, requires a theoretical framework within which to structure and test these higher ordered inference statements. It is precisely at this juncture that, if persuaded by this discussion, one might see the efficacy in assuming the process-oriented approach to understanding motor skill development. This approach, now evident in the research on adult motor skill performance, has yielded important insights into motor skill by focusing on the underlying mechanisms or processes which control and regulate skillful movement (see Stelmach, 1978, for a review). Clearly, a similar benefit might be provided by the process-oriented approach to those in motor development, particularly if we define our focus for study as motor *skill* development.

Patently, this definitional constraint and the call for process-oriented research in motor development is neither new nor unique (Clark, 1976; Wade, 1976; Williams, 1973). It is offered here to preface the discussion that follows with a clearer focus of the phenomenon to be explained. As forwarded earlier, the study of motor skill development is viewed as the study of the lawful relationship between antecedent and subsequent changes in motor skill behavior across the lifespan. Constraining the definition to motor skill behavior focuses inquiry on understanding the mechanisms underlying motor skill behavior and how they change or control the change we see in motor skill development.

## RESPONSE MECHANISMS: PROCESSING RESPONSE DECISIONS

A skilled motor act is the result of the central nervous system's sequence and timing of the commands to the musculoskeletal system. In the section to follow, a brief review of the organizational mechanisms or processes which are postulated to control the motor apparatus in the execution of a motor skill is offered. The purpose of this review is to provide a framework within which to examine the response-processing mechanisms and to provide a background to the later discussion of the developmental role these mechanisms may play.

Prior to the initiation of a response, a number of decisions must be made by the mover. Most theoretical formulations of the mover's decisions include perceptual decisions: those decisions required to identify the environmental stimuli. Not until recently has attention been focused on the decisions required to select and organize the response required (for reviews, see Klapp, 1978 and Glencross, 1979). Of those models of human performance which have considered the processing of response decisions, differing views of the processes exist. General accord does seem to exist, however, with regard to at least two general types of response-processing mechanisms. One of the mechanisms included in most models is a response-selection mechanism. After the perceptual mechanism has identified the environmental stimulus, a decision must be made to select a response to that stimulus. The response may be to move the right index finger or to wiggle the right thumb, or, in fact, it may be decided not to move at all. In other words, this first class of response decisions identifies what movement is necessary to match the perceived environmental stimuli.

The second response-processing mechanism, response programming, organizes the response selected such that the neuromuscular apparatus can be mobilized to achieve the selected response. For example, if in the prior stage of processing it was determined that the right index finger was to be moved, then the response-programming mechanism must operationalize this decision. The nervous system must provide an answer to accomplish the selected response. It is not enough to select a response. If that were the case, we would all be able to select and, therefore, perform front somersaults or back handsprings. But the reality of the matter requires that the nervous system also specify the commands necessary to execute the response selected. Clearly, for many of us, it is not selecting a response that presents the difficulty, but rather programming the response selected.

The conceptualization of a dual mechanism for response-decision processing is that following the perceptual identification of an environmental event, a response is selected to match the environmental demand. Following response selection, the motor system must organize and prepare the response selected. The latter process is referred to as response programming. Evidence that response programming is a separate mechanism from response selection comes from two sources. First, evidence comes from work by Theios and Walter (1974). They had subjects perform a binary classification task in which either stimulus-response (S-R) pairs were repeated or the responses alone were repeated independent of a particular stimulus. Theios and Walter found that in successive trials where the response alone was repeated independent of any S-R pair repetition, subjects' response latencies decreased 8 msec with each successive response repetition. If the repetition was of a particular S-R pair, the response latency decreased 48 msec. In a later paper, Theios (1975) argued that these findings supported the notion of two separate response-decision stages, one sensitive to response repetitions (response programming) and one sensitive to stimulus-response repetitions (response selection).

Additional support for this conclusion comes from an experiment I recently completed (Clark, 1979). Using a reaction time-movement time (RT-MT) task, subjects performed under one of two levels of stimulus-response compatibility and one of two levels of movement complexity. Using Sternberg's logic (1969), if the two variables, compatibility and complexity, each affect one of the two stages (i.e. compatibility affecting response selection and complexity affecting

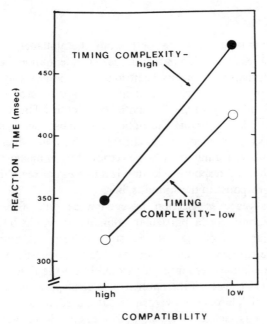

FIGURE 1    Mean reaction time (in msec) for performance under two levels of timing complexity and compatibility

response programming), then a finding of additivity would support the two-stage model of response-decision processing. If the effect of the two variables is interactive, then they would be presumed to affect the same stage of processing. The results of the experiment were interpreted as support for the two-stage model. As Figure 1 shows, subjects performing under low compatibility and high movement complexity were slower in their times to initiate their movements. More importantly, the combined effect of compatibility and complexity was additive.

Taken together, the two experiments would suggest a dual mechanism for response-decision processing. The first mechanism, *response selection*, is responsible for deciding on the response to be made. The second mechanism, *response programming*, is responsible for organizing and preparing the response to be executed. Each mechanism or process is viewed as experimentally independent of the other. Both mechanisms may well contribute to the changes observed in motor skill development. In the next two sections each mechanism will be considered separately in an attempt to describe the role it might have in the developmental changes observed in motor skill behavior across the lifespan.

### Response Selection

If an individual is typing, reading, or printing the alphabet, the perception of the letter 'b' will result in different responses dependent upon the task demands. Once the perceptual decision has been made that indeed this is a 'b,' rather than a 'd,' or any other letter, it is then necessary to process the response-selection decision. Should I type 'b,' say 'b,' or print 'b'? The response-selection mechanism must decide among the options. To most theorists, the response-selection process is a memory-dependent process in which the response appropriate to a given stimulus must be retrieved from memory. For example, in typing the letter 'b,' response selection is a process of searching memory for the appropriate response to the stimulus 'b.'

If one views response-selection processing as one of remembering the appropriate response for a particular stimulus, it would be predicted that repeated presentations of the specific stimulus-response pair will facilitate responding time (Mowbray and Rhoades, 1959). Similarily, the spatial compatibility of the stimulus-response pair would affect the time to respond (Fitts and Seeger, 1953). Clearly, if the natural or logical spatial mapping of stimulus and response (which have been overpracticed) is used, an individual will be able to make the response-selection decision more easily. However, if a transformation must be done prior to selecting the correct response, i.e. translate the response paired with a stimulus into quite another response, then the time taken for response-selection processing will increase. For example, Allusi, Strain, and

Thurmond (1964) had subjects name the presented number or name the next number in the arithmetic order. Subjects who had to name the next number required more time to respond than those who had to name the number itself. Further, it would be predicted that if more than one response has been paired with a stimulus then the subject will have more difficulty selecting the particular response necessary for that particular task (Theios, 1975).

In summary, the response-selection mechanism described here is one dependent on the relationship between the environmental event and the response required. If the event and response have been paired together often and few other responses have been paired with that stimulus, then response selection will undoubtedly be quicker and easier. If, however, the pairing is new or requires a transformation, the individual will require more time and perhaps commit more errors in selecting the response. Relative to response programming, the response-selection mechanism may be viewed as a mechanism which uses the environmental information to put the response programming mechanism in the 'right ball park.' It will select the response: 'type "b";' 'print "b";' or 'say "b".' The response-programming mechanism must provide the motor organization to complete the response selected.

## Developmental Considerations in Response Selection

Getting into the 'right ball park' may well prove a formidable task for a young child. Selecting a response is often more time-consuming and more often incorrect for the young child than for her older counterpart. Given the nature of response selection – i.e. a translation mechanism between perception and action – the less experienced, less practiced mover will undoubtedly have a more difficult task identifying the response to be initiated. Since the developmentally young are less experienced and less practiced movers, the results of an experiment I conducted a few years ago (Clark, 1976) are not particularly surprising. This experiment sought to determine if indeed there were age-related differences in response-selection processing. To that date, there had been no evidence to support such a conclusion. Children (six- and ten-year-olds) and adults performed a two-choice reaction-time task under one of two levels of spatial S-R compatibility (high and low) and one of two levels of response discriminability (high and low). For the present discussion, the results of the effect of spatial S-R compatibility on RT performance are relevant since the compatibility of the stimulus and the response directly affects the selection time for a response to its paired stimulus. As expected, all three age groups were slowed when performing under the low-compatibility condition where the left light was paired with the right-positioned response, and vice versa for the right light. More importantly, the six-year-olds were slowed more by lower compatibility than the ten-year-olds and adults, and the ten-year-olds were slowed more than the adults. This differential slowing is shown in Figure 2. The effect of S-R compatibility on RT performance is clearly different for the three age groups. The time taken to respond to the low-compatible S-R pair was much greater for the younger than older subjects. Assuming that S-R compatibility affects the response-selection mechanism (Theios, 1975; Clark, 1979), then the finding of this experiment can be interpreted as support for age-related differences in the response-selection mechanism.

Additional support for developmental differences in response selection can be found in a number of choice reaction-time experiments done with children. Unlike the simple reaction-time task, where response-selection decisions may be bypassed (Klapp, 1978), the choice reaction-time task affords an opportunity to observe the effect of such variables as the number of S-R pairs, or the amount of practice with certain S-R pairs on the response-selection mechanism. For example, previous research with adults has shown that increasing the number of stimulus-response pairs in a task increases the time taken to respond. This relationship, known as Hick's Law, predicts that as information transmitted increases (usually represented by increasing the

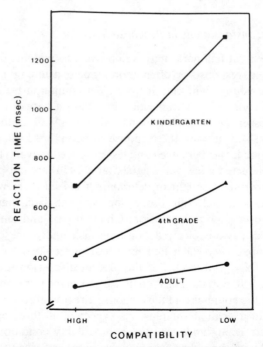

FIGURE 2    Right middle finger mean reaction
time (in msec) of three age groups under two
levels of spatial S-R compatibility

number of S-R pairs), reaction time increases linearly (Hick, 1952). It has been argued that the locus of this rise in RT is centered on the response-selection mechanism (Sternberg, 1969; Theios, 1975; Fairweather and Hutt, 1978). If response selection is developmentally different across the lifespan it might be expected that increasing the number of choices (i.e. the number of S-R pairs) might differentially affect RT performance across age. In fact, Fairweather and Hutt (1978) have shown this to be the case. They had children (ages five to eleven years) perform two-, four-, and eight-choice reaction-time tasks. Their results indicated that as ensemble size increased from two- to eight-choice S-R pairs, the difference between the youngest and the oldest subjects increased differentially. In other words, while Hick's Law fitted the data at each age, the slope of the regression line decreased significantly as age increased.

Insight into the nature of the developmental differences in response selection may be found in those studies which have examined the effect of practice on the choice reaction-time performance of children. It might be argued that response selection requires more time for the developmentally young because they have had less practice with the various stimulus and response pairings. If the young children are given more practice on the task it may eliminate the age-related differences. Such an argument was forwarded by Fairweather and Hutt (1978). In the experiment discussed above, they had the children perform 100 trials of the two-, four-, and eight-choice reaction-time tasks on five consecutive days. While practice reduced RT performance for all subjects, it did not differentially reduce the younger children's performance as one might like to argue.

Morin and Forrin (1965) asked a similar question, but framed the issue differently. They argued that by contrasting tasks on which younger subjects have had less experience with those tasks in which both younger and older subjects are essentially novices, they should be able to demonstrate the effects of prior experience on the slope of the regression line in Hick's Law. They assumed third-graders had had more experience with numeral naming than their first-grade counterparts. As a control, they used the task of naming shapes, presumably a task on which both age groups had equalized experience. As expected, with an increase in information on the shapes task, the RT slopes increased for both age groups. Third-graders were generally faster, but increasing the information or choices did not differentially affect the performance of the two groups. The hypothesis for the numeral-naming task was not confirmed. Slopes for *both* first- and third-graders were flat, i.e. unaffected by stimulus information. This was an unexpected finding, but perhaps one confounded by a methodological flaw (Wickens, 1974). Wickens has pointed out that Morin and Forrin's stimulus set size which supposedly contained two, four, or eight digits to be named actually represented an effective stimulus set size of eight. It seems Morin and Forrin had selected set samples of two and four digits, but had selected the digits from a set ranging across eight numbers.

Earlier research by Fitts and Switzer (1962) on adults had demonstrated that in effect this made the set size eight, not two or four. This 'subset familiarity' phenomenon may well have affected the Morin and Forrin findings.

Allusi (1965) replicated the Morin and Forrin study with appropriate sets and found that increasing the information in numeral naming affected the youngest group, the five-year-olds, more than the older groups (seven-, nine-, and eleven-year-olds). The older groups were unaffected by increases in the number of stimuli within the set, a finding similar to that found with adults (Allusi, Strain, and Thurmond, 1964). Thus, age-related differences in response selection are, at least in part, due to previous experience with the S-R pairs. The only strong evidence contrary to this conclusion would be that found in the Fairweather and Hutt (1978) experiment. Recall that they found no age-related differential effect for practice (over 100 trials a day for five days). However, it may well be that their subjects did not have enough practice. Fairweather and Hutt themselves suggest that the data for the youngest subjects had not asymptoted at the end of the five days of practice.

It is also possible that the children are selecting the response in qualitatively different ways than are older children and adults. One such processing difference is suggested by the work done on perceptual or identification processing. Research on adults has shown that the stimulus is identified through a parallel search strategy (e.g. Blake, 1976). This strategy permits the simultaneous scanning of more than one possibility at a time and thus results in a shorter search time than a serial search where one looks at one item at a time. A number of studies (Liss and Haith, 1970; Blake, 1974, 1976) have pointed to the possibility that developmental differences in perceptual processing are a result of the younger children's use of the less efficient serial search rather than the faster parallel search strategy. Such processing-strategy differences may also be evident in response selection processing. To date, however, no evidence is available to shed light on the viability of this explanation.

Another possible explanation of age-related differences in response-selection processing is a subject's strategy in reaction-time tasks. For example, Theios (1975) suggests that a subject in a choice reaction-time task sets up a limited capacity serial buffer in short-term memory. This buffer contains the most likely S-R pairs, i.e. those to be used in the experimental task. This short-term memory (STM) buffer would reduce the need for the more time-consuming long-term memory (LTM) search for such pairings. Developmentally, it may well be that the younger children cannot establish this STM buffer; or can establish it but do not; or can establish it but cannot maintain it. In any case, the result is that the child must rely on a LTM search for the response paired with a particular stimulus, while the older child or adult utilizes the quicker STM search.

Some suggestion that differences in the use of a STM buffer strategy may contribute to response-selection processing differences in the developmentally young is offered by an experiment we recently conducted (Clark and Moore, 1980). What we hoped to demonstrate was that young children (four- and five-year-olds) could preselect their response prior to stimulus onset and that once selected they could maintain the precued response for a brief duration (up to five seconds). If they could preselect a response, we argued, they must be bringing the response 'up front,' i.e. employing a STM buffer. In addition, by requiring them to delay the initiation of the response for one, three, or five seconds, we also could provide evidence regarding their ability to maintain the response in the STM buffer.

The experiment employed a precuing technique in which the child was told in advance what light was going to come on and therefore what response would be required. Three precue conditions were used: precue-blocked; precue-mixed; and no precue. The precue-blocked condition was equivalent to a simple reaction-time task in which the same S-R pair is precued across the trial block. In the precue-mixed condition, the S-R pair was precued but unlike the precue-blocked condition, the S-R pair was randomly varied within the trial block. Presumably the precue-mixed condition required the child to reselect a response with each change in precue information, a situation which may not exist in the blocked-precue condition. The no-precue condition was a two-choice reaction-time task in which no precue information was provided. Three precue intervals (one, three, and five seconds) were randomized within each condition. All children performed under each condition − randomized in presentation across three consecutive days.

The results of the experiment for a group of four- and five-year-old children and for adults are presented in Figure 3. Across precue intervals, the precue conditions (both block and mixed) were statistically different from the no-precue condition, though not from each other. In both the blocked- and mixed-precue condition, it would seem that the children, like the adults, were able to use the precued information to reduce their response latencies. Further, performance for the children was best when the precue interval was one second. For example, under the precued-mixed condition with a one-second precue interval, the youngsters' mean RT was 502 msec whereas when the interval was three or five seconds RT performance was 572 msec and 587 msec, respectively. This would seem to suggest that performing under longer precue intervals made it difficult for the children to maintain the preselected response. The finding would appear to support the notion that young children (four- and five-year-olds) are capable of using precued information to preselect a response; however, they seem to have difficulty in maintaining this response for intervals of three seconds or longer.

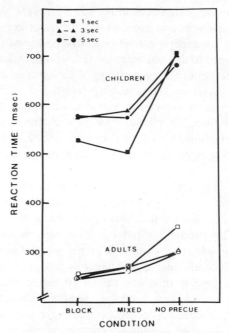

FIGURE 3    Mean reaction time (in msec)
of four- and five-year-olds and adults
under three levels of response uncertainty
and three preparatory intervals

## Summary

In sum, an attempt has been made to describe the mechanism which selects a motor response. This response-selection mechanism is viewed as getting the motor system into the 'right ball park.' Developmentally, the evidence would suggest that the response-selection mechanism is responsible for at least some of the observable changes we see in motor skill behavior. Clearly, the young child requires more time to select a response, and in many cases selects the inappropriate response. Response-selection errors and increased selection-processing time may well account for motor skill development changes. However, it is not the only response-processing mechanism that might contribute to these changes. In the next section, we shall examine another response mechanism which may also contribute to the developmental changes observed in motor skill behavior.

**Response Programming**

If response-selection processing gets the mover 'into the ball park' with the correct environmentally appropriate response, the response-programming mechanism must take this selected response and operationalize it, i.e. mobilize the motor apparatus with the correct spatial, temporal, and force parameters necessary to execute the intended response. Several conceptualizations of the programming process have been forwarded. Kerr (1978), for example, has argued that response programming is comprised of two processes, response selection and response preparation. Unlike the response-selection process described previously where the response *per se* is selected, Kerr's response-selection process selects the appropriate *motor control* parameter values. The motor control values for a key-press response, for example, might be to flex the forefinger and to stabilize the wrist, elbow, and shoulder joints. After these parameters are selected, the response is organized and prepared. For Kerr, the latter process, response preparation, involves the elaboration and translation of the motor control parameters into a format appropriate to the neuromuscular system.

Sternberg and his colleagues (Sternberg *et al.*, 1978) offer a somewhat different conceptualization of the response-programming process. In a series of converging experiments, they provide a picture of response programming as a three-stage process. The first stage retrieves the selected response's program, the second 'unpacks' the program, and the third stage issues the sequence of commands that control the program. The retrieval stage is the stage of processing in which the subprogram for a given response unit is located through a self-terminating search. Experimentally, the retrieval stage was shown to be influenced by the number of units in the set and by the serial position of the unit in the search order. The 'unpacking' stage which follows the retrieval stage begins to decode and assemble the unit's constituents. The processing time for unpacking depends on the number of constituents in the unit (i.e. the length of the subroutine). After unpacking, the commands to prepare and execute the response are issued. This final processing stage was influenced by the size of the unit but not the serial position of the unit or the number of units.

Left unclear by conceptualizations such as those offered by Kerr and Sternberg is the nature of the response program that is retrieved, stored or parameterized. What is contained in the program? Is each movement separately stored? Clearly, an incredible memory load would be imposed on the central nervous system if each movement in an individual's action repertoire must be stored. One conceptualization of the 'program' which is stored for a motor skill is offered by Schmidt's schema theory (1975; and Shapiro and Schmidt, this volume). Schema theory described motor skill performance as the result of schema rules which generate the motor skill rather than retrieve it. Such a conceptualization of motor-control processing may solve the storage problem, but it presents its own enigma. In the schema style of response programming, an enormous amount of working space is required for computation. If the schema is stored and used centrally, then, it very well could impose a computational load that would appear to occupy more processing capacity than has been observed in the automatic, smoothly timed motor behavior of the skilled performer. Perhaps schema theory, as proposed by Schmidt, is an adequate theoretical framework for explaining and predicting *discrete* motor skill learning but as a theoretical framework for understanding the rapid, *continuous* movement required in so many motor skills, it would appear inadequate.

An alternative conceptualization offered by Bernstein (1967) and more recently by Greene (1972) might afford a more workable solution to both the storage and working space problem. The style of response programming they suggest for the motor-control system would be one whereby subsystems having many degrees of freedom are governed by a central control system having but a few degrees of freedom. Within such a model, some measure of control is assigned to peripheral mechanisms freeing the central system of constant vigilance and considerable computation and retrieval. Such a response-programming system is made possible by having the central executive system make use of the lower level organizations which control individual movement components. The control system might be envisioned as a multistage computing system in which each level controls the level below it, thus reducing the executive system's degrees of freedom.

Essential to such a style of control is the notion of *co-ordinative* structures (Easton, 1972). If at each joint in the body there exists a given number of degrees of freedom (i.e. representing all possible movements at that joint), and if the central response-programming mechanism were required to specify the movements at each joint (i.e. specify the degrees of freedom) for a given action, the computational task would overwhelm the central programming system. It is argued, instead, that the response-programming mechanism specifies the lower level organizational units (i.e. the co-ordinative structures) in the order and time it requires them. The central control system permits the unit's control over their own individual elements. These lower level organizations may be built-in structures such as reflexes (Easton, 1972; Turvey, 1977), inherent patterns (Knott and Voss, 1968), or may be gradually built into the system in functional sets specific to repeated movement requirements. In any case, these lower level organizations are recruited by the executive system and the co-ordinative structures, themselves, specify the interaction of the muscles within their units.

If the individual segments are being controlled within their functional and structural units, then it is the central executive system which must organize the co-ordinative structures both spatially and temporally. To have a co-ordinated skillful act, the individual units must be recruited and fitted together at precisely the right moment and in the proper sequence. It is the responsibility of the response programming mechanism to select the appropriate co-ordinative structures and to program the units into a single act under restricted temporal and spatial constraints. To understand the response-programming mechanism, then, requires understanding not only the units used, but also the process by which these units are recruited and fitted together.

In summary, the response-programming mechanism presented here is a mechanism which prepares and organizes the motor system to execute the selected motor response. The style of control suggested is one proposed by Bernstein (1967) in which the motor-control system is viewed as a multistaged system whereby the subsystems having many degrees of freedom are governed by a central executive system having but a few degrees of freedom. In the proposed control system, the executive selects the co-ordinative structures, orders up the units one after another, and modulates the units temporally. Details of the movement requirements are relegated to lower levels of control. The response-programming mechanism then, is one with multiple levels of computing, in which each successive computation brings the movement response closer and closer to an approximation of the environmentally determined response. In the next section, we will examine the developmental implications of such a response-programming system and attempt to determine its role in the development of motor skills.

### Developmental Considerations

Once the child selects the response for her purpose, she then must control her neuromuscular system to organize and execute the selected response. In the sections which follow, consideration will be given to the developmental consequences of both the co-ordinative structures and the programming process of the response-programming mechanism. The basic issues to be explored, as we consider each of these components of response programming, are to what extent they themselves change developmentally and to what extent they affect a change in the observable motor skill behavior. To begin, we will focus on the fundamental unit of the motor control system: the co-ordinative structure (see Kugler, Kelso, and Turvey, this volume).

*Co-ordinative structures.* A co-ordinative structure or collective is that unit of motor control which governs a group of muscles as it operates over one or more body joints. Further, a co-ordinative structure is constrained to act as a single unit which may be recruited as such by a central command signal. A co-ordinative structure is one which provides the control system with one-degree-of-freedom control over a unit containing many possible degrees of freedom.

The obvious advantage of this type structure to a developing motor-control system is the immediate parsimony such a unit affords. If the developing child can specify a one-degree-of-freedom act, it would free that child's processing capacities for other decisions including possible modifications of the existing units of control. A key developmental issue regards the origin and growth of the co-ordinative structures. How does a co-ordinative structure arise and how does it evolve?

One possible explanation for the origin of a co-ordinative structure is that it comes with the system; that is, the co-ordinative structures is a built-in, inherent unit to the human motor system. The reflexes of the newborn infant are suggestive of such inherent units (Easton, 1972). Clearly, the reflexes constitute prefabricated means-ends relationships between specific stimuli and response patterns. Their fixed, wired-in relationships might well serve as the basic units of the motor control system. Later, volitional motor skill may be orchestrated from the reflexive base as the co-ordinative structures are modified and blended together under the executive system's control.

Although intuitively appealing, empirical evidence that reflexes form the co-ordinative structures of the motor control system is sparse. Easton (1972) argues that research by Hellebrandt (Hellebrandt, Schade, and Carns, 1962) offers clear support for the position that reflexes are available and operating in voluntary motor skill behavior. Hellebrandt and her colleagues demonstrated that in the neurologically intact and normally functioning individual, stress could evoke reflexive behavior thought to have disappeared in infancy. If reflexes are still available to the adult as Hellebrandt's data would suggest, then, argues Easton, why would the nervous sytem rewire or redundantly wire muscle collectives to achieve the same goal as that already achieved with a particular reflex?

Perhaps more compelling evidence for the role of reflexes as co-ordinative structures comes from the work done on locomotion. Recent work (Shik and Orlovski, 1976; Grillner, 1975) has shown that the movements of the lower segments are organized into flexor-extensor synergies which are constrained to operate as a unit. At birth, the newborn infant can be shown to exhibit well-co-ordinated 'walking.' If held in an upright posture, with the feet just in contact with a surface, the infant will demonstrate a rhythmical stepping pattern in which the movements of both limbs are synchronized and co-ordinated. This walking reflex can be evoked in the infant for the next three or four months – although it may disappear as early as two months (Peiper, 1963). Further, it is argued by most developmentalists that in order for voluntary walking to occur, the walking reflex must disappear (Milani-Comparetti and Gidoni, 1967). Relevant to our discussion here on the role of reflexes as the co-ordinative structures of the system is the evidence provided by two studies (Andre-Thomas and Dargassies, 1952; Zelazo, Zelazo, and Kolb, 1972) on the relationship between the walking reflex and later voluntary walking behavior. The design of both studies was essentially the same: exercise the walking reflex in one set of babies from birth on while a control group receives no such practice; compare the groups on the age of onset of independent voluntary walking. If there is a relationship between the antecedent reflex and the subsequent congruent voluntary behavior, then one might suggest that the reflex is serving as co-ordinative structure for later walking behavior. Indeed, the results of both studies would tend to support such an argument. In each study, the group that was exercised on the walking reflex had an earlier onset of walking than did the nonexercised group. The suggestion, then, is that there is a developmental relationship between the antecedent reflex behavior and the subsequent congruent voluntary behavior. Given that there is such a coupling between the behaviors, it might be argued that reflexes serve as the built-in, preadapted co-ordinative structures of the response-programming system.

Another suggestion which also argues that the origin of the co-ordinative structures is inherent, is offered by Knott and Voss (1968) and recently extended to motor development by Shambes and Campbell (1973). Their conceptualization is that the human movement system has basic inherent motor patterns which underlie *all* movement activity. Though developed as a framework for therapeutic treatment, Knott and Voss' proprioceptive neuromuscular facilitation (PNF) technique is based on the premise that all movements are comprised of cross-diagonal inherent movement patterns. According to Knott and Voss, there are two fundamental cross-diagonal patterns for the upper and lower limbs. For example, the first diagonal pattern of the upper and lower extremity consists of proximal joint (shoulder or hip) flexion, adduction, and external rotation. The most distal joints (wrist or ankle) exhibit the same joint actions as the proximal joint, with the intermediate joint (elbow or knee) either flexed or extended. This first diagonal pattern also includes the reciprocal actions: extension, abduction, and internal rotation. The underhand throwing pattern may be viewed as an example of the first diagonal pattern where the forward throwing action involves shoulder flexion, adduction, and external rotation, elbow extension, and wrist flexion, adduction, and external rotation. Although Knott and Voss (1968) did not refer to their inherent patterns as co-ordinative structures, clearly these patterns, as proposed, are functional fixed relationships which are hypothesized to govern the actions of muscle collectives. One might argue, then, that if such cross-diagonal patterns do exist in the motor system, then they may serve as co-ordinative structures for that system.

Although developmentally it seems advantageous to have the motor system come with built-in co-ordinative structures, it must also be obvious from the foregoing review that little is known about the origin or nature of such structures. For example, reflexes and inherent patterns seem constraining and inflexible for the versatility demanded by most voluntary motor skill. Are the co-ordinative structures modifiable? If so, in what ways may modifications be made? Clearly, to understand the nature of response programming, we must understand the fundamental unit of programming and its development.

*Programming.*    If the co-ordinative structures serve as the 'units' of the action system, we need to see when and how these units are incorporated into the movement expression of the action system. Response programming becomes the process by which the co-ordinative structures are recruited, assembled, and activated into an organized whole. Several elements of the programming process are of particular importance to a developmental theory of motor skills. The first such element is the nature of the programming language. As with any language, the programming language of the motor-control system may be viewed as comprising words (perhaps co-ordinative structures) and sentences (syntactical organization) into which the words are placed. As Turvey (1977) points out, the analogy between linguistics and movement provides a useful contrast for a theory of action. For example, the universal and phylogenetic character of motor skill behavior argues well for the inherency of a 'deep structure' (Chomsky, 1965) for the programming of movement such as that hypothesized in language. Clearly there are far too many combinations and configurations of muscle actions to be produced anew or remembered from past experiences. The notion of a deep structure underlying the generation of movement sequences, analogous to the deep structure underlying language, affords the same theoretical parsimony and deployability, namely, that the observable movement skill is the result of an abstract and generative structure, which is capable of producing an infinite number of possible movements in much the same way as the deep structure of language produces an infinite number of sentences. Hence, it is the deep structure which determines the ordering and sequencing of the co-ordinative structures as they are recruited for a particular action.

If one accepts the foregoing analogy, then it is obvious that our developmental questions regarding response programming must focus on how the child acquires the deep structure of movement, and how this structure may change with movement experience. Is, for example, the deep structure inherent to the human species and its appearance prompted and modified by environmental interaction? Recent evidence in language development would seem to suggest that syntactical organization may well be a uniquely human process not manifested by the trained apes who use American Sign Language (Terrace *et al.*, 1979). Is there an inherency and constancy to the syntax of action? How does the child '. . . determine the nature of the underlying deep structure from a limited experience with surface structure' (Turvey, 1977, p. 214)? Our understanding of the language of response programming may well be augmented by drawing from the extensive research on language development. The possible benefit of such an approach awaits future assessment.

Another aspect of the programming process which bears examination is the process of modularization. Modularization provides the substitution of units (i.e. modules) for each other, or the reorganization of units for the solution of a new movement problem. Modular flexibility permits adaptability in programming necessary to a control system which must operate under ever-changing environmental conditions. Closely associated with the notion of modularization is the concept of timing. Once the correct sequence of units is found, the moment for activation and precise duration of each unit must be regulated. To attain the high degree of temporal precision required in most motor skills, the response-programming mechanism must maintain control over the temporal constraints of the unfolding movement action.

There are several developmental studies which provide insight into the nature of modularization in response programming. In each (Connolly, Brown and Bassett, 1968; Elliott and Connolly, 1974; Todor, 1975, 1979), the research has shown that developmentally movements begin as individual discrete components and are slowly phased together into a smoothly functioning and precisely timed act. Once the child has the correct components in their proper place in the sequence, that child still requires more time than her older counterpart to switch from one component to the next. Except for the evidence that such changes occur, we have little information with regard to the nature of change. Clearly more research is necessary if we are to understand modularization and timing control in response programming.

## Summary

In summary, the discussion of response programming has focused on two aspects: co-ordinative structures and the programming process itself. One clear perspective would seem to have emerged – namely, that response programming is the process of a developing biological system. Our scientific heritage for rejecting nativism may well have shortened our vision with regard to the inherencies of this developing biological being. Our present theoretical positions in motor development, it would seem, need to take account of our biological heritage without resorting to low-inference statements of the obvious and observable. More pointedly, we have described the developmental sequence for the fundamental movement skills (see Wickstrom, 1975, for a review); it would seem now that our task is to explain their development. The response-programming process described here might well serve as a conceptual framework within which to attempt such an explanation.

## CONCLUSION

In conclusion, this chapter has attempted to describe the role of two possible response mechanisms in the development of motor skill behavior. Clearly, these mechanisms which select and regulate the neuromuscular interactions, play an important part in the observable motor behavior of the newborn, five-year-old, or adult. Empirical evidence bearing on the developmental role of response mechanisms is clearly lacking. A great deal has yet to be learned about these mechanisms and their role in motor skill development. It is hoped that the review offered here will further promote future investigation of these mechanisms and contribute to the ever-expanding knowledge of motor skill development.

## NOTES

1. Appreciation is expressed to Beth Kerr, Sally Phillips, and Elliot Saltzman for their constructive comments on an earlier draft of this chapter.
2. It should not be misconstrued that the only proper individuals for analysis in motor skill development are the highly skilled performers and their ontogenetic history. Rather it is argued that all individuals seek to be skillful in their movement. This point is made particularly clear if we assume a means-ends principle whereby a skillful motor act is one which accomplishes a specified end with the necessary means. Admittedly, individual differences in the degree to which the end is achieved will be obvious. Some will set a world record with their body projection (i.e. long jump) while others will merely jump the brook! The important point to be remembered however, is that for both the world-class athlete or the average person control and co-ordination of the body is the goal, and this is the same goal for motor skill development.

## REFERENCES

Allusi, E. (1965). Interaction of S-R compatibility and rate of gain of information, *Perceptual and Motor Skills*, **20**, 815–816.

Allusi, E. A., Strain, G. S., and Thurmond, J. B. (1964). Stimulus-response compatibility and the rate of gain of information, *Psychonomic Science*, **1**, 111–112.

Andre-Thomas, S., and Dargassies, St. A. (1952). *Etudes neurologiques surle nouveau-né et le jeune nourrison*, Paris: Masson et Olivier Perrin.

Bernstein, N. (1967). *The Co-ordination and Regulation of Movements*, New York: Pergamon.

Blake, J. (1974). Developmental change in visual information processing under backward masking, *Journal of Experimental Child Psychology*, **17**, 133–146.

Blake, J. (1976). Parallel processing of position and form information in young children, *Perception & Psychophysics*, **20**, 403–407.

Chomsky, N. (1965). *Aspects of the Theory of Syntax*, Cambridge, Mass: MIT Press.

Clark, J. E. (1976). Age-related differences in response decision processing, unpublished doctoral dissertation, University of Wisconsin-Madison.

Clark, J. E. (1978). Memory processes in the early acquisition of motor skills, in M. Ridenour (ed.), *Motor Development: Issues and Applications*, Princeton, NJ: Princeton Book Co.

Clark, J. E. (1979). Compatibility and complexity in response decision processing, in G. C. Roberts and K. M. Newell (eds.), *Psychology of Motor Behavior and Sport – 1978*, Champaign, Ill.: Human Kinetics.

Clark, J. E., and Moore, J. (1980). Young children's use of precued information in selecting and maintaining a preselected response, paper presented at the North American Society for Psychology of Sport and Physical Activity, Boulder, Colorado, May.

Connolly, K., Brown, K., and Bassett, E. (1968). Developmental changes in some components of a motor skill, *British Journal of Psychology*, **59**, 305–314.

Easton, T. A. (1972). On the normal use of reflexes, *American Scientist*, **60**, 591–599.

Elliott, J., and Connolly, K. (1974). Hierarchical structure in skill development, in K. J. Connolly and J. S. Bruner (eds.), *The Growth of Competence*, New York: Academic Press.

Fairweather, H. (1978). Choice reaction times in children: error and post-error responses, and the repetition effect, *Journal of Experimental Child Psychology*, **26**, 407–418.

Fairweather, H., and Hutt, S. J. (1970). The development of information processing and reaction times in normal school children, *Bulletin of the British Psychological Society*, **23**, 61.

Fairweather, H., and Hutt, S. J. (1978). On the rate of gain of information in children, *Journal of Experimental Child Psychology*, **26**, 216–229.

Fitts, P. M., and Seeger, C. M. (1953). S-R compatibility: spatial characteristics of stimulus and response codes, *Journal of Experimental Psychology*, **46**, 199–210.

Fitts, P. M., and Switzer, G. (1962). Cognitive aspects of information processing: I. the familiarity of S-R sets and subsets, *Journal of Experimental Psychology*, **63**, 321–329.

Fowler, C. A., and Turvey, M. T. (1978). Skill acquisition: an event approach with special reference to searching for the optimum of a function of several variables, in G. E. Stelmach (ed.), *Information Processing in Motor Control and Learning*, New York: Academic Press.

Glencross, D. J. (1979). Output and response processes in skilled performance, in G. C. Roberts and K. M. Newell (eds.), *Psychology of Motor Behavior and Sport – 1978*, Champaign, Ill.: Human Kinetics.

Greene, P. H. (1972). Problems of organization of motor systems, in R. Rosen and F. Snell (eds.), *Progress in Theoretical Biology* (Vol. 2), New York: Academic Press.

Grillner, S. (1975). Locomotion in vertebrates: central mechanisms and reflex interaction, *Physiological Reviews*, **55**, 247–304.

Halverson, L. E., Roberton, M. A., and Harper, C. (1973). Current research in motor development, *Journal of Research and Development in Education*, **6**, 56–70.

Hellebrandt, F. A., Schade, M., and Carns, M. L. (1962). Methods of evoking the tonic neck reflexes in normal human subjects, *American Journal of Physical Medicine*, **41**, 89–139.

Hick, W. E. (1952). On the rate of gain of information, *Quarterly Journal of Experimental Psychology*, **4**, 11–26.

Kerr, B. (1976). Decisions about movement direction and extent, *Journal of Human Movement Studies*, **3**, 199–213.

Kerr, B. (1978). Task factors that influence selection and preparation for voluntary movements, in G. E. Stelmach (ed.), *Information Processing in Motor Control and Learning*, New York: Academic Press.

Klapp, S. T. (1977). Response programming, as assessed by reaction time, does not establish commands for particular muscles, *Journal of Motor Behavior*, **9**, 301–312.

Klapp, S. T. (1978). Reaction time analysis of programmed control, in R. Hutton (ed.), *Exercise and Sport Science Reviews* (Vol. V), Santa Barbara, CA: Journal Publishing Affiliates.

Knott, M., and Voss, D. E. (1968). *Proprioceptive Neuromuscular Facilitation*, New York: Harper & Row.

Liss, P., and Haith, M. (1970). The speed of visual processing in children and adults: effects of backward and forward masking, *Perception and Psychophysics*, **8**, 396–398.

Milani-Comparetti, A., and Gidoni, E. A. (1967). Pattern analysis of motor development and its disorders, *Developmental Medicine and Child Neurology*, **9**, 625–630.

Morin, R. E., and Forrin, B. (1965). Information processing: choice reaction times of first- and third-grade students for two types of associations, *Child Development*, **36**, 713–720.

Mowbray, G. H., and Rhoades, M. V. (1959). On the reduction of choice-reaction times with practice, *Quarterly Journal of Experimental Psychology*, **11**, 16–23.

Peiper, A. (1963). *Cerebral Function in Infancy and Childhood*, New York: Consultants Bureau.

Roberton, M. A. (1977). Stability of stage categorizations across trials: Implications for the 'stage theory' of overarm throw development, *Journal of Human Movement Studies*, **3**, 49–59.

Schmidt, R. A. (1975). A schema theory of discrete motor skill learning, *Psychological Review*, **82**, 225–260.

Seefeldt, V. (1974). A researcher's view: Motor development, in L. E. Halverson and M. A. Roberton (eds.), *Elementary school physical education: Progress – Problems – Predictions*, Madison, WI: Women's Physical Education Alumnae Association, University of Wisconsin.

Shambes, G., and Campbell, S. (1973). Inherent movement patterns in man, *Kinesiology*, **III**.

Shik, M. L., and Orlovski, G. N. (1976). Neurophysiology of locomotor automatism, *Physiological Reviews*, **56**, 465–501.

Stelmach, G. E. (ed.) (1978). *Information Processing in Motor Control and Learning*, New York: Academic Press.

Sternberg, S. (1969). The discovery of processing stages: extensions of Donder's method, *Acta Psychologica*, **30**, 276–315.

Sternberg, S., Monsell, S., Knoll, R. L., and Wright, C. L. (1978). The latency and duration of rapid movement sequences: comparisons of speech and typewriting, in G. E. Stelmach (ed.), *Information Processing in Motor Control and Learning*, New York: Academic Press.

Terrace, H. S., Petitto, L. A., Sanders, R. J., and Bever, T. G. (1979). Can an ape create a sentence? *Science*, **206**, 891–902.

Theios, J. (1975). The components of response latency in simple human information processing tasks, in P. M. A. Rabbitt and S. Dornic (eds.), *Attention and Performance V*, New York: Academic Press.

Theios, J., and Walter, D. G. (1974). Stimulus and response frequency and sequential effects in memory scanning reaction times, *Journal of Experimental Psychology*, **102**, 1092–1099.

Todor, J. I. (1975). Age differences in integration of components of a motor task, *Perceptual and Motor Skills*, **41**, 211–215.

Todor, J. I. (1979). Developmental differences in motor task integration: A test of Pascual-Leone's theory of constructive operators, *Journal of Experimental Child Psychology*, **28**, 314–322.

Turvey, M. T. (1977). Preliminaries to a theory of action with reference to vision, in R. Shaw and J. Bransford (eds.), *Perceiving, Acting, and Knowing*, Hillsdale, NJ: Lawrence Erlbaum.

Wade, M. G. (1976). Developmental motor learning, in J. Keogh and R. S. Hutton (eds.), *Exercise and Sport Sciences Reviews*, (Vol. 4), Santa Barbara, CA: Journal Publishing Affiliates.

Wickens, C. D. (1974). Temporal limits of human information processing: a developmental study, *Psychological Bulletin*, **81**, 739–755.

Wickstrom, R. L. (1975). Developmental kinesiology: maturation of basic motor patterns, in J. H. Wilmore and J. F. Keogh (eds.), *Exercise and Sport Sciences Reviews* (Vol. 3), New York: Academic Press.

Williams, H. G. (1973). Perceptual-motor development as a function of information processing, in M. G. Wade and R. Martens (eds.), *Psychology of Motor Behavior and Sport*, Champaign, Ill.: Human Kinetics.

Zelazo, P., Zelazo, N. A., and Kolb, S. (1972). 'Walking' in the newborn, *Science*, **176**, 314–315.

Zigler, E. (1963). Metatheoretical issues in developmental psychology, in M. Marx (ed.), *Theories in Contemporary Psychology*, New York: Macmillan.

The Development of Movement Control and Co-ordination
Edited by J. A. S. Kelso and J. E. Clark
© 1982, John Wiley & Sons, Ltd

CHAPTER 6

# Developing Knowledge About Action

KARL M. NEWELL AND CRAIG R. BARCLAY

## 1 INTRODUCTION

Relationships between knowledge and action are apparent at both theoretical and operational levels of analysis. From a conceptual perspective, knowledge and action can be viewed, at one and the same time, as both the product and/or process of the organism-environment interaction. This paradox has contributed to the ambiguity that exists as to whether an action should be defined by its consequences or whether the consequences should be defined by the action. From an operational perspective the relationship between knowledge and action appears equally equivocal. We can do things that we do and do not know about, and conversely, we can know things that we can and cannot do. It is apparent, therefore, that the relationship between knowing and doing is a very intricate and intimate one, and at the heart of any attempt to elucidate the concepts of knowledge and action.

The concept of action has been given rather short change in psychological theory despite the leads provided by philosophical lines of enquiry (for recent summaries, see Care and Landesman, 1968; Mischel, 1969). To be sure there have been contributions to action within the field of psychology. For example, Thorndike's (1931) theory of learning was very much concerned with the acquisition of acts, and from a different orientation, Piaget (1971, 1976, 1978) has elaborated at length on the relationship between knowledge and action. These contributions, however, represent exceptions rather than the rule. With little concern for action then, it should not be surprising that psychological theorizing about knowledge is bereft of relationships to action. Thus, we have theories about every conceivable knowledge domain – objects, events, images, situations, meanings, etc. – except action. A representative reflection of this bias by omission can be found in a recent major text on the acquisition of knowledge (Anderson, Spiro, and Montague, 1977) in which less than half-adozen of some 400 pages focus on knowledge and action and these are contained in principally one source (Rumelhart and Ortony, 1977).

Nevertheless, during the last decade there have been a number of suggested changes in orientation to psychological theory, together with shifts of conceptualization in related areas such as speech which, when viewed collectively, indicate that the barriers to linking accounts of knowledge and action may at last be in a position to be broken down. First, there are growing arguments for a continuous, almost circular, relationship between perception and action (e.g. Neisser, 1976; Trevarthen 1978; Turvey, 1977). This view not only helps promote the concept of action *per se*, but in addition, the role of action in perception; a stark contrast to the traditional theories of perception which are promulgated on the basis of a static organism. Second, and related to the previous point, there are moves afoot to recognize the active organizational processes of the organism in perceiving and acting and postulations of the complementary reciprocal nature of the organism-environment interaction (e.g. Bandura, 1978; Bronfenbrenner, 1977; Fowler and Turvey, 1978). Third, notions about action are slowly but surely moving away from the ideas of S-R psychology which have dominated conceptualizations of the initiation and control of movement for most of the twentieth century (cf. Adams, 1971). The revival of the schema notion as the knowledge structure for action reflects this shift in viewpoint (Pew, 1974a; Schmidt, 1975, 1976). Fourth, new approaches to the problem of speech production are being established against a background of a general theory of action (Fowler, 1977; Fowler *et al.*, 1980). The foregoing lines of theorizing do not all hold common domain assumptions but, taken together, they reflect the significance of action in other aspects of human behavior together with a changing orientation to the study of action *per se*.

Our essay is not a statement of a theory of the development of action skills, but rather an attempt to formalize an orientation toward theorizing about some of the significant issues in the development of knowledge about action. In one sense, this paper represents a metatheoretical treatment of seemingly divergent and incompatible viewpoints. The basic phenomena to be examined is the development of cognitive control in action. A traditional assumption, following Piaget, is that thought is internalized action and that the earliest action results from the exercise of pre-existing reflexes. Through experience and maturation it is clear that reflexes become increasingly under the control of the individual and that actions are used in purposeful ways to solve motor problems. We examine issues related to these long-standing ideas together with the role that a person's knowledge of his or her own action may play in the development of purposeful motor behavior. An important theme emerging from the paper is that many of the observed differences in action between children of varying chronological ages are principally due to the experiential factors of knowledge and strategies rather than the traditionally held developmental views of capacity.

The paper is molded around three related issues. The first section discusses problems in the representation of knowledge and action. At the outset, we did not want to get drawn into this issue which, after all, is a major bone of contention in its own right. However, as we began to piece together our ideas about the process of acquiring knowledge about action and the role that maturation plays in this process, we began to recognize the need for a firm grasp on *what* it is about action that is represented. The opening section lays out ideas relative to the product of knowledge about action rather than the process of acquiring that knowledge.

We recognize the difficulties inherent in drawing the distinction between product and process. In the first place, inferences about the processes in knowledge acquisition can only be advanced from the basis of products. Furthermore, what is a product at some particular moment in time could be merely part of the ongoing process, and this problem is magnified when different levels of analysis to issues in the representation of knowledge are considered. The distinction between product and process should be treated, therefore, from a heuristic perspective and probably from a relative rather than an absolute position.

The process of acquisition is the domain of the second section which centers on the acquisition of knowledge about action. Acquisition is viewed in the general vein of the effects of time and practice upon knowledge and action. Developmental or age-dependent influences on the acquisition of knowledge and action is the thrust of Section 3. Sections 2 and 3 also consider, from their respective orientations, knowledge about one's own action system, or as it is often expressed, 'knowing' about knowledge (Brown, 1975; Flavell and Wellman, 1977; Tulving and Madigan, 1970) and action. This aspect was included to extend notions of metacognition to the action domain and to provide a comprehensive analysis of the problems inherent in the development of knowledge about action.


## 2   REPRESENTATION OF KNOWLEDGE ABOUT ACTION

Traditionally, knowledge refers to the product that is stored in memory as a consequence of our innate disposition or invariant tendency to interact adaptively with the environment. The product is a result of organism-environment interactions and its scope is as broad as our imagination in defining knowledge domains. Consequently, knowledge has taken on the burden of representing various things as it were: for example, objects, situations, events, semantics, and so on. On this view, memory is the retention of these 'things' and the acquisition, storage, and retrieval of these things have been the operations of principal concern to cognitive psychologists. Although this interpretation of what knowledge is has developed in large part outside the domain of action it is one which is not incompatible with most notions of the representation of action. For example, representations of movements reflect another knowledge class that has been viewed as being stored in memory (cf. Stelmach, 1974).

Theoretical accounts of the nature of each knowledge domain have generally fallen somewhere between two contrasting and extreme interpretations. One polar position indicates that representation is peculiar to or isomorphic with each 'thing' stored in memory. S-R psychology with its stimulus-response bonds was a prime example of this orientation. The constrasting position holds that as a consequence of mental transformations, representations of the 'things' are far removed from any one-to-one correspondence, to the extent that they are abstract representations. This latter orientation is the fundamental premise of a good number of recent cognitive accounts of knowledge representation which are epitomized, for example, in the concept of schema. It appears commonplace in the action domain to regard these specific and generic representations of knowledge as reflections of traditional and modern interpretations, respectively. Unfortunately, or fortunately, depending upon one's stance, nothing could be further from the truth. Like many polemics, the origins of perspectives are rarely unequivocal and depend as often as not on the thoroughness of one's backdrop into history.

Whatever the antecedents to current theorizing there is no doubt that the last two decades have witnessed a dramatic growth in the theoretical and empirical activity relating to the construct of memory (Tulving, 1979), together with changes in orientation to the nature of memory representation. The current 'zeitgeist' has it that knowledge is stored in terms of generic concepts rather than in a more direct one-to-one correspondence. The nomenclature for the knowledge structure tends to vary but each has a number of common core elements. Thus, we can compare the traditional ideas on plans (Miller, Galanter, and Pribram, 1960) to the current versions of scripts (Schank and Abelson, 1977); definitions (Norman, Rumelhart, and LNR, 1975); schemata (Rumelhart and Ortony, 1977), prototypes (Rosche, 1975), and descriptions (Norman and Bobrow, 1979); but there is a central feature to all of these accounts of knowledge representation. They are all knowledge structures which represent generic concepts at various levels of abstraction.

The above accounts of knowledge representation, emerging as they predominantly are from the recently self-styled discipline of cognitive science, have as yet little direct application to the concept of action. And yet, this orientation to the issue of representation bears a number of resemblances to those recently developed in the motor skills domain. The similarity stems from both the nomenclature for the knowledge structure-schema (Pew, 1974a; Schmidt, 1975, 1976), and the basic interpretation of the nature of the representation of knowledge about action. The conceptualization behind these schema approaches to the representation of knowledge and action is the focus of the next section.

## 2.1 Schemata and Representation of Action

Schemata as the knowledge structures for action have been appealing for two principal reasons. First, and perhaps foremost, is the issue of response generalization and novelty. How is it that one can produce what approaches an infinite variety of actions from a finite action experience? Schemata with their generalized rule prototypes for classes of actions intuitively appear to provide the answer to this question. Second, schemata seem to handle quite readily the assumption that the storage capacity of the human memory system is limited. The retention of generalized rules for action is presumed drastically to reduce the number of items stored in memory. As we shall point out, these respective problems of so-called novelty and storage may not be as acute as generally perceived, and even if they were, the current versions of schemata hold several limitations in their attempts to handle them.

The modern ideas of schema representation for action stem in large part from Bartlett (1932) and his well-hackneyed example of the problems facing the tennis player in stroke production. Bartlett's view of memory was that of a constructive-reconstructive system, in that the tennis player, for example, never produces a backhand which is an identical replica of previous strokes, but by the same token, the backhand produced is not entirely novel either. Bartlett's account of memory representation was comprehensive in that it applied to all knowledge domains including action. It is probably true, however, to say that his conceptual orientation to memory representation is more popular today than it was at the time of the publication of the book in 1932.

The concept of schema for action lay dormant for a good number of years and it is only in this last decade that it has been revitalized as a viable account of knowledge structures. One interpretation of schema is in relation to posture and the notion of a general body schema (e.g. Gross, Webb, and Melzack, 1974), an orientation compatible with the earlier views of Head (1926). This use of schema in essence provides some reference against which one's postural, locomotive, or manipulative actions are assessed. In modern day parlence it is synonymous with a recognition schema (e.g. Schmidt, 1975).

The more general usage of schema, however, relates to the representation for recall or what might more appropriately be called the production of skilled action. There are currently two constrasting, although not necessarily contrary, orientations to this interpretation. One approach stems from cognitive psychology (e.g. Piaget, 1971; Rumelhart and Ortony, 1977), while the other derives from the motor skills literature (e.g. Pew, 1974a; Schmidt, 1975, 1976). These orientations to schema differ in focus not so much on what the fundamental characteristics of schema are, but rather on the nature of the knowledge about action that is represented in the schema structure. Thus, although there is general agreement that schemata are prototypes of action there is a difference in emphasis on what the variables or features represent in these generic concepts.

The idea that there are schemata for both the recognition and production of actions is explicitly outlined in the Schmidt (1975) theory of motor learning. The background to this distinction can be found in the closed-loop human performance accounts of motor control in which some reference or template is designated for the evaluation of feedback, together with mechanisms for subsequent error detection and correction procedures. Adams (1971), in providing a learning theory perspective to closed-loop accounts of human performance, argued on a number of grounds that the processes of recall and recognition must be independent, and as a consequence, designated separate mechanisms for these operations. Schmidt (1975) has essentially followed this logic with the additional requirement that the memory representation for recall and recognition is in a schema mode, rather than some direct representation.

While it seems to be the case that we can recognize movements that we cannot produce and produce movements that we cannot recognize this does not necessarily dictate that the knowledge representation for these action processes is distinct. It could be that the processes of perception and action, which both presumably engage knowledge schemata, are not equally accessible. If this were the case, the constancy function for perception could be isomorphic with the one for action (Turvey, 1977). On this view, the schema which recognizes, for example, the infinite variety of 'A's' in different handwriting styles, is also responsible for the production of the different ways in which one can produce the letter 'A.' Considerable conceptual and empirical activity needs to be engaged in to support such a view, which for the present merely holds the intuitive appeal of parsimony. Certainly, such a prediction is compatible with Neisser's (1976, p. 56) postulation that schema is a pattern *of* action as well as the pattern *for* action.

The major distinction between current interpretations of schema for action rests very much on the level of detail seen to exist in the structure. The cognitive science approach has focused principally on the representation of the act itself (e.g. Rumelhart and Ortony, 1977), without recourse to the details of movement *per se*. In contrast, the motor skill learning orientation gives principal emphasis in schema representation to details of the response specifications (e.g. Schmidt, 1975), such as the kinematic and kinetic features of the movement. Of course, these interpretations of schema are not mutually exclusive, but the gulf between them is wide, and the motor skills approach in particular is much narrower than it should be. The need for a link between the two orientations, even with their current assumptions, is eminently self-evident. Unless there is some conceptual action peg on which to hang response specifications the act will not be completed!

Given that schema prototypes for action are designed to allow response generalization it follows that the orientation one takes to designating the variables of the schema leads directly to predictions of what it is that is transferred to allow generalization. If it is essentially the act itself that is postulated as the schema, then it is transfer at this general level that should take place. For example, if there is a schema for grasping then one should observe generalization of grasping across various tasks involving a grasp, independently it would seem, of the details determining the precision of the grasp. If, however, it is details of the response specifications that are the variables in the schema, then it is at this level that transfer should take place (Schmidt, 1975), particularly with the same act. Empirical examinations of response generalization have typically, if unwittingly, followed these two levels of analysis to the transfer issue.

Response generalization of the act to different situations has been examined principally from the developmental viewpoint (cf. Ginsberg and Opper, 1969; Piaget, 1971). For example, observations have been made of the change from a power to a precision grip through differentiation of the motor response and the subsequent generalization of this latter more elegant grasp through childhood (e.g. Connolly, 1973). The transfer of the precision grip to a variety of situations is an example of the broader schema class. In contrast, the motor skills literature has focused on the generalization of response parameters to essentially the same act (e.g. Newell and Shapiro, 1976). Specifically, it has usually been the same old right arm moving a lever in the same direction along a linear trackway, but with different response specifications. Despite the recent surge of research activity on the generality issue promoted by Schmidt's (1975) schema theory of motor learning, the evidence in favor of a schema account of transfer of response specifications is meager (Newell, 1981; but see Shapiro and Schmidt, this volume, for a more favorable interpretation).

Instead of continuing to search for the benefits of variable practice on response specifications, maybe we should recognize that the equivocal findings are actually telling us something. That message could be that there are different levels of response generalization; a broad class of generalization that reflects the transference of the act to a range of circumstances and a narrow range of response generalization that reflects the transference of details relative to the precision of the movement pattern. The former seems inherently more symbolic than the latter and probably less influenced by the degree of physical practice.

Viewed in this light, it is instructive to close this appreciation of schema and classes of transfer with a recent finding on the effects of mental practice on motor skill learning. It seems that mental practice facilitates the production of an appropriate action (broader schema class) but only actual practice alone facilitates the acquisition of the response specifications (narrower schema class) which are to be imposed upon the movement pattern (Minas, 1978).

Although kinematic features, for example, of simple discrete movements appear to be rehearsable or codeable (Stelmach, 1974), this does not dictate that kinematic features of action are stored in memory or are parameters in a motor program. In other words, simply because these are the features of movements which are observable and conveniently measurable this might not be the appropriate grain of analysis at which to examine representation. While actions take place in time and space, and can be constrained by temporal and spatial demands, these movement parameters or their derivations could well be consequences of an action rather than features of the motor program. On this view, a dynamic perspective of response organization would seem far more appropriate (Bernstein, 1967), and as a result, response details would not be the appropriate level of analysis for schema representation. To show that the system *can* code response specifications when required to do so under the artificial constraints of the experimenter's laboratory requirements (as in the motor short-term memory research) does not necessarily dictate that the system *does* store movement details in other more natural demands of everyday life.

The distinctive approaches to classes of schemata and action can be placed at different positions of an abstract to concrete continuum. On this view, the process of intention to action passes from an abstract representation of the act through successive stages of differentiation to the point where some specific movement or sequence of movements is produced so that some particular consequence or set of consequences is achieved. The motor skills approach to schema is simply at a more advanced stage in the differentiation process, or farther down the line, as it were. The idea of successive stages of differentiation from intention to action does not imply that entry into this continuum has to be at the most abstract level. Indeed, it would seem that reflexive behavior and highly automated responses bypass this level of cognitive control in the differentiation process.

The implications of a time-based continuum of differentiation from intent to action bring to the forefront several interrelated questions. Are schemata for actions and other knowledge domains distinctive knowledge structures? Are there distinct schemata for action at the different stages of the differentiation process, or is perhaps the same structure rearranged depending on the task at hand? If many schemata exist, how do they conflate to produce the infinite adaptive varieties of skilled action?

If schemata are viewed as independent knowledge structures then the first question leads us directly into the storage issue, with the 'things' now stored in memory being schemata. Given the variety of actions that humans perform and the range of details required of the response specifications, the number of schemata required to conduct our everyday affairs would be very large. And when the schemata for other domains are considered such as those presumed for our range of behaviors (Schank and Abelson, 1977) together with perception (Neisser, 1976) and comprehension (e.g. Rumelhart and Ortony, 1977), it would seem that the storage problem still exists, even though it has been reduced by a considerable factor through the prototype formulation. Thus, rather than attempting to retrieve some memory trace specific to a particular movement, one is attempting to retrieve, for example, an action schema. Does memory consist of a library of schemata each representing some stereotype of a knowledge domain? This seems an unlikely explanation of the representation of knowledge, but not because of the limitations of the human storage capacity, a claim which has always been advanced on the basis of a default argument. There is no physiological or psychological evidence that the capacity of the human long-term memory system can be exceeded through a lifetime of interactions with the environment. Indeed, long-term memory failures may well be more a problem of accessibility rather than of availability (Tulving and Pearlstone, 1966).

The notion that the process of action revolves around the retrieval and subsequent sticking and cutting, as it were, of schemata, seems too rigidly structured and at the same time rather pedestrian. It is the case that one can break up actions into movement pattern sequences which appear to be subsets or subroutines of the whole action (Bruner, 1970), and that learning the parts of an action can transfer to the acquisition of the complete action sequence (e.g. Knapp and Dixon, 1952). These occurrences, do not, however, dictate that the rules which link and co-ordinate movement sequences should be usefully viewed as analogues to syntax in language (e.g. Goodnow and Levine, 1973; Ninio and Leiblich, 1976), or the rules of transformational grammar (Bruner, 1973), despite their apparent similarity. The compartmentalizing of knowledge structures is based in large part upon the problems of comprehension and the retrieval of the ideas retained which are all processes, at least in the way they are studied, that are typically divorced from action. Such an approach might be appropriate for comprehension which is highly symbolic and can be made explicit to a large degree. In contrast, much of our everyday motor activity belies explicit accounts of its construction, leaving, as often as not, the intention and goal as the only aspects of action which can be articulated. A tacit level of knowledge representation (Polanyi, 1958) seems more in order for skilled action and yet we actively attempt to make it explicit.

The distinction between explicit and tacit knowledge parallels in a number of respects that made between voluntary and involuntary levels of control. The boundaries between these levels of control, however, are not rigid (Hilgard, 1977), and a more thorough investigation of this seemingly intangible area is clearly required to explicate the relationships of knowledge and action. In the meantime, we are left with the rather unsatisfactory traditional generalization that skilled actions are largely automatic and under minimal influence of cognitive activity, whereas the early stages of skill learning are characterized by explicit cognitive involvement (Fitts and Posner, 1967; Adams, 1971).

## 2.2   Schemata and Motor Programs

The transformation of knowledge into action represents a major problem for theorists of skill acquisition. The generally accepted view, even if it is only implied, is that it involves the differentiation of the schema into an appropriate movement configuration for the action at hand. If schemata represent the abstract, what is it that supplies the muscles with the movement specification for the act? The currently prevailing answer to this question is the motor program. The modern conceptualization of the motor program (Keele, 1968) is that it is muscle-specific and it contains all of the details necessary for the movement to run its course uninfluenced by peripheral feedback. More recent versions (Pew, 1974a; Schmidt, 1976) postulate a generalized capacity for the motor program while some propose that the program itself is not muscle-specific (e.g. Klapp, 1977). Taking the latter view literally, forces the conclusion that motor programs are nothing more than schemata under a different guise.

One way around this semantic polemic is to argue that the motor program is at some intermediate stage of differentiation from the schema to the production of movement. That is, the motor program could be at the stage where the details of the response parameters are imposed upon some action already established to complete the act. This intermediate version of the motor program in the intention to action continuum leaves open the question of what we call the final command issued to the functional groupings of muscles, assuming of course, that we want to give it a label.

In a sense then, what the motor program is, and particularly whether it is muscle-specific, depends basically upon the stage in the differentiation process where one wants to place it. In short, the structure of the motor program becomes a matter of definition. Our bias is to reserve the motor program as the construct for the final stage of differentiation (Newell, 1978) and thus by definition it includes parameters which are muscle-specific. There are no apparent conceptual advantages from this approach, merely the recognition that motor processes are involved in action and more importantly, that organization of the musculature is a significant factor in skilled action (see for example, Glencross, 1974; Waterland, 1970) a fact that can be underplayed, if not overlooked, in discussions focusing on the role of cognition in action. This view is also compatible with Keele's (1968) original definition of the motor program, although this endorsement does not include the rider that it is uninfluenced by peripheral feedback – a notion which is clearly wrong (Evarts *et al.*, 1971).

## 2.3 Schemata as Knowledge Structures and Attunements to the Environment

The accounts of schemata for action, which have been outlined briefly, suggest a very static organism in relation to the interaction with the environment (e.g. Schmidt, 1975). The emphasis has been on schemata as memory records or products of the organism-environment interaction. The former view implies that schema is an end result rather than a process or set of procedures that are engaged in throughout the perceiving-acting cycle. This static or passive view of schema has even led to the question of where schema might be located in the brain.[1] The process view of schema, however, suggests it is the 'set' that all the brain mechanisms have as they interact together in the perception-action cycle, rather than designating it as any specific mechanism.

Recently, it has been proposed that the growth of knowledge represents a remodeling of the knowledge structure as a whole, rather than an accumulation of pieces or even prototypes of knowledge (Bransford, Nitsch, and Franks, 1977). This view stems from the strong version of direct perception in which perceptual learning is a matter of differentiation rather than enrichment or construction (Gibson and Gibson, 1955). The ability to differentiate or pick up information with experience comes not from a broader and stronger collection of memory metaphors, but rather from an improved attunement of the system to various environments. It is this attunement to the environment which determines that information is picked up through perception and this process has been likened to the notion of stage-setting (Bransford and Franks, 1976).

This view suggests the primacy of perceiving in accounts of what has traditionally been called memory (Turvey and Shaw, 1979). Learning becomes no longer a matter of accumulating records in memory, but rather it rests on the development of a more appropriate postural orientation of the system to organism-environment interactions. The end product of this attunement is the understanding that certain econiches afford certain acts (Gibson, 1977). Although Gibson and his followers would be wary of constructionist nomenclature, the term schema, when viewed from the process point of view, seems very analogous to the stage-setting idea; that is, schema may be represented by the organism's current level of attunement to the environment.

While the direct perception argument highlights the significance of the organism-environment interaction and the limitations of the traditional constructionist focus to the organism alone, there seems a potential for the Gibsonian position to swing the emphasis the other way. That is, to focus principally on the environment and stimulus characteristics at the expense of the organism. There are heuristic merits in providing the strong position to one's theoretical viewpoint, but the direct perception position in doing this could undermine its adherence, at least in the way in which it is interpreted, to the organism-environment interaction. The concept of schema as an active entity is only possible when the organism-environment interaction is recognized. Schema seems a relatively passive construct when the organism alone is considered and irrelevant or unnecessary when the environment alone is considered.

What is suggested here is an active schema which is continually being tailored by organism-environment interactions, but not just as a consequence of the environment attuning the organism. It would seem necessary for both top-down, knowledge to action, and bottom-up, perception to knowledge, influences on the schema development. When the environment is stable how else can the organism produce different actions and attempt different acts but through conceptually driven procedures? An overriding issue is the establishment of common principles through which different sources can activate and tune schemata.

Our view is that a schema is not only the product of the organism-environment interaction but also the cognitive 'set' or processing rule for understanding and acting in subsequent interactions. The exercise of a schema is the process through which future knowledge is acquired. This position suggests that the acquisition and representation of knowledge are interdependent complementary processes. Therefore, schemata are end products (at any point in time) represented in a cognitive system as well as process tendencies for acting. Thus, we agree with Neisser (1976) that some rapprochement needs to be made between the constructionist views of current cognitive psychology and the nonmediatory direct perception position to provide an adequate explanation of the organism-environment interaction.

## 3   THE ACQUISITION OF KNOWLEDGE ABOUT ACTION

The acquisition of knowledge refers to the process of accumulating information about specific events, tasks, and situations as well as general conceptualizations and attunements to the environment. The acquisition process is assumed to follow, in some form, principles of learning. These traditional principles, however, may not account for the complex structural arrangements of schemata. That is, while learning may explain the acquisition of pieces of information, it is not clear how these pieces are organized in meaningful structural units which afford the schema through which new information is accommodated.

Within the developmental literature, the only reasonable growth mechanism proposed is that of assimilation and accommodation (Piaget, 1952). Unfortunately, while learning principles appear too limited to account for the acquisition of knowledge, assimilation and accommodation are too vague to specify the exact nature of the acquisition process (see Broudy, 1977; Brown, 1979, for a more complete discussion of these issues). Although no new formulations of an accommodation mechanism are proposed, it seems that a major theoretical effort is needed in developmental psychology to instantiate the parameters of such a process.

In reference to action, it is assumed that knowledge is acquired about the utility of various actions for meeting different motor task demands. In the simplest case, knowledge results from the success or failure of an action to solve a motor problem. In this section we are not directly concerned with the acquisition of action *per se*, but with potential types of knowledge one might develop about the action process; thus, our major focus is on the metacognitive aspects of action.

## 3.1   Types of Knowledge about Action

One way to approach the theoretical issue of acquiring knowledge about action is to attempt to provide an answer to the following question: 'What can a person know or come to know about his/her own actions?' This question has been broached in other knowledge domains such as verbal learning (Tulving and Madigan, 1970) and has led to the development of a taxonomy of types of knowledge, such as that outlined by Flavell and his associates for the study of memory (Flavell and Wellman, 1977). The general thrust of this line of enquiry is metacognition or knowing about knowing as it as often been labeled (e.g. Brown, 1975).

Metacognition can be defined broadly as a person's knowledge about his own or others' psychological, social, and physical behavior and abilities. This knowledge is acquired by interacting with the environment in a purposeful and intentional way. One aspect of this knowledge is the person's awareness of the association between movement and its consequences – action. We discuss this relationship through applying some of Flavell's notions about metacognition to action. This approach serves principally a heuristic function since there have been no systematic attempts to develop a taxonomy of types of knowledge for the action domain. Nevertheless, Flavell's taxonomy provides a useful frame of reference for outlining what types of knowledge might develop in relation to action. In general, it would seem that an awareness of one's own actions involves at least two major types of knowledge: sensitivity to those situations requiring a skilled action; and knowledge of variables or factors which affect the outcome of action.

Sensitivity to different situations includes knowledge not only of the fact that action is required but also an understanding of the movement or sequence of movements that will complete the act. Stated differently, sensitivity cues the individual to organize an appropriate schema or orientate to an environmental cue and subsequently tailor it to the specific problem at hand. This suggests that sensitivity accounts, in part, for flexibility and generalizability since the person modulates the schema through the movement produced to meet differing task demands. For example, if a person is skilled in throwing, he must know the degree of force required by the task to determine how hard the ball must be thrown to hit the target. Therefore, this sensitivity is not only knowledge about environmental demands, but also represents an awareness of the means-end nature of action.

More specifically, any sensitivity to a motor act requiring skilled action involves at least two related elements. One element involves an understanding of the nature of the problem to be solved or a knowledge of how the characteristics of the task must be manipulated to meet an identified goal. This does not necessarily mean that the task characteristics or nature of the problem are evaluated correctly, but it does suggest that the person is alerted to the fact that he must do something purposeful and voluntary. The person knows, although not in these terms, that an instantiated schema is needed even if he has no idea as to an appropriate solution or plan to be used. Nevertheless, knowledge or sensitivity to the task results in the generation of a schema which, through action, results in a motor response or series of motor responses until successful adaptation to the task occurs.

The second element involves the person's awareness of the context in which the task is presented, where context refers to the situational cues or stimuli which define the parameters of the task demands (e.g. Bransford and Johnson, 1972). As an illustration in the action domain, a task could be presented in a competitive or noncompetitive context. These two settings would probably motivate the individual to perform somewhat differently. The point to be stressed is that context determines to a large degree the action needed to perform successfully. Context is viewed as a separate element from task features since the former deals with the way a task is presented and not the specific characteristics of the task. This is not to say, however, that task context and features be considered in isolation of each other since the awareness category of knowledge about action involves an appreciation of the context by task-feature relationship. Obviously, the same task (holding characteristics constant) presented in two different contexts could result in different task demands, e.g. playing basketball for fun instead of money.

According to Flavell and Wellman (1977) the second major category of metacognitive knowledge is variables; that is, the person's knowledge of the factors affecting skilled performance. This category includes three related elements: person, task, and strategy variables.

The person variable represents a knowledge of oneself or others as skilled in certain actions and involves two dimensions. The first dimension is traits or the person's knowledge of his or other's enduring physical structures, e.g. knowing the morphological constraints of the human action system. This knowledge of structure relates to Bernstein's (1967) notion that physical attributes can be characterized in terms of the number of degrees of freedom allowed by structural limitations. A representative case is an agonist-antagonist muscle pair which has one degree of freedom around a hinge joint. Flexibility in movement is achieved, however, since the muscles need not be maximally flexed or extended. Over time, through maturation and experience, the person presumably acquires knowledge about the degrees of freedom afforded by his various physiological structures. This knowledge influences the person's choice of a specific structure or group of structures to complete the act, e.g. using your arm and hand to propel a ball instead of your leg and foot.

The second dimension of the person variable is states, which refers to the individual's knowledge of his ongoing action. For example, through proprioceptive and exteroceptive feedback, a person is capable of monitoring the consequences of a response as well as knowing when the act is completed. This monitoring of ongoing action results in the continuation or termination of movement(s) relative to whether the perceived goal of the act is reached. This knowledge which is the outcome of monitoring the states of action not only plays an evaluative role but also updates the schema or provides the basis for formulating a different rule if the person is unsuccessful. In this characterization, states is somewhat analogous to the notion of an 'executive' in information-processing models (e.g. Atkinson and Shiffrin, 1968; Bower, 1972).

Consider next the task variable. This variable refers specifically to the person's knowledge of task characteristics that affect the difficulty and complexity level of the act and reflect an individual's perception of the nature of the task. For example, the person is capable of deciding whether one task is harder or easier than another as a function of the nature of the movement(s) to be performed. It seems that knowledge of task characteristics is acquired through two sources: (i) actual experience on the specific task, and/or (ii) generalized (constructed) knowledge from experience on a class of tasks with similar characteristics. This later source of knowledge should result to a large degree from an elaboration of information already learned. In one sense, the generalization of knowledge is the reorganization of existing schemata to meet a new task demand. Generalized knowledge could also result from inferences based on information available from a specific task and its demands, in which case the person goes beyond the available knowledge or information given.

The last variable considered here is strategy, which refers to a person's approach to problem-solving. This is assumed to reflect knowledge of the movement configurations which can be invoked voluntarily to complete the act in a skillful manner. The repetition of a specific action pattern represents one type of strategy and suggests a number of features of knowledge about one's problem-solving approach. One such feature is that the person, through practicing a motor skill, can organize an appropriate schema or level of attunement for the desired response. Also, as the individual executes a strategy repeatedly, information pertinent to the act accumulates, and based on this feedback and the monitoring of knowledge of results, the person adjusts, analyzes, revises, or selects a new strategy. Thus, two features of skill are apparent: (i) behavior useful in acquiring an appropriate action pattern and (ii) responses which, through feedback, allow the person to modify his behavior.

Apparently, knowledge is also acquired about specific strategies useful for solving specific tasks, as well as knowledge about general strategies useful for solving a class of similar tasks. These types of strategies are viewed not as independent but as falling along some continuum of specifity. Obviously, few strategies are exclusive to a single task, and certain strategies can be used on a greater variety of tasks. This suggests that a person presented with a different task will perform using a generalized strategy which becomes more specific, through feedback, to the demands of the task.

In the above discussion, it was implied that an understanding of skilled action requires an analysis of the interrelationship of the sensitivity and variables categories of metacognition. While no attempt is made here to consider all possible combinations of different types of knowledge, an overview of the interactive process is described which permits analysis of action from a metacognitive viewpoint.

Consider the case where an individual is presented with an unfamiliar task but one to which he can perform some response. The person is given instructions regarding the expected goal and outcome, and asked to complete the act. Initially, the person responds to the instructions or task demands through his knowledge that the situation requires skilled effort; that is, the person is aware of the task to be solved and the context within which it is presented. Since the task is unfamiliar, no specific strategy is known. Thus, the person must evaluate his repertoire of available strategies in light of the task demands and make an initial trial and error response. Depending on the temporal duration of the response, the person monitors the execution given the selected strategy and evaluates the response relative to the actual behavioral effect. After the response is completed, the person evaluates the entire situation – strategy, response, and outcome before making the next response. In this way, on subsequent responses, the individual's expectations (knowledge) of the situation and factors or variables affecting performance develop until the problem is solved or the person gives up. This characterization of the initial acquisition phase is similar to what Gentile (1972) has described as getting the idea of the response.

In summary, the two categories of metacognitive knowledge, sensitivity and variables, function dynamically in the case of the skilled performer, allowing the individual to adapt to the environment. The description of metacognition outlined above did not include a discussion of specific perceptual factors in the task or situation, nor did this description attempt to cover the material on possible structural limitations within the individual. However, any complete understanding of knowledge about skilled action must include these factors.

# 4   DEVELOPMENTAL ISSUES IN KNOWLEDGE AND ACTION

## 4.1   Measurement Considerations

Although the focus of this book is developmental issues in the motor development of children from birth through maturity, the term development, and the work conducted under this umbrella, is slowly taking on a broader perspective to include human development throughout the lifespan. This latter connotation is the orientation that we will follow, although we will give emphasis to changes in knowledge and action in the childhood period. This section has two main thrusts. Initially, we focus on the relative contribution of capacity, strategy, and knowledge factors in the development of knowledge and action. This is followed with a discussion of the idea that development follows some invariant order both within and between periods of change.

Historically, developmental changes in behavior, meaning performance differences between younger and older subjects, have been attributed to maturational or chronological age (CA) effects. Recently, however, the pervasiveness of this interpretation has been questioned which has led developmental psychologists to a methodology that considers two additional factors which potentially cause behavior change over time (Bijou and Baer, 1963a, b; Schaie, 1965; Wohlwill, 1970). These factors are environmental or time-of-testing effects and events acting at the time of a person's birth or cohort effects. In the motor skills literature no attempt has been made to distinguish cohort and secular trends.

In the typical developmental study various-aged subjects are tested on some task at a specific point in time; that is, a cross-sectional design is used. With this methodological approach, however, any age effect found cannot be unequivocally attributed to maturation since the subjects not only differ in CA but also in the point in time when they were born. In other words, the age change observed may not represent maturational effects at all since the older subjects come from a different cohort group than the younger subjects. In most studies, therefore, the age (maturation) factor is inextricably confounded with the cohort factor.

To avoid the possible confounding of age and cohort, a longitudinal design can be used. In this approach, cohort is held constant by selecting subjects born at the same point in time and testing them repeatedly as they age. Unfortunately, while this approach eliminates some of the problems of a cross-sectional study, any age-related performance differences may be confounded with the effects of a changing environment. In the longitudinal study, the subjects are getting older, physically, which takes time! To sort out the relative contribution of maturational and environmental variables to age-related performance differences a cross-sequential experiment design has been proposed which combines both the longitudinal and cross-sectional approaches (Goulet and Baltes, 1970; Goulet, Hay, and Barclay, 1974; Schaie, 1965). With this design, the analysis of maturational and environmental causation is desirable and more importantly possible.

The major purpose of opening our discussion on developmental issues in the acquisition of knowledge and action, with a brief treatise of methodological issues, is to point out that clean manipulations of the appropriate variables need to be made if any worthwhile distinction between experiential and maturational contributions to performance is to be addressed. Most research on the acquisition of skilled action has failed to account for these experimental design problems. This, as we will see throughout the remainder of the paper, makes inferences tenuous relative to teasing out the relative contribution of maturational (capacity) and environmental (strategy, knowledge) influences.

## 4.2   Capacity, Strategy, Knowledge, and Metacognition

One basic phenomenon that needs to be explained from a lifespan developmental perspective is the almost universal finding across a wide variety of tasks that performance reflects an inverted curvilinear function with age. Specifically, the relative contributions of the key variables which are instrumental in determining this relationship need to be established. The title to this section indicates some of the most influential factors and we continue with a discussion of their relative contribution to age-related differences in skilled action. Before elaborating on the contribution of these factors to performance, we need to be explicit on the meaning of the terms capacity, strategy, and knowledge. Definition of these factors should not only explicate their meaning, but in addition, indicate why they have been and continue to be the major general factors seen to determine the age-by-performance relationship.

Capacity refers to the collective potential of the various structural features of the organism. For example, age covaries with physical parameters of the human system, such as height, strength, etc. (e.g. Tanner, 1962), particularly, in the span from birth to adolescence. Less obvious structural limitations are the changes in brain activity with ontogeny (e.g. Bergstrom, 1969), together with changes in the speed with which nerve impulses can be transmitted around the organism (e.g. Schulte *et al.*, 1969). These illustrations should be sufficient to indicate the potential range of capacity differences that exist between age groups and to point up the fact that many of them are not immediately apparent at first sight. In sum, capacity or structural factors are seen as direct reflections of maturational (biological) influences.

In contrast, strategy and knowledge fall more under the domain of environmental or experiential factors. Strategies can be viewed as classes of knowledge or schemata which are specific to the organism-environment interactions at hand. In essence, strategies determine the procedure or sequence of actions that will be performed in a situation and reflect an instantiated schema (Rumelhart and Ortony, 1978). This leaves knowledge as the general concepts or uninstantiated schemata as we discussed in the initial section of the paper on representation. This distinction between strategies and knowledge follows to some degree what Piaget (1970) has referred to as operative and figurative knowledge, and what is often referred to elsewhere as procedural and declarative knowledge.

## Capacity

Without doubt the principal focus of researchers investigating developmental trends in skilled action has been the issue of capacity. The pioneering early work on motor development by Gesell (1929), McGraw (1935), Shirley (1931), Halverson (1931) and others examined and plotted the time course of the onset of certain phylogenetic skills, with the emphasis of explanation for the action difference over age being maturation (physical capacity) rather than experiential. The tenor of this work was that maturation reflects the development of the central nervous system following the principles of cephalo-caudal and proximo-distal development (Gesell, 1929). Maturation affords the inhibition of primitive and postural reflexes and the acquisition of the fundamental actions of locomotion such as crawling, walking, and hopping, together with the prehensile skills of reaching and grasping.

While it is likely that maturation and hence capacity arguments account for the lion's share of performance variance in the onset of phylogenetic skills, some recent work has demonstrated that the experiential factors of strategy and knowledge can also play a role in their development. For example, Zelazo, Zelazo, and Kolb (1972) have shown that exercising the stepping reflex during the first and second months of life can accelerate the onset of self-controlled walking in infants, and corresponding findings have been demonstrated for crawling by Lagerspetz, Nygard, and Stranduick (1971). Similarly, Bower (1974) has demonstrated the role of experience in facilitating the onset of reaching and grasping skills. These illustrations suggest then, that even with the so-called fundamental actions of locomotion and prehension, experience can modify the imposition of cognitive control on the primitive and postural reflexes, and by implication, the contribution of the strategy and knowledge factors to this process.

Although most of the research on motor development has been descriptive in orientation and focused on the initiation of the phylogenetic skills, there has been an increased emphasis on explanation for performance differences observed over age, especially during the last decade. The central outcome of this work is that capacity is also seen to be the key factor in the development of ontogenetic or 'socially desirable' skills. This research reflects in large part ideas and paradigms of the information-processing approach (e.g. Connolly, 1970a) and the neo-Piagentian influences (e.g. Pascule-Leon's, 1970 notion of M-space). The capacity referred to here is not, strictly speaking, limitations with respect to physical structure but rather postulated differences in so-called mental capacity. Thus, the elevation of performance through adolescence and the decrease in performance in senility is often ascribed to some changes in mental capacity.

The information-processing approach provides the basis for the postulation that there might be age-dependent capacity limitations with respect to the number of bits of information that can be processed or maintained in working memory for some unit time (Wickens, 1974). For example, age-related differences in decision times are often attributed to capacity changes in one or another mental operation along the information-processing continuum. This has been postulated at both the birth through adolescence (e.g. Connolly, 1970b; Morin and Forvin, 1965) and elderly (Welford, 1958) ends of the lifespan continuum, and between populations of different mental ages (MA) (Baumeister and Kellas, 1968). In the same vein, the interaction of chronological age (e.g. Kerr, 1975) and mental age (e.g., Wade, Newell, and Wallace, 1978) with index of difficulty in the Fitts' law movement paradigm, has also been principally ascribed to capacity limitations.

Mental capacity limitations have also been invoked to explain age-related differences in the acquisition of a motor skill. Kay (1970) for example, discusses improvements in ball-catching ability with age on the basis of developmental differences in information processing. The more recent findings that older children can effectively handle more precise levels of information feedback (Newell and Kennedy, 1978) and utilize less KR processing time (Barclay and Newell, 1980) than younger children, also fall nicely in line with the capacity hypothesis of the information-processing approach. Indeed, it seems a self-fulfilling prophesy, that laboratory findings demonstrate that older children perform better than their younger counterparts.

It should be clear from the introduction to this section that exclusive capacity arguments for the differences in performance levels with age are inappropriate when the experimental design lacks the appropriate controls.

This is not to eliminate the potential of capacity factor to age-performance relationships but rather to indicate that CA as well as MA merely correlate with the performance differences in the above studies and are not necessarily causal independent variables. To our knowledge, no study on the acquisition or control aspects of action has included a design which allows separation of age, cohort, and time effects. This design limitation, in itself, should suggest reservations to the capacity argument for the age-related performance effects, particularly with ontogenetic skills. Furthermore, when this limitation is considered in conjunction with the potential contributions of environmental influences and the growth of knowledge and strategic behaviors on skilled action, we can see that capacity becomes an even less convincing explanation for age-related performance differences. This reservation is bolstered by the fact that motivational and attitudinal factors may also contribute to the CA and MA performance differences in experiments conducted under the information-processing paradigms (Wickens, 1974; Zigler, 1969).

A striking example which supports the proposal that the role of capacity may be overplayed as an explanatory construct in performance differences due to CA comes from a recent developmental study on memory for chess positions (Chi, 1978). Chi showed that ten-year-old children who were expert chess players could remember chess positions better than skilled but less knowledgeable adult chess players, but only when the chess positions to be remembered were meaningful and not randomly determined. Yet, when the stimuli (i.e. digits) were more familiar to the adults, typical developmental trends were found. This is a nice illustration of the role that knowledge plays in performance and suggests that many of the memory performance differences usually observed with age may be due to strategic and knowledge-based differences. There is a growing body of empirical evidence to support the knowledge factor in developmental differences (e.g. Brown et al., 1973; Chi, 1977). An even stronger argument for this claim could be made if one could equate experience with the stimuli and task at hand over age and still obtain the same results.

There are a number of suggestions from the human performance literature that experiential factors can overcome performance deficits usually attributed to capacity limitations. With respect to decision time, Mowbray and Rhoades (1959) showed that adult's reaction time (RT) to a four-choice task equalled RT to a two-choice task after 42,000 trials of practice. And in a somewhat different context, work from our labtoratory has demonstrated a reduction of both RT and movement time (MT) in a Fitts' law aiming task, with severely retarded young adults, given that appropriate training procedures were employed. The performance of these mentally retarded people did not reach the level of the normal control group, but who is to say that this would not be the case, given even more practice and possibly different training procedures (Gold, 1975). Following the influential paper of Atkinson and Shiffrin (1968)

RT is often viewed as a measure of a limitation of predominantly a structural or capacity nature and, as a consequence, impervious to practice or strategic influences. The above findings, however, together with others of the same vein, tend to confirm Simon's (1972) suggestion that there is a fine line between capacity and strategic limitations, particularly when developmental issues are considered (see also Flavell, 1970 for a discussion of the same issue in memory development). The question then, of what can and cannot be trained in skilled action remains a relatively empirical issue (Welford, 1976).

Certainly, anecdotal evidence suggests that experience plays a tremendous role in developing action skills in the young. Children can be highly skilled in a variety of activities from everyday socially desirable acts to the more specialized sporting and musical domains. Yet somehow, when it comes to laboratory tasks, younger children always perform at a lower level than older children. It does not seem too adventurous to suggest, therefore, that many of the inferences advanced upon the basis of laboratory findings may well underestimate the capabilities of children in the acquisition of various skilled actions, and as a consequence, provide a false base upon which to build mental capacity explanations. Given the similar degrees of pertinent experience on a task, how different would be the performance of younger children?

The verbal learning literature suggests that one of the major difficulties facing younger children is the spontaneous implementation or adoption of an appropriate strategy for the task at hand (Brown, 1975; Flavel, 1970). Laboratory examinations of developmental issues in motor skill learning rarely allow subjects very much practice time and the experimenters usually do not provide strategic prompts. And yet, as indicated previously, we often attribute performance differences which correlate with age as being due to capacity limitations. The problem is that although the results are often compatible with a capacity hypothesis, and may in part be determined by capacity factors, the findings are also in line with respect to strategy implementation and general differences with respect to knowledge of organism-environment interactions. Indeed, given the fact that many laboratory skill acquisition tasks minimize structural or physical capacity differences between age groups, the experiential factors of strategy and knowledge would seem to account for a larger part of the performance variance between age groups than is usually accredited.

## Strategy

As we have indicated, strategy represents a decision rule or problem-solving approach and represents the instantiation of knowledge. The verbal learning literature suggests that with increasing age children adopt a more strategic role in maintaining their own performance (e.g. Flavell, 1970). Indeed, the spontaneous use of strategies and the flexible adjustment of these behaviors to a variety of task demands is one of the factors that distinguishes young children from adolescents and adults. There are a variety of strategic behaviors that children can adopt in most motor skill learning situations, particularly in open skills. Unfortunately, we have little knowledge of the organizational processes employed by the child in motor skill acquisition (see Wade, 1976 for a recent review of the scanty evidence available).

It is perhaps not surprising then, to find minimal empirical work in response strategies given that the thrust of the motor developmental literature revolves around capacity arguments. Thus, it appears that the conceptual bias of researchers has elminated the experiential factors of strategy and knowledge as contributors to skill development rather than the traditional techniques of strong inference. A more balanced assessment of the basic factors contributing to motor skill development is clearly warranted, particularly in light of the obvious role of strategies in skill acquisition.

## Knowledge

The concept of knowledge is used in different ways depending on the content area under study. For example, a philosopher may regard knowledge in the sense of the collective awareness people have about some cultural phenomena, whereas a psychologist may assume that knowledge is isomorphic to some specific experience like learning-to-learn. In a broad sense then, knowledge is the representation thought synthesis of one's varied experiences. Reconsidering Bartlett's (1932) example of the tennis play, the notion of nonspecific knowledge implies the tendency to respond in a prototypical fashion without much regard for the details of the movement. This use of knowledge further implies the accumulation of semantic features of an information-processing system which, at any point in time, represents the organism's current level of attunement to the environment (e.g. Collins and Loftus, 1975; Turvey and Shaw, 1979). Unfortunately, many theoretical treatments of knowledge in this sense assume that knowledge exists and ignore how the system acquired what is known (Neisser, 1976). In part, the problem set for cognitive science must not only include a consideration of how knowledge is organized, structured, and used but also how it is acquired.

Ther term knowledge is also used in a narrow sense, that is, knowledge is the representation of what one has learned about specific aspects of unique situations or tasks. In this sense, knowledge is context- as well as task-specific, so that what is known about a given task is not generalizable to other, even similar problems. In this regard, knowledge is synonymous with what is typically meant by learning in the short sense of the word. In the area of motor skills attention has been given to the problem of specifying how movement information is represented in the system. In fact, some of the arguments focus on what features of the action are coded in the cortex (e.g. Evarts, 1967; Walshe, 1943).

There is little evidence, however, on the possible role extant knowledge plays in the acquisition of an action. A notable exception is an early experiment by Judd (1908) which showed that *a priori* knowledge influences the production of an action. In this study, knowledge of the rule of refraction facilitated the acquisition of hitting targets under different water levels, but only after some degree of physical practice. A more recent replication of this study (Hendrickson and Schroeder, 1941) found immediate performance benefits from a knowledge of action principles, suggesting an intricate relationship between knowing and doing.

Polanyi (1958) has suggested that knowledge of the rule for completing various acts may be tacit and so complex as to not be useful in the acquisition of skill. On the other hand, knowledge for action may be useful even if it is at some tacit level of representation and the performer is not aware of its influence. Consider a tracking study by Pew (1974b). Subjects learned to track a stimulus pattern over a series of days after which time the stimulus pattern was changed except for one segment of it which was retained, although presented backwards. The results showed that subjects tracked this reverse segment much better than the new portions of the overall pattern, even though they were not aware that a segment of the original pattern was present in reversed form. Thus, it appears that knowledge of the act does not have to be explicit to facilitate performance, although on some occasions the performer may be able to articulate aspects of his knowledge relative to the task at hand.

*Metacognition*

As mentioned earlier, metacognition refers to what a person knows or could come to know about his own system. In specific reference to action, metacognition relates to a person's knowledge about the process of how he relates a movement to its consequences. A general issue is the child's increasing sensitivity for when a situation requires that he uses an intentional skilled effort to meet the task demands. There are few data on this issue, but the general finding emerging from a variety of situations is that young children tend to externalize the responsibility for their success and failure at the task at hand. In other words, they seem to have little or no comprehension of the effort demanded of them by the task. Elliot and Connolly (1974) have provided some evidence of this in a motor skills context, but to highlight the point we will draw on some observations recently gathered in our laboratory with three- and four-year-old children. In one task, the child's goal was to roll a ball a certain distance to a target. On completion of a set of trials, we asked each child a series of questions in an attempt to ascertain just how he went about learning the task and why he was or was not performing very well. With respect to the latter question, several times we received answers such as 'silly ball' or 'the ball is sleep.' Carey (1974) has argued that expressions such as these represent a sense of 'powerlessness' on the part of the child. She claims this phenomenon is more pronounced in young children, although even adults will display tendencies of powerlessness given an appropriately novel and difficult task. The main point, however, is that young children are often not aware that they control their own behavior, and that it is their own intentional efforts that determine success and failure on a particular task (Kopp, 1979).

There are very few studies that have investigated a child's awareness of the variables that relate to himself in a motor skills context. Perhaps the only study to apply metacognitive notions directly to action is a dissertation by Markman (1973). She asked four-year-old children to estimate their memory span for a list of digits, and in addition, what their performance would be on a standing long jump and a task requiring them to carry as many marbles as they could in one hand from one location to another. She found that the children clearly overestimated their memory span for the verbal items, yet with the physical activities, the children were almost as accurate as adults in assessing what the level of their own performance would be. These findings led Markman to con- clude that there are developmental differences in the rate with which metacog- nition strategies appear with respect to verbal skills and motor skills. This is rather a premature conclusion because the differences obtained in children's knowledge about their own capacity in verbal and motor skills may be due to the fact that the physical skills of jumping and carrying marbles are ones that the children had previous experience of, and as a consequence, were able to give a better estimate of their own performance. Given a relatively novel and more difficult task than those employed by Markman, we may see similar developmental differences in a child's knowledge of motor ability, as Markman, Flavell and others have observed in other contexts. In addition, the motor tasks employed in the Markman study seem to tap the child's knowledge of the limitations of his own physical system, rather than the processes which are instrumental in the production of a skilled action.

Attentional processes represent one class of mental operations that appears to be developmentally sensitive. By way of example, we will confine our discus- sion to the concepts of selective attention and the attention demands required to control an ongoing response. It is generally recognized that prior to the initiation of a movement the performer evaluates information contained in the environment so that an appropriate action plan may be formulated. Consider- ing the variety of sensory stimuli that are available to the performer, and that these stimuli may change as a function of time, as in an open skill (Poulton, 1957), it is necessary that the performer selectively attend to only the cues directly relevant to the act at hand. This process of selective attention is very sensitive to developmental differences. Not only do young children fail to scan the stimulus array selectively, but they are often unaware of how to undertake such an operation unless guidance is provided (Day, 1975). In contrast, adults tend to know, or learn very quickly, the task-relevant features and focus their attention appropriately (Mackworth and Bruner, 1970; Zaporozhets, 1965). The fact that young children fail to appreciate the necessity of selectively processing information in the ambient array has a number of implications for eventual production of the response. The significant point to be made here, however, is that selective attention is a process which the child becomes more and more aware of, and as a consequence employs increasingly in the task situation.

In the same vein, it is apparent that as the child matures and gains mastery of a skill, he also gains knowledge of situational demands that determine whether he pays more or less attention to the ongoing movement. Connolly (1970a) has provided some anecdotal evidence on this issue. He related a story of when he took his three-year-old daughter to the local restaurant for a meal. As soon as her attention was drawn from the act of eating, she lost control of the spoon with the result that the food did not reach the intended goal. In other words, some secondary activity in the surrounding distracted or divided her attention when it was necessary for this child to focus fully on the eating behavior if no accidents were to occur. In contrast, his four-year-old daughter was carrying a tray of crockery from the drawing room to the kitchen at home one day, and as she passed by him, Connolly started to talk to her. Immediately, she said to her father in a rather emphatic manner, 'Don't talk to me.' The implication that Connolly drew, and one that seems most reasonable, is that the older daughter seemed to have some knowledge that in order to carry the tray successfully from point A to point B, her full attention on this project was required. Lane (1979) has provided direct evidence of this developmental trend in showing that as children get older they are able to differentiate meaningfully whether a task is primary or secondary as a function of pay-off manipulations. In the same way, adults are often aware of this limitation and make attempts to insure that their attention is focused appropriately when needed. For example, one of us (KMN) often finds himself leaning over to turn the car radio down or off as he leaves the interstate to enter a busy traffic area, which ties in rather nicely with the fact that driving in towns is more attention-demanding than driving on the interstate (Brown and Poulton, 1961).

The gist of these few examples is that as the child gets older, he shows increased knowledge of the attentional demands of skill situations and is flexible enough to adjust his behavior appropriately. Whether the maturing child shows an increased propensity generally for flexibly handling the attentional demands of response production, or whether this behavior is specific to the motor task and/or skill level of the performer remains an empirical question.

Connolly (1970a) proposed that his three-year-old daughter lost control of the spoon because she had not developed the appropriate motor program or subroutine of the act. As a consequence, the movement required some form of feedback control by the child, probably in the form of visual monitoring. The implication is that until a child has reached the stage of preprogramming an action or a sequence of actions, he has to monitor relevant feedback signals and initiate changes in response output where appropriate. This means that the child has to give much more mental capacity or effort to the primary motor task (Kahneman, 1973; Kerr, 1973) with the result that the limit on control capacity is reached more rapidly when time sharing is required. Interestingly, Birch (1976) has shown that seven-year-old children are distracted more by the same secondary task than ten- and thirteen-year-old children, as evidenced in a larger decrement in primary task performance. However, would these apparent developmental differences in attention result if the younger and older children were equated initially with respect to primary task performance? It may be the case that the performance differences in the Birch (1976) study do not reflect a fundamental capacity shift but rather are due to experiential factors which in turn led to different primary task performance levels. Evidence from more recent studies subscribes toward this latter point of view (Birch, 1978; Lane, 1979; see Wickens and Benel, this volume, for amplification).

The central point to be drawn from the above examples is not that the child's information-processing ability may develop as a function of CA, but rather that the child's knowledge or cognizance of the processes pertaining to his own and indeed other persons' action skills also develops. It should be recognized that knowledge about a process pertinent to the production of a response may not develop at the same rate or point in time as the use of that process by the child in the skills situation. For example, it is possible that a child may selectively attend to the relevant stimuli without being aware that he is doing this or why. Thus, actual performance may not provide an accurate picture of the child's awareness of his own information-processing system.

In the same way that a child develops knowledge about his own system and the processes that control it, he apparently also develops an awareness of task or situational variables. In essence this reflects a child's cognizance of the nature of the input factors and includes knowledge of task variables that affect the difficulty level of the motor problem. There are many task parameters that make certain motor skills more difficult than others and certain situations within a skill more difficult. For example, the temporal limitations imposed upon a baseball batter vary as a function of the speed of the pitch; the performance of the same skill in an open as opposed to a closed situation; the use of the nonpreferred hand in comparison to the preferred hand, and so on. This knowledge may arise from experience in the specific motor skill or may be generalizable from skills of a similar class. In addition, certain task information may be more difficult for the younger child to comprehend, and as a consequence even practice in the task will not generate immediate cognizance of the role some task variables play. Indeed, sometimes the exact rules that govern performance on a task are not known even to adults, as Polanyi (1958) has pointed up on the case of bicycle riding. It would seem, however, that a workable understanding of task variables is necessary if schema is to be instantiated appropriately (Judd, 1908).

We have briefly outlined the case where the maturing child gains increased control over his actions, and just as importantly, that he strategically employs this control according to the task demands. It should be apparent that if a veridical picture is to be painted from the outline presented, a considerable research effort needs to be made. As this starts to occur, we will hopefully begin to realize whether this phenomenon of a child's knowledge of the processes controlling his own motor behaviors – a kind of 'metamotorial' knowledge if you will – is a real phenomenon in motor development, or whether it represents merely an epiphenomenon or theoretical explanation in general of something to explain!

In summary, the relative contributions of capacity, strategy, knowledge, and metacognitive factors will vary according to age group and skill together with the task at hand (Flavell, 1970). Capacity clearly plays a strong role in the exercise of phylogenetic skills but its role becomes less as age increases and in the acquisition of ontogenetic skills. Indeed, with more appropriate experimental analysis, it might well become apparent that the traditional developmental variable of maturation is less significant in the acquisition of skilled actions than current evidence suggests. In fact, age may best be considered as a selection variable instead of a true manipulatable independent variable (Wohlwill, 1973).

## 4.3    Invariants

One of the most important theoretical issues in developmental psychology has centered around the notion of invariance, and specifically the idea that we may have invariant tendencies to respond in certain ways over the lifespan. This notion is generalizable to the hypothetical case where the organism acquires action skills through an unchanging perceiving-acting-knowing cycle. In this regard, unchanging refers to the possibility that the same process accounts for the development of knowledge about action independent of chronological age. In view of the preceding section, it is noteworthy that any invariant process is not tied directly to the specific features of a given strategy. That is, depending on the task the same strategy may assume different forms. While strategies and knowledge highlight potential areas of individual differences (in the sense that these experimentally sensitive variables represent the organism's current developmental level), the components of the organism's 'cognitive' repertoire may be acquired via the invariant tendency with which one perceives, acts, and knows.

The notion of an invariant has been traditionally characterized in three principal ways.[2] First, theories of behavior and learning have used invariant to mean the ordered arrangement of behavior or skill (e.g. Gagne, 1965; Piaget, 1952), such that the child is thought to progress through various stages of development. This is the most widely held view of invariance in motor development and is epitomized in the description of the development of phylogenetic motor skills (e.g. Bayley, 1935; Shirley, 1933). In some fundamental skills, invariance may be witnessed within components of an action rather in terms of the whole action (Roberton, 1977; and this volume). A similar characterization of an invariant order is reflected in the traditional idea that complex learning is the compilation of simple (S-R) responses. The essential feature of this theoretical posture is that one stage of an adaptive state follows another more basic stage in the same order for every individual. This notion is based primarily on the assumption that development is explained by (biological) maturation. That is, the child develops physically, which mediates a certain level or stage of cognitive development, which implies that basic competence is required *before* the child can adaptively respond. The logical consequence of this theoretical position is that it is impossible to train a specific action skill if the child is not maturationally ready.

Second, invariant has been used to mean what Werner (1948) has referred to as the 'orthogenetic principle.' That is, 'whenever behavior change occurs it proceeds from a state of relative globality and lack of differentiation to a state of increasing differentiation, articulation and hierarchic integration' (p. 125). While this notion was applied originally to ontogenetic change over the lifespan, it has come to imply also, that independent of age or stage, behavior change occurs in a characteristic way — greater and greater differentiation or focusing. For example, the apparent random to systematic nature of visual scanning strategies follows a similar developmental progression as that apparent in verbal rehearsal strategies (Barclay, 1979; Mackworth and Bruner, 1970; Zaporozhets, 1965). With experience or practice children (young or old) become more efficient in the use of certain strategies. The thrust of this view is that behavior is modifiable through experience and suggests that intervention into the child's environment can produce significant changes, especially in the areas of strategies and knowledge (cf. Siegler, 1978). Indeed, recent interpretations of this hypothesis suggest that development is explained in large part by experience through practice.

Third, invariant is used to mean what Piaget (1952) terms 'invariant function,' that is prototypical tendencies for coping with the environment displayed by all species, including man. For Piaget, when an organism, specifically a child, is presented a task, the content or task characteristics and demands are organized and adapted to. This adaptation occurs through the complementary assimilation and accommodation process which in turn results in structural (schema) change and equilibrium. If the content of the task cannot be assimilated to existing structures, then the structures change, thereby accommodating the content. This notion of invariant as a tendency to respond in certain ways suggests that whatever the task or age of the person, organization and adaptation are high probability responses to environmental stimulation which accounts for the developmental progression (or structural change) through a hierarchy of stages. Each stage of development is thus characterized by a qualitative shift from an earlier stage in the way that content is processed.

Piaget's theoretical posture is not unlike that taken here since it is proposed that the acquisition of knowledge results from an interaction with the environment through perception and action which provides information upon which knowledge is constructed. The construction of knowledge could be explained in Piagetian terms since knowledge is represented in schemata which are acquired and modified through the invariant functions. This knowledge subsequently affects how the child deals with future environmental events since acquired knowledge determines, to some degree, the way in which the child orders the environment. It is our interpretation also that assimilation and accommodation not only represent the adaptation process as an invariant function, but also, these processes mediate the developmental stage a person is in at any point in time. Our emphasis, however, unlike that of Piaget, is more on the effects that experience rather than maturation has on development, except with respect to exercise of phylogenetic skills in infants.

The position here is that regardless of age, maturational level or stage, the growing child deals with the environment in an invariant manner analogous to Piaget's concepts of organization and adaptation. The comparison between Piaget's invariants and our characterization of the acquisition and representation of knowledge is not, however, direct. Since for us what accounts for the greater proportion of developmental differences is not maturation *per se*, but rather the type of tasks and experiences the child is faced with. This suggests that if the task were adjusted to the child's level of competence the manner in which the child processes information and acquires a skill would in large part be independent of CA. Clearly, experimental work needs to establish whether and to what extent age-related differences in ontogenetic action skills can be minimized with appropriate experiences.

## 5    SUMMARY

In this paper we have described certain issues which must be considered in the construction of a theory of motor development. A broad range of ideas were discussed, from the nature of representation to the mechanics of experimental design. Although the advancement of a theory of knowledge about action would undoubtedly be premature, there are emerging trends which would seem to provide the backbone to any theory that might be developed. We have tried to highlight some of these here together with their limitations with respect to theory development.

One major issue was the problem of how knowledge might be represented in the information-processing system. The fundamental concerns were the nature of representation and the structure/organization of knowledge. In one sense, knowledge is the product of the organism-environment interaction. If this assumption is made then knowledge is equivalent to the organism's current level of adaptation. In another sense, knowledge is the process through which the organism interacts with the environment. Given this view, knowledge represents a set of procedures for adaptation. Regardless of whether knowledge is an architectural feature of the system or a tendency to adapt in a certain way, it affords the degree to which the organism adjusts to changing environmental processes.

We have argued that the field of motor development has overplayed the significance of capacity in action development at the expense of knowledge and strategy variables. This bias does not appear to have been based upon empirical findings but rather on the narrow focus given to performance differences over age, probably as a consequence of the early emphasis of the 1920s and 1930s toward physical capacity as the overriding explanatory construct. Of course, it remains to be determined what the relative contribution of capacity, strategy, and knowledge might be in motor skill development but there is sufficient evidence to indicate that experimental factors contribute more than is often recognized. What needs to be understood is that time or CA may not be equated satisfactorily with experience. There are a number of obvious experimental tactics, some of which were mentioned in the body of the paper, that can be and need to be adopted if we are to separate the relative contributions of these factors to the development of skilled action will undoubtedly provide insights on a more general level to the nature-nurture interaction.

In closing, it is probably appropriate to offer a caveat with respect to our ideas of knowledge about action, and in particular, our notions about the role of metacognition. The concern relates to the distinction between tacit and explicit knowledge and more generally the role of cognition in action. First, as we indicated previously, much of our knowledge about action is apparently tacit. By requesting subjects to be explicit on knowledge about action, an erroneous conceptualization could emerge, independent of the normal attendant problems of interview or questionnaire techniques. Second, in pursuing ideas about knowledge and action which can be made explicit, we might be developing theoretical constructs on the basis of what individuals *can* know about skilled action rather than what they *do* know. This concern is a more limited version of a general reservation about enquiry into cognition and skilled action which, through initial biases and subsequent experimental techniques, may be developing theory on the basis of what the system *can do* rather than on what it actually *does do* in the majority of everyday activities.

The above concern should not be taken merely as a typical call for ecological validity (of which it is in part), but rather as a feeling that current experimental tactics of cognitive psychology may, as it were, be putting too much cognition into the system. Demonstrating the limitations of a system can be and often is a useful line of enquiry for theory development. The problem is that the findings of such approaches are often then taken as representative of the usual mode of control, when in actual fact they merely reflect elements of the potential capacity of the system. The reservations expressed above relate to the ideas and experimental tactics of cognitive psychology in general. We raise them here in closing because an issue such as knowledge about action is implicitly, if not explicitly, taken as appropriately analyzed at a cognitive level and, therefore, could potentially invite such misleading approaches. One of the challenges for cognitive psychology is to establish domain assumptions which reduce the degrees of freedom to be controlled by executive functioning (Bernstein, 1967), so that in the long run some compatibility might be established with biological or physical theories of action.

## NOTES

1. This view is exemplified in a recent witty but telling observation of our colleague M. G. Wade who, after reading a manuscript of one of our other not-to-be-mentioned colleagues, observed '... you know, people talk about schema as if it were situated $12\frac{1}{2}$ miles southeast of Peoria.' A more serious discussion of the issue of localization of function may be found in Luria (1966, Chapter 1).
2. The ethological literature also discusses the notion of invariants as fixed action patterns (Eibl-Eibesfeldt, 1970), where a response is said to be constant in form and is associated with a releasing stimulus. Once the response is initiated it continues to completion, regardless of whether the eliciting stimulus remains present.

## REFERENCES

Adams, J. A. (1971). A closed-loop theory of motor learning, *Journal of Motor Behavior*, **3**, 111–150.

Anderson, R. C., Spiro, R. J., and Montague, W. E. (eds.) (1977). *Schooling and the Acquisition of Knowledge*, Hillsdale: NJ: Lawrence Erlbaum.

Atkinson, R. C. and Shiffrin, R. M. (1968). Human memory: A proposed system and its control processes, in K. W. Spence and J. T. Spence (eds), *The Psychology of Learning and Motivation: Advances in research and theory* (Vol. II), New York: Academic Press.

Bandura, A. (1978). The self system in reciprocal determinants, *American Psychologist*, **33**, 344–358.

Barclay, C. R. (1979). The executive control of mnemonic activity, *Journal of Experimental Child Psychology*, **27**, 262–276.

Barclay, C. R., and Newell, K. M. (1980). Children's processing of information in motor skill acquisition, *Journal of Experimental Child Psychology*, **30**, 98–108.

Bartlett, F. C. (1932). *Remembering: A study in experimental and social psychology*, Cambridge: Cambridge University Press.

Baumeister, A. A., and Kellas, G. (1968). Reaction time and mental retardation, in N. R. Ellis (ed.), *International Review of Research in Mental Retardation* (Vol III), New York: Academic Press.

Bayley, N. (1935). The development of motor abilities during the first three years, *Monographs of the Society for Research in Child Development*, **1** (1).

Bergstrom, R. M. (1969). Electrical parameters of the brain during ontogeny, in R. J. Robinson (ed.), *Brain and Early Behavior*, New York: Academic Press.

Bernstein, N. (1967). *The Coordination and Regulation of Movements*, New York: Pergamon.

Bijou, S. W., and Baer, D. M. (1965a). *Child Development: A systematic and empirical theory* (Vol. I), New York: Appleton-Century-Crofts.

Bijou, S. W., and Baer, D. M. (1965b). *Child Development: Universal stage development* (Vol. II), New York: Appleton-Century-Crofts.

Birch, L. L. (1976). Age trends in children's time-sharing performance, *Journal of Experimental Child Psychology*, **22**, 331–345.

Birch, L. L. (1978). Baseline differences, attention, and age differences in time-sharing performance, *Journal of Experimental Child Psychology*, **25**, 505–513.

Bower, G. H. (1972). A selective review of organizational factors in memory, in E. Tulving and W. Donaldson (eds.), *Organization and Memory*, New York: Academic Press.

Bower, T. G. R. (1974). *Development in Infancy*, San Francisco: Freeman.

Bransford, J. D., and Franks, J. J. (1976). Toward a framework for understanding learning, in G. Bower (ed.), *Psychology of Learning and Motivation*, (Vol. 10), New York: Academic Press.

Bransford, J. D., and Johnson, M. K. (1972). Contextual prerequisites for understanding: Some investigations of comprehension and recall, *Journal of Verbal Learning and Verbal Behavior*, **11**, 717–726.

Bransford, J. D., Nitsch, K. E., and Franks, J. J. (1977). Schooling and the facilitation of knowing, in R. C. Anderson, R. J. Spiro, and W. E. Montague (eds.), *Schooling and the Acquisition of Knowledge*, Hillsdale, NJ: Lawrence Erlbaum.

Bronfenbrenner, U. (1977). Toward an experimental ecology of human development, *American Psychologist*, **32**, 513–531.

Broudy, H. S. (1977). Types of knowledge and purposes of education, in R. C. Anderson, R. J. Spiro, and W. E. Montague (eds.), *Schooling and the Acquisition of Knowledge*, Hillsdale, NJ: Lawrence Erlbaum.

Brown, A. L. (1975). The development of memory: Knowing, knowing about knowing, and knowing how to know, in H. W. Reese (ed.), *Advances in Child Development and Behavior* (Vol. 10), New York: Academic Press.

Brown, A. L. (1979). Theories of memory and the problems of development: Activity, growth, and knowledge, in L. S. Cermak and F. I. M. Craik (eds.), *Levels of Processing and Human Memory*, Hillsdale, NJ: Lawrence Erlbaum.

Brown, A. L., Campione, J. C., Bray, N. W., and Wilcox, B. L. (1973). Keeping track of changing variables: Effects of rehearsal training and rehearsal prevention in normal and retarded adolescents, *Journal of Experimental Psychology*, **101**, 123–131.

Brown, I. D., and Poulton, E. C. (1961). Measuring the spare 'mental capacity' of car drivers by a subsidiary task, *Ergonomics*, **4**, 35–40.

Bruner, J. S. (1970). The growth and structure of skill, in K. J. Connolly (ed.), *Mechanisms of Motor Skill Development*, London: Academic Press.

Bruner, J. S. (1973). Organization of early skilled action, *Child Development*, **44**, 1–11.

Care, N. S., and Landesman, C. (1968). *Readings in the Theory of Action*, Scarborough, Ontario: Fitzhenry and Whiteside.

Carey, S. (1974). Cognitive competence, in K. Connolly and J. Bruner (eds.), *The Growth of Competence*, New York: Academic Press.

Chi, M. T. H. (1977). Age differences in memory span, *Journal of Experimental Child Psychology*, **23**, 266–281.

Chi, M. T. H. (1978). Knowledge structures and cues, in R. S. Siegler (ed.), *Children's Thinking: What Develops?* Hillsdale, NJ: Lawrence Erlbaum.

Collins, A. M., and Loftus, E. F. (1975). A spreading-activation theory of semantic processing, *Psychological Review*, **82**, 407–428.

Connolly, K. J. (1970a). Response speed, temporal sequencing and information processing in children, in K. J. Connolly (ed.), *Mechanisms of Motor Skill Development*, New York: Academic Press.

Connolly, K. J. (1970b). Skill development: Problems and plans, in K. J. Connolly, (ed.), *Mechanisms of Motor Skill Development*, London: Academic Press.

Connolly, K. J. (1973). Factors influencing the learning of manual skills by young children, in R. A. Hinde and J. Stevenson-Hinde (eds.), *Constraints on Learning*, London: Academic Press.

Day, M. C. (1975). Developmental trends in visual scanning, in H. W. Reese (ed.), *Advances in Child Development and Behavior* (Vol. 10), New York: Academic Press.

Eibl-Eibesfeldt, T. (1970). *Ethology: The biology of behavior*, New York: Holt, Rinehart and Winston.

Elliott, J., and Connolly, K. (1974). Hierarchial structure in the development of skill, in K. Connolly and J. Bruner (eds.), *The Development of Competence in Childhood*, London: Academic Press.

Evarts, E. V. (1967). Representation of movements and muscles by pyramidal tract neurons of the perceptual motor cortex, in M. D. Yahr and D. P. Purpura (eds.), *Neurophysiological Basis of Normal and Abnormal Motor Activities*, New York: Raven.

Evarts, E. V., Bizzi, E., Burke, E., DeLong, M., and Thach, W. T. (1971). Central control of movement, *Neurosciences Research Program Bulletin*, **9**, No. 1.

Fitts, P. M., and Posner, M. I. (1967). *Human Performance*, Belmont, CA: Brooks/Cole.

Flavell, J. H. (1970). Developmental studies of mediated memory, in H. W. Reese and L. P. Lisitt (eds.), *Advances in Child Development and Behavior* (Vol. 5), New York: Academic Press.

Flavell, J. H., and Wellman, H. M. (1977). Metamemory, in R. V. Kail and J. W. Hagen (eds.), *Developmental Perspectives on Memory and Cognition*. Hillsdale, NJ: Lawrence Erlbaum.

Fowler, C. A. (1977). *Timing Control in Speech Production*, Bloomington: Indiana Linguistics Club.

Fowler, C. A., Rubin, P., Remez, R. E., and Turvey, M. T. (1980). Implications for speech production of a general theory of action, in B. Butterworth (ed.), *Language Production*, New York: Academic Press.

Gagne, R. M. (1965). *The Conditions of Learning*, New York: Holt, Rinehart, & Winston.

Gentile, A. M. (1972). A working model of skill acquisition with application to teaching, *Quest*, **17**, 3–23.

Gesell, A. (1929). Maturation and infant behavior pattern, *Psychological Review*, **36**, 307–319.

Gibson, J. J. (1977). The theory of affordances, in R. Shaw and J. Bransford (eds.), *Perceiving, Acting, and Knowing: Toward an ecological psychology*, Hillsdale, NJ: Lawrence Erlbaum.

Gibson, J. J., and Gibson, E. J. (1955). Perceptual learning: Differentiation or enrichment? *Psychological Review*, **62**, 32–41.

Ginsberg, H., and Opper, S. (1969). *Piaget's Theory of Intellectual Development*, Englewood Cliffs, NJ: Prentice-Hall.

Glencross, D. J. (1974). Pauses in repetitive speed skill, *Perceptual and Motor Skills*, **38**, 246.

Gold, M. W. (1975). Vocational training, in J. Wortis (eds.), *Mental Retardation and Developmental Disabilities: An annual review* (Vol. 1), Mazel: Brunner.

Goodnow, J., and Levine, R. A. (1973). The grammar of action: Sequence and syntax in children's copying, *Cognitive Psychology*, **4**, 82–98.

Goulet, L. R., and Baltes, P. B. (eds.) (1970). *Life Span Developmental Psychology: Research and theory*, New York: Academic Press.

Goulet, L. R., Hay, C., and Barclay, C. R. (1974). Sequential analysis and developmental research methods: Descriptions of cyclic phenomena, *Psychological Bulletin*, **81**, 517–521.

Gross, Y., Webb, R., and Melzack, R. (1974). Central and peripheral contributions to localization of body parts: Evidence for the central body schema, *Experimental Neurology*, **44**, 346–362.

Halverson, H. (1931). An experimental study of prehension in infants by means of systematic cinema records, *Genetic Psychology Monographs*, **10**, 107–286.

Head, H. (1926). *Aphasia and Kindred Disorders of Speech* (Vol, 1), New York: Macmillan.

Hendrickson, G., and Schroeder, W. H. (1941). Transfer of training in learning to hit a submerged target, *Journal of Educational Psychology*, **32**, 205–213.

Hilgard, E. R. (1977). *Divided Consciousness: Multiple controls in human thought and action*, New York: Wiley.

Judd, C. H. (1908). The relation of special training to general intelligence, *Educational Review*, **36**, 28–42.

Kahneman, D. (1973). *Attention and Effort*, Englewood Cliffs, NJ: Prentice-Hall.

Kay, H. (1970). Analyzing motor skill performance, in K. J. Connolly (ed.), *Mechanisms of Motor Skill Development*, London: Academic Press.

Keele, S. W. (1968). Movement control in skilled motor performance, *Psychological Bulletin*, **70**, 387–403.

Kerr, B. (1973). Processing demands during mental operations, *Memory and Cognition*, **1**, 401–412.

Kerr, R. (1975). Movement control and maturation in elementary-grade children, *Perceptual and Motor Skills*, **41**, 151–154.

Klapp, S. T. (1977). Reaction time analysis of programmed control, in R. S. Hutton (ed.), *Exercise and Sport Sciences Reviews* (Vol. 5), Santa Barbara, CA: Journal Publishing Affiliates.

Knapp, C. G., and Dixon, W. R. (1952). Learning to juggle II. Study of whole and part methods, *Research Quarterly*, **23**, 398–401.

Kopp, C. B. (1979). Perspectives on infant motor system development, in M. H. Bornstein and W. Kessen (eds.), *Psychological Development from Infancy: Image to intention*. Hillsdale, NJ: Lawrence Erlbaum.

Lagerspetz, K., Nygard, M., and Stranduick, C. (1971). The effects of training in crawling on the motor and mental development of infants, *Scandinavian Journal of Psychology*, **12**, 192–197.

Lane, D. M. (1974). Developmental changes in attention-deployment skills, *Journal of Experimental Child Psychology*, **28**, 16–29.

Luria, A. R. (1966). *Higher Cortical Functions in Man*, New York: Basic Books.

Mackworth, N. H., and Bruner, J. S. (1970). How adults and children search and recognize pictures, *Human Development*, **13**, 149–177.

Markman, E. M. (1973). Factors affecting the young child's ability to monitor his memory, unpublished doctoral dissertation, University of Pennsylvania.

McGraw, M. B. (1935). *Growth: A study of Johnny and Jimmy*, New York: Appleton Century.

Miller, G. A., Galanter, E., and Pribram, K. H. (1960). *Plans and the Structure of Behavior*, New York: Henry Holt.

Minas, S. C. (1978). Mental practice of a complex perceptual-motor skill, *Journal of Human Movement Studies*, **4**, 102–107.

Mischel, T. (1969). Scientific and philosophical psychology: A historical introduction, in T. Mischel (ed.), *Human Action*, New York: Academic Press.

Morin, R. E., and Forvin, B. (1965). Information-processing: Choice reaction times of first- and third-grade students for two types of associations, *Child Development*, **36**, 713–720.

Mowbray, G. H., and Rhoades, M. U. (1959). On the reduction of choice reaction times with practice, *Quarterly Journal of Experimental Psychology*, **11**, 16–23.

Neisser, U. (1976). *Cognition and Reality*, San Francisco: Freeman.

Newell, K. M. (1978). Some issues on action plans, in G. E. Stelmach (ed.), *Information Processing in Motor Learning and Control*, New York: Academic Press.

Newell, K. M. (1981). Skill learning, in D. H. Holding (ed.), *Human Skills*, New York: Wiley.

Newell, K. M., and Kennedy, J. A. (1978). Knowledge of results and children's motor learning, *Developmental Psychology*, **14**, 531–536.

Newell, K. M., and Shapiro, D. C. (1976). Variability of practice and transfer of training: Some evidence toward a schema view of motor learning, *Journal of Motor Behavior*, **8**, 233–243.

Ninio, A., and Lieblich, A. (1976). The grammar of action: 'Phrase structure' in children's copying, *Child Development*, **47**, 846–849.

Norman, D. A., and Bobrow, D. G. (1979). Descriptions: An intermediate stage in memory retrieval, *Cognitive Psychology*, **11**, 107–123.

Norman, D. A., Rumelhart, D. E., and the LNR Research Group (1975). *Explorations in Cognition*. San Francisco: Freeman.

Pascual-Leone, J. (1970). A mathematical model for the transition rule in Piaget's developmental stages, *Aca Psychologica*, **32**, 310–345.

Pew, R. W. (1974a). Human perceptual-motor performance, in B. J. Kantowitz (ed.), *Human Information Processing: Tutorials in performance and Cognition*, Hillsdale, NJ: Lawrence Erlbaum.

Pew, R. W. (1974b). Levels of analysis in motor control, *Brain Research*, **71**, 393–400.

Piaget, J. (1952). *The Origins of Intelligence in Children*, New York: International Universities Press.

Piaget, J. (1970). *Structuralism*, New York: Harper Row.

Piaget, J. (1971). *Biology and Knowledge*, Chicago: University of Chicago Press.

Piaget, J. (1976). *The Grasp of Consciousness: Action and concept in the young child*, Cambridge MA: Harvard University Press.

Piaget, J. (1978). *Success and Understanding*, Cambridge, MA: Harvard University Press.

Polanyi, M. (1958). *Personal Knowledge: Towards a post-critical philosophy*, London: Routledge & Kegan Paul.

Poulton, E. C. (1957). On prediction in skilled movements, *Psychological Bulletin*, **54**, 467–479.

Roberton, M. A. (1977). Stability of stage categorization across trials: Implications for the 'stage theory' of overarm throw development, *Journal of Human Movement Studies*, **3**, 49–59.

Rosche, E. (1975). Universals and cultural specifies in human categorization, in R. Brislin, S. Bochern, and W. Lonner (eds.), *Cross-cultural Perspectives on Learning*, New York: Sage-Halsted

Rumelhart, D. E., and Ortony, A. (1977). The representation of knowledge in memory, in R. C. Anderson, R. J. Spiro, and W. E. Montague (eds.), *Schooling and the Acquisition of Knowledge*, Hillsdale, NJ: Lawrence Erlbaum.

Schaie, K. W. (1965). A general model for the study of developmental problems, *Psychological Bulletin*, **64**, 92–107.

Schank, R. C., and Abelson, R. P. (1977). *Scripts, Plans, Goals and Understanding*, Hillsdale, NJ: Lawrence Erlbaum.

Schmidt, R. A. (1975). A schema theory of discrete motor skill learning, *Psychological Review*, **82**, 225–260.

Schmidt, R. A. (1976). The schema as a solution to some persistent problems in motor learning theory, in G. E. Stelmach (ed.), *Motor Control: Issues and trends*, New York: Academic Press.

Schulte, F. J., Linke, I., Michaelis, R., and Nolte, R. (1969). Excitation, inhibition and impulse conduction in spinal motoneurones of preterin, term and small-for-dates newborn infants, in R. J. Robinson (ed.), *Brain and Early Behavior*, New York: Academic Press.

Shirley, M. M. (1931). *The First Two Years: A study of twenty-five babies, Vol. 1, Postural and locomotor development*, Minneapolis: University of Minnesota Press.

Siegler, R. S. (ed.) (1978). *Children's thinking: What develops?* Hillsdale, NJ: Lawrence Erlbaum.

Simon, H. A. (1972). On the development of the processor, in S. Farnham-Diggory (ed.), *Information Processing in Children*, New York: Academic Press.

Stelmach, G. E. (1974). Retention of motor skills, in H. J. Wilmore (ed.), *Reviews of Exercise and Sports Sciences* (Vol. II), New York: Academic Press.

Tanner, J. (1962). *Growth at Adolescence*, 2nd Eds Oxford: Blackwell.

Thorndike, E. L. (1931). *Human Learning*, New York: Century.

Trevarthen, C. (1978). Modes of perceiving and modes of acting, in H. L. Pick and E. Saltzman (eds.), *Modes of Perceiving and Processing Information*, Hillsdale, NJ: Lawrence Erlbaum.

Tulving, E. (1979). Memory research: What kind of progress? in L. G. Nilsson (ed.), *Perspectives on Memory Research: Essays in honor of Uppsala University's 500th Anniversary*, Hillsdale, NJ: Lawrence Erlbaum.

Tulving, E., and Madigan, S. A. (1970). Memory and verbal learning, *Annual Review of Psychology*, **21**, 437–484.

Tulving, E., and Pearlstone, Z. (1966). Availability versus accessibility of information in memory forwards, *Journal of Verbal Learning and Verbal Behavior*, **5**, 381–391.

Turvey, M. T. (1977). Preliminaries to a theory of action with reference to vision, in R. Shaw and J. Bransford (eds.), *Perceiving, Acting, and Knowing: Toward an ecological psychology*, Hillsdale, NJ: Lawrence Erlbaum.

Turvey, M. T., and Shaw, R. (1979). The primacy of perceiving: An ecological reformulation of perception for understanding memory, in L-G. Nilsson (ed.), *Perspectives on Memory Research: Essays in honor of Uppsala University's 500th Anniversary*, Hillsdale, NJ: Lawrence Erlbaum.

Wade, M. G. (1976). Developmental motor learning, in J. Keogh and R. S. Hutton (eds.), *Exercise and Sport Science Reviews* (Vol. IV), Santa Barbara, CA: Journal Publishing Affiliates.

Wade, M. G., Newell, K. M., and Wallace, S. A. (1978). Decision time and movement time as a function of response complexity in retarded persons, *American Journal of Mental Deficiency*, **83**, 135–144.

Walshe, F. M. R. (1943). On the mode of representation of movements in the motor cortex, with special reference to 'convulsions beginning unilaterally' (Jackson), *Brain*, **66**, 104–139.

Waterland, J. C. (1970). The harmonies of movement recorded electromyography, *Perceptual and Motor Skills*, **31**, 1001–1002.

Welford, A. T. (1958). *Aging and Human Skill*, Oxford: Oxford University Press.

Welford, A. T. (1976). What can be trained? *Journal of Human Movement Studies*, **2**, 53–63.

Werner, H. (1948). *Comparative Psychology of Mental Development*, Chicago: Follet.

Wickens, C. D. (1974). Temporal limits of human information processing: A developmental study, *Psychological Bulletin*, **91**, 739–755.

Wohlwill, J. F. (1970). The age variable in psychological research, *Psychological Review*, **77**, 49–64.

Wohlwill, J. F. (1973). *The Study of Behavioral Development*, New York: Academic Press.

Zaporozhets, A. V. (1965). The development of perception in the preschool child, in P. H. Mussen (ed.), *European Research in Cognitive Development: Monographs of the society for research in child development*, **30** (2 Whole No. 100).

Zelazo, P., Zelazo, N., and Kolb, S. (1972). 'Walking' in the newborn, *Science*, **177**, 1058–1059.

Zigler, E. (1969). Developmental versus different theories of mental retardation and the problem of motivation, *American Journal of Mental Deficiency*, **73**, 536–556.

The Development of Movement Control and Co-ordination
Edited by J. A. S. Kelso and J. E. Clark
© 1982, John Wiley & Sons, Ltd

# CHAPTER 7

# A Model for Movement Confidence[1]

NORMA S. GRIFFIN AND JACK F. KEOGH

The confidence or assurance with which an individual approaches a movement situation should be an important determinant of what an individual will choose to do and how adequate the movement performance will be. The level of confidence of an individual likely will influence how information about a movement situation is processed and utilized, thus leading to important changes in movement skill development. A working model will be presented to describe movement confidence as both a consequence and a mediator in an involvement cycle. The model provides a framework around which the functioning of movement confidence can be traced and existing literature can be organized. Several developmental concerns will be discussed in the concluding portion of the paper. Before the model is presented, we want to provide some general comments about movement confidence, and introduce sensory experiences of moving as an important and integral aspect of movement confidence. Our preliminary comments also are intended to illustrate the importance of movement confidence in studying movement skill development.

## MOVEMENT CONFIDENCE

Confidence is a general term, often used in a nonspecific way, to indicate an individual sense of competence (Connolly and Bruner, 1974) or efficacy (Bandura, 1977). Harter (1978) recognized that a sense of competence or effectiveness might be different for cognitive, social, and physical (movement) situations. As a general definition, we are viewing movement confidence as an individual feeling of adequacy in a movement situation. Movement confidence needs to be studied as a type of confidence. The study of movement confidence should be expanded beyond the ability notion of competence to include the evaluation an individual makes of sensory experiences directly related to

213

moving. We also wish to emphasize that movement confidence involves a cognitive evaluation of self in relation to task demands. The evaluation process, as an outcome or consequence, produces a sense of movement confidence that then mediates or influences several aspects of participation in movement situations. Movement confidence will be traced through an involvement cycle, illustrated in Figure 1, to identify movement confidence as both a consequence and a mediator.

Movement confidence is viewed as a consequence of a personal (performer) evaluation of self in relation to the demands of a movement situation. The product of the evaluation is a two-factor personal assessment, one a factor we are calling MOVCOMP (MOVement COMPetence: personal skill in relation to task demands) and the second a factor we are calling MOVSENSE (personal expectations of sensory experiences related to moving). Perceived MOVCOMP and perceived MOVSENSE interact to produce a sense or state of movement confidence. Movement confidence then functions to mediate or influence variables which affect three aspects of participation: (i) participation choice, whether to become involved or not; (ii) participation performance, how the individual will do whatever the individual chooses to do; (iii) participation persistence, whether to continue involvement now and in the future. The involvement cycle likely will be a positive spiral for the confident individual, more likely to seek and choose participation and to perform and behave in ways that are satisfying to the individual. The involvement cycle likely will be a negative spiral for the unconfident individual, less likely to seek and choose participation and less likely that participation performance and behavior will be satisfying to the individual.

The involvement cycle is similar to what is proposed in general explanations of competence (Coelho, Hamburg, and Adams, 1974; White, 1978), achievement motivation (Atkinson, 1964), intrinsic motivation (Deci, 1975) and causal attributions (Weiner, 1974). An individual, when approaching a situation, will generate expectations that will influence choice, intensity (performance), and

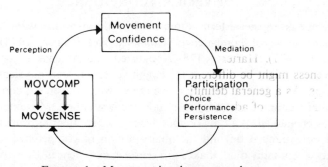

FIGURE 1    Movement involvement cycle

persistence. We are proposing an important additional consideration for movement situations in terms of the sensory experiences which are directly related to
moving. A wide range of sensory experiences is possible when a person moves,
including muscle aches, perspiration, and breathing hard. Moving also may
lead to the sensing of speed, changes in body position, and the pain of injury.
When an individual evaluates a movement situation, sensory experiences of
many kinds are expected, depending upon what the individual is considering as
a plan of action. The individual will evaluate the expected sensory experiences
as desirable or undesirable. The individual may seek particular sensations of
moving and may avoid others or at least may be a reluctant and tentative
participant.

Perceived MOVCOMP unquestionably is an important influence on
participation but MOVSENSE also needs to be considered as an important
influence. It seems likely that early movement skill development will be
influenced more by MOVSENSE than MOVCOMP in that the sensory
experiences of moving are primary when attempting new movement tasks.
Infants and young children in learning to walk and jump must learn what are
the expected sensory experiences related to moving in these different ways as
well as determine their personal preferences for such sensory experiences.
Sensory experiences related to moving sometimes become effects to be sought
in their own right, thus becoming important parts of the outcomes to be
achieved.

Sensory experiences related to moving are an integral part of all movement
activities, although the extent and intensity of sensory experiences generally
will be greater when the body mass is displaced more. Doing a forward roll
involves more muscle activity sensations and a considerable change in body
position sensations, in contrast to sitting while moving a lever or using a pair of
scissors. Also, it is important to differentiate between how we feel about
moving and how movement makes us feel, a distinction that is seldom made.
Enjoying a particular sensation of moving, such as moving fast, is not the same
as exercise making one feel relaxed or exhilarated, or competition being exciting. The recent study by Bain (1979) illustrates the wide range of values that
might be related to how movement makes us feel.

A distinction needs to be made between MOVCOMP and MOVSENSE
which can be done by viewing them as related to different aspects of movement
performance: movement and moving. Achievement outcomes (MOVCOMP)
are effects produced by the total action or movement (e.g. doing a forward
roll). Sensory outcomes (MOVSENSE) are sensory effects produced by the
moving, independent of any achievement outcomes (e.g. the sensation of
turning upside down). It is difficult to articulate a single term or concise phrase
which connotes both the complex evaluation process and the product we are
identifying as MOVSENSE. The essence of the factor is movement sensations.

The evaluation process involves projecting oneself into the moving before it occurs, identifying expected sensory experiences directly related to the anticipated moving, and determining the personal desirability of the anticipated sensory experiences. The product is MOVSENSE, the anticipated moving sensations which are parallel to but different from MOVCOMP.

Personal feelings about movement and moving have not been studied in a systematic and continuous manner. Movement concept (Caskey, 1973) and movement satisfaction (Tanner, 1969) have been used as constructs in studying how participants feel about their movements, generally their movement skill or competence. The general research approach for studies of this nature is illustrated in the one published study (Maul and Thomas, 1975) which was located. No models or conceptual frameworks have evolved from this line of work and no effort has been made logically or experimentally to examine these constructs (Shavelson, Hubner, and Stanton, 1976).

Movement confidence is multidimensional and goes beyond the limits of this paper to include personal-social aspects of participation in many kinds of movement situations. The initial formulation of our model is focused on movement competence and sensations of moving as the basic concerns in studying movement skill development.

## MOVEMENT CONFIDENCE MODEL

A model for movement confidence will be presented in two parts. Movement confidence will first be described as an outcome or a *consequence* of a personal evaluation process. Movement confidence will then be described as a *mediator* to influence several aspects of participation, particularly movement performance. Although the two parts of the model are discussed separately to provide a clearer picture of each part, the model covers the total involvement cycle presented in Figure 1. The overall concern in the model is the manner and extent to which movement confidence is important in explaining various aspects of participation in specified movement situations. The first step will be to identify what is movement confidence in terms of how changes in two major elements of a personal evaluation process will lead to expected changes in movement confidence. The second step will be to indicate the relationship of changes in movement confidence to changes in participation performance.

### Movement Confidence as a Consequence

As an individual approaches a movement situation, a personal evaluation is made, probably in the general manner described in Figure 2. The personal evaluation process has three phases, as identified in the top of Figure 2, occurring somewhat in a sequence to produce a level of movement confidence for the

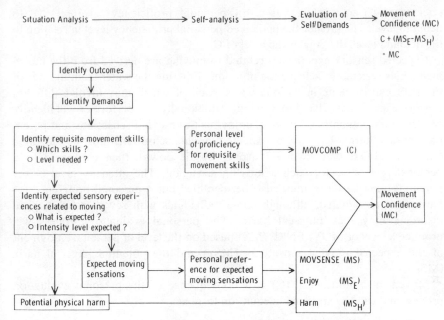

FIGURE 2    Personal evaluation of a movement situation to produce a level of movement confidence

particular movement situation. The movement situation is analyzed to identify
what the individual perceives as the outcomes to be achieved. The perceived
outcomes are then analyzed to identify the situation demands in terms of what
are the movement skills needed to achieve the outcomes and what are the
expected sensory experiences related to moving (when doing the requisite
movement skills). A self-analysis is made to check personal levels of
proficiency and preference. The analysis of self is compared to the perceived
situation demands which produces a level of movement confidence for the
particular movement situation. The personal evaluation process will be
examined in detail to derive a general equation as a formal definition of movement confidence.

Assuming that an individual has identified the outcome to be achieved, a
movement skill must be selected as the means of achieving the desired
outcome. Some estimate also must be made of the proficiency level needed. If I
am preparing to enter the water from the side of the pool, I must decide
whether to enter feet first or head first, with many other options possible. Also,
how precisely or skillfully must I make the entry, perhaps to avoid others? A
check must be made of my personal level of proficiency for the various water-
entry skills I am considering. A level of MOVCOMP (C) is established for the

selected water-entry skill, based on personal proficiency level relative to demand level. The greater the perceived personal proficiency level in relation to the demand level, the greater the level of C.

Expected sensory experiences related to moving are derived from the movement skills selected to achieve the outcome. Entering the water from the side of the pool can be done in various ways, each of which may involve different sensory experiences related to moving. Additionally, the performer will identify two different outcomes of moving, enjoyment of moving sensations and potential physical harm. The level of expected moving sensations must be identified (e.g. a head-first dive involves turning upside down), then compared to a personal preference for such a moving sensation. The intensity level of the potential physical harm must also be identified but a personal preference for harm is not evaluated, although some individuals with severe psychological disorders may seek physical harm. The personal evaluation process will produce a level of MOVSENSE (MS) based on the level of personal enjoyment of the expected moving sensations $(MS_E)$ and the potential physical harm $(MS_H)$.

Movement confidence (MC) is a consequence of the personal evaluation process and can be expressed in equation form as:

$$C + (MS_E - MS_H) = MC.$$

The general sense of the equation is that MOVCOMP (C) is modified by MOVSENSE $(MS_E - MS_H)$ to produce a state of confidence for a particular movement situation. As noted earlier, confidence often is used in a nonspecific way as a sense of competence or efficacy. This would be expressed for movement situations as $C = MC$, which would be a redundancy in that a measure of competence would be a measure of movement confidence. We are adding MOVSENSE, which expands movement confidence to a fuller meaning beyond the limited sense of movement competence. Our equation provides a beginning point to express the general nature of relationships which can be tested. Refinements and additions can be made but it is important to begin with a simple, manageable set of relationships.

$MS_E$ and $MS_H$ are proposed for simplicity as additive in relation to MOVCOMP (C). However, it seems likely that $MS_H$ is more complicated than is represented in the equation. $MS_H$ is an identification of the expectation for physical harm, including the level of seriousness and the probability of occurence. Each individual in a movement situation should recognize the same potential physical harm and what the harm would mean in terms of pain and injury. However, the probability of physical harm should be lessened as C increases. Thus, $MS_H$ should vary as C varies. On entering the pool from a 10-meter board, pain and injury are possible but less likely if the performer is more skillful, presumably more competent. $MS_H$ is recognized at this point only as lowering the level of movement confidence or having no effect if no physical harm is perceived as possible. The more complex interaction with level of competence needs to be resolved along with the recognition that physical harm must be evaluated in terms of both seriousness and probability.

Considering the general equation, changes in MOVCOMP (C) and MOVSENSE ($MS = MS_E - MS_H$) will produce changes in movement confidence (MC), somewhat in the manner illustrated in Figure 3. If MS is zero, enjoyment of moving sensations is neutral and no physical harm is perceived. The equation then reduces to $C = MC$ which is illustrated by the diagonal line $MS^0$ in Figure 3. A change in C will be reflected directly in a change in MC. The diagonal $MS^0$ provides a point of reference for considering changes in level of MC when MS is positive or negative.

If MS is positive, MC will be increased beyond the level predicted by C, as illustrated by the upper line $MS^+$ in Figure 3. The effect of $MS^+$ on MC is additive but not to provide a simple, linear increase. At a lower level of C, MC could be at a relatively higher level if an individual had a very high level of MS. A very high level of MS would mean a low level of $MS_H$, that no physical danger is likely, and a high level of enjoyment ($MS_E$) is anticipated for the moving sensations. Moving sensations could become an important outcome to be achieved such that an individual would have a moderate level of movement confidence in the movement situation even though low in C. As C increases, particularly to reach very high levels, the addition of MS may have a negligible effect on MC. Positive MS is a more important determinant of MC at lower levels of C than at higher levels of C.

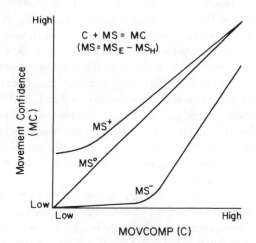

FIGURE 3   Level of movement confidence (MC) in relation to MOVCOMP (C) and three levels of MOVSENSE (MS)

If MS is negative, the lowering of MC may be quite marked. A very negative MS means that an individual expects the moving sensations to be unpleasant and perceives a high expectancy of physical harm. As illustrated in the lower line $MS^-$ in Figure 3, the level of MC will decrease at a relatively greater rate than the decrease in C until a zero level of MC is reached, even though the level of C may be in a middle range. A high level of C may be sufficient to maintain MC above the zero floor level but a very negative level of MS will be an important determinant of level of MC.

The relationship of MOVCOMP (C) to movement confidence (MC) is assumed to be direct and linear. The relationship of MOVSENSE (MS) to MC is more complicated because different combinations of $MS_E$ and $MS_H$ must be considered. Even if $MS_E$ and $MS_H$ are added separately in the equation, rather than summed to provide a measure of MS, certain levels of these two elements of MS may interact to produce equivocal expectancies for the individual, thus for the researcher. An individual may like the moving sensations but may expect a high probability of sustaining a serious injury. Such combinations will need to be considered when formulating more precise predictions of levels of movement confidence.

A general set of predictions about level of movement confidence begins with the expectation that level of movement confidence (MC) is predicted by level of MOVCOMP (C). If MOVSENSE (MS) is positive, MC will be increased more when C is at a lower rather than at a higher level. If MS is neutral (zero), level of MC will be determined by level of C. If MS is negative, MC may be lowered quite markedly.

Change in movement confidence also can be achieved by changing important aspects of the movement situation demands. Returning to the personal evaluation process in Figure 2, perceived demands of the situation and a self-analysis are combined in one evaluation to determine a level of MOVCOMP (MC) and in a second evaluation to determine a level of MOVSENSE (MS). Assuming that the perception from each self-analysis is stable and changes only with active participation, then C and $MS_E$ cannot vary markedly or quickly unless the perceived demands are changed. The same reasoning holds for $MS_H$ in terms of identifying physical harm in the movement situation. Situation demands can change quite rapidly only if the *perceptions* of the individual in the same situation can be changed and if the *situation* is changed in significant ways.

Abrupt changes in level of movement confidence may be expected when an individual is participating in a new or unfamiliar situation. Initial perceptions of the demands of a movement situation may be quite naive, either positively or negatively, such that initial participation may produce a rather quick change in perceived demand and level of movement confidence. The first trip down a slide may be perceived as fast but just right. After one trip, some children will find the moving not as fast as anticipated, whereas others will confirm their anticipation or will realize that the moving was faster than they anticipated. Familiarity can produce a marked change in perceived level of demand, either positively or negatively, with a corresponding change in level of movement confidence.

Demands of the movement situation can be changed directly by the participant or others. The participant can lower situation demands, for example, by going slower and holding the hand of another person or can raise situation demands by going faster and not accepting the support of others. Another person, such as a parent or a teacher, can also alter the skill and sensory experience demands by changing aspects of the movement situation. The important point is that movement situation demands can be changed more rapidly than the more stable self-analysis. This general point has considerable application for parents and teachers in arranging appropriate developmental experiences (Griffin and Keogh, in press).

Movement confidence as a consequence or an outcome has been discussed in terms of an immediate situation. Movement confidence must also be considered in terms of achievement of long-term rather than immediate objectives. An individual might have a long-term sense that in time he/she can be effective and assured in this type of movement situation. The participant likely will have a higher than expected level of movement confidence in the immediate movement situation, probably with a high level of MOVSENSE and a low level of MOVCOMP. The long-term perspective of individuals must eventually be considered in the personal evaluation process.

## Movement Confidence as a Mediator

### Participation

The participation phase of the involvement cycle is elaborated in Figure 4 and will be described briefly as a basis for identifying the mediation role of movement confidence in relation to participation choice, performance and persistence. The left side of Figure 4 traces the participation of an individual whereas the right side of Figure 4 indicates nonparticipation, which may occur at several decision points. As a general observation, participation provides information which is added to an individual's experiences for future use in the personal evaluation process. If an individual chooses not to participate, participation information will not be created which means that information about the demands of the movement situation and related self-analyses will not change, at least not as a direct result of movement participation. One participation experience is diagrammed in Figure 4 with all participation information and noninformation returning to the individual for use in evaluation of subsequent participation opportunities.

Participation choice, whether to become involved or not, will be determined

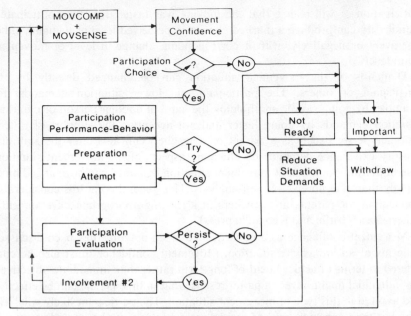

FIGURE 4     Participation phase of the movement involvement cycle

by many factors, including the importance or value an individual attaches to participation at a particular time and personal attributes which are more general dispositions. An example is the decision not to participate, noted in the right side of Figure 4, because involvement at this time is not important even though the individual may be confident in this movement situation. We are limiting our discussion in this paper to active participation, however eager or reluctant the participant may be. We will deal only with active participation because our primary concern is the functioning of movement confidence as a mediator to influence movement performance. Participation persistence, as the third aspect of participation, is essentially the same as participation choice, except the participant must now decide whether or not to participate again. We will include some discussion of participation persistence because it relates directly to learning and development of movement skills, thus to a long-term perspective of movement confidence.

Assuming that an individual decides to participate, some preparation for the movement attempt is often necessary. The participant might do the preparation activities, such as climbing the ladder to the diving platform, but decide not to attempt the movement or dive. If not participating beyond preparation, the individual would enter the negative cycle at the right of Figure 4 and would add only limited participation information for the next personal evaluation process.

If the participant does decide to attempt the movement, the level of achievement may be influenced by the level of movement confidence. The influence upon achievement is our primary concern and will be elaborated after all portions of Figure 4 have been reviewed. It is important to note that the movement behaviors of the participant, as differentiated from movement performance achievements, may also be influenced by the level of movement confidence. For example, the participant may hesitate or make unnecessary movements in ways that are viewed as behavioral manifestations or indicators of lack of movement confidence, a topic to be discussed in a later section. Movement behaviors are included in Figure 4 by noting 'Performance-Behavior' as participation outcomes.

The negative or right side of Figure 4 is entered if an individual decides 'No' instead of 'Yes' at any of the three decision points. If the decision not to participate is that the individual is 'not ready,' two options are possible. The participant may withdraw, which limits the amount and kind of participation information available for subsequent personal evaluation processes. The second option is to reduce situation demands, as noted in the previous section, by changing perceptions of the immediate demands or changing the demands. Reduction of situation demands may also occur passively, perhaps as a function of time wherein changes in physical structure-function, personal-social behavior and movement skills may alter the personal evaluation processes. When the level of MOVCOMP and/or MOVSENSE is increased, the movement situation may be approached again. A decision of 'No' at later points in participation will involve the same two options but with different amounts and kinds of participation information available.

## Movement Confidence and Movement Performance

The basic proposition in our model is that movement confidence is a mediator, as diagrammed in Figure 5, in the processing of information related to movement performance. The proposition begins with the assumption that performance of movement skills is determined in large part by the processing of internal and external information, along the lines described by Marteniuk (1976) for adults and with considerations for children as suggested by Keogh (1981). Looking at Figure 5 but ignoring the role of movement confidence for the moment, perceptual and cognitive processing operations will evaluate available information, will create additional information, and will make decisions about the what, when, and how of the movement situation. If an individual decides to participate, the level of movement performance will be affected by the nature and quality of the information processing output, both preceding and during movement execution.

An important determinant of movement performance adequacy is attention

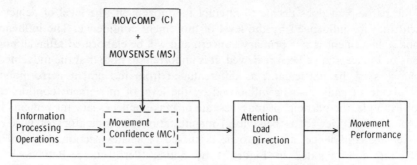

FIGURE 5    The role of movement confidence as a mediator in the processing
of information related to movement performance

in terms of load and direction. Attention load can be increased in many ways, including the addition of more information (e.g. more participants), an increased rate of presentation of information (e.g. participants move faster), and the presence of unknown information (e.g. new participants). Attention direction is what the participant selects as the information of importance, sometimes resulting in using the wrong information or excessive focusing of attention (e.g. watching the new participant while neglecting known participants). As information load increases and attention is misdirected, by whatever means, a point will be reached where the performance of an individual will be adversely affected.

We are proposing that the level of movement confidence will have an influence upon information-processing operations in terms of contributing directly to attention load and direction, thus indirectly to the achievement of desired movement outcomes. The level of movement confidence may influence specific processing operations, the effects of which can be traced by monitoring changes in attention load and direction. This is a general statement that must be applied to the relevant processing demands in different types of movement situations.

Movement confidence can add information to be processed and can direct and narrow attention to a particular aspect of the movement situation. The general effect is to change attention in terms of amount to be processed and what is processed, as well as what is not processed. If a skier does not anticipate enjoying the sensations of moving down a ski slope (low $MS_E$), attention will be directed to the moving sensations and away from the environmental information of where to turn and where other skiers are. A similar focusing of attention is expected for the less competent skier (low C) who might watch his skis instead of the slope ahead and the more fearful skier (negative $MS_H$) who might watch the nearby trees and skiers instead of attempting to avoid them.

Direction of attention in each of these examples is narrowed and probably intensified, which will increase attention load.

Movement confidence, attention load and direction, and level of movement performance are proposed as having a neutral relationship which becomes negative at critical points. Mid-range levels of attention load should produce optimal opportunities for an individual to perform well in terms of the individual's usual or expected performance level. As attention becomes inappropriately directed and load increases, a point will be reached where performance may decrease markedly. Level of movement confidence is predicted as having a similar relationship to attention load and direction. Until level of movement confidence decreases to a critical point, attention load and direction will not be altered significantly. When level of movement confidence decreases below a critical negative level, attention load will be increased and attention will be narrowed, possibly misdirected, thus leading to a lowering of performance level.

This current discussion of the model deals primarily with the negative aspects of movement confidence, both as a consequence and as a mediator. It is more difficult to conceptualize the production of high levels of movement confidence and how increases in movement confidence to a high level will facilitate performance, except that performance will be smooth and not disrupted to produce a relatively good outcome. It seems reasonable that a positive level of movement confidence is important, particularly as movement situations become more complex and competitive. The positive aspect of movement confidence is intrinsic within our model but predictions for positive levels of movement confidence will not be considered at this time. The predictions for neutral and negative levels of movement confidence do not extend in a logical continuum to positive levels. A similar point was made earlier in noting that MOVSENSE (MS) probably has a different and less predictable relationship with MOVCOMP (C) in producing movement confidence as MS and C values increase to high, positive levels (see MS$^+$ line in Figure 3).

## EVALUATION AND CLARIFICATION OF THE MODEL

The evaluation and clarification of this working model of movement confidence will involve the testing of several general predictions which will depend upon the measurement of key components. The general predictions and related measurement problems will be reviewed to provide a summary of the model as it is now proposed. Additionally, behavioral manifestations of movement confidence will be discussed in a second section to suggest another way to look at the influence of movement confidence in a movement situation, and to argue for the importance of movement confidence as having a reality in the minds of observers who can influence the performance and behavior of movement participants.

### Predictions and Related Measurement Problems

A general representation of our working model of movement confidence is provided in Figure 5. It is also necessary to include Figure 2 for an elaboration of the establishment of a level of movement confidence and Figure 3 for the graphic representation of related predictions. The model is limited at this time to movement situations in which outcomes and demands are related to movement achievements and moving sensations, and does not include personal-social outcomes and demands. The model is intended to be sufficiently general in structure that the model can be expanded to include more complex movement situations. Predictions about participation choice and persistence also are not included at this time in an effort to simplify the initial work with the model. Predictions are further limited to the negative aspects of movement confidence, both as a consequence and a mediator.

The first general set of predictions relates to the equation for movement confidence: $C + (MS_E - MS_H) = MC$. Three elements of the equation – C, $MS_E$ and $MS_H$ – must be measured, then evaluated in terms of their power to predict MC, as measured in a separate way. The general predictions diagrammed in Figure 3 could be evaluated to learn how changes in MOVSENSE (MS) interact with changes in MOVCOMP (C) to produce changes in movement confidence (MC). Also, interrelationships among the three elements can be examined (e.g. whether or not potential for physical harm is perceived as less when perceptions of competence increase). Familiarity and changes in outcome demands are predicted as having immediate and marked effects on level of movement confidence, which could be examined when adequate measures of the three elements are established.

The second general set of predictions relates to predicting the mediational function of movement confidence, as diagrammed in Figure 5. Using the measure of movement confidence derived from the general equation, changes in level of movement confidence can be studied in relation to changes in attention load and direction. The study of this general relationship then must be extended to determine if changes in movement confidence and attention are predictors of changes in movement performance, along the lines of the neutral to negative effects suggested in the previous section. Measures of attention load and direction will be needed, as well as movement performance measures appropriate to specific movement situations.

The immediate evaluation difficulty is to measure the three elements of the equation (C, $MS_E$ and $MS_H$) and establish a separate, criterion measure of movement confidence (MC). Measures of attention (load and direction) and movement performance, which are not needed until MC can be measured adequately, exist in various forms that can be adapted for use in studying movement confidence. Measures of perceived competence are available but only Harter (1978; in press) has a measure of physical (movement) confidence. Her measure is general in nature (e.g. 'do really well at sports') and not useful in the more limited way we are defining movement confidence. Two general approaches seem promising in identifying and measuring the three elements of the equation but the criterion measure of movement confidence is a more elusive problem.

The measurement of C, $MS_E$ and $MS_H$ depends on how an individual perceives the demands of a movement situation in relation to a self-analysis (see Figure 2). If individuals evaluate a number of movement situations, C, $MS_E$ and $MS_H$ should vary, particularly if the movement situations are selected to represent a wide range of movement and moving demands. Individuals could be asked to identify perceived demands and make self-ratings in ways that would provide measures of the three elements. Interview techniques also might be used as another approach, with the words and phrases of individuals used in a content analysis. Different elements or different emphases within elements might be identified in this manner.

A technique used by Bandura (1977) in measuring self-efficacy might be adapted as a second approach. Bandura measures self-efficacy by arranging a list of similar tasks and asking people to indicate those tasks they feel they could perform. As a movement example, Feltz, Landers, and Raeder (1979) used Bandura's technique to prepare a self-efficacy measure of diving tasks, ranging from jumping feet-first from the side of the pool to doing a modified back-dive from a one-meter board. Lewis (1974) used a sixteen-item list with children in which tasks ranged from approaching the water to doing a prone float. A Bandura-list is a task analysis to identify variations of a movement task, particularly when modifying skill difficulty and physical harm. This technique could be used to have individuals sort items in relation to the three elements. As another approach, the examiner could manipulate the items to study shifts in selections related to differences in demands, which have been previously identified by the examiner.

It is important to note that we are not seeking general trait measures of the three elements in our equation. Our concerns in this phase of our work are the identification of the elements that will predict level of movement confidence and how changes in these elements affect the level of movement confidence for different movement situations. Therefore, we need techniques to measure these elements as they are manipulated by changing movement and moving demands. The Bandura technique is an example of the type of procedure which is needed.

The external criterion of movement confidence will be a difficult matter to resolve, as is generally the case in trying to establish construct validity. One possibility is to identify observable behavioral manifestations which are accepted as indicators of movement confidence. Some preliminary work along these lines is discussed in the next section.

### Behavioral Manifestations of Movement Confidence

Although movement performance is the focus of our model, behaviors other than movement skill may be influenced by movement confidence. For example, an individual lacking in movement confidence might stop and look around when approaching the side of the pool to enter the water. Behaviors which are a normal part of a movement situation may be important indicators of movement confidence to others who are observing the participant. If behaviors change in a way to be different from what is expected for a particular movement situation, we might be observing behavioral manifestations of movement confidence.

A study was undertaken to look at two aspects of children's behaviors while performing three similar movement tasks (Griffin, Keogh, and Spector, 1979). The first concern was whether or not movement confidence was perceived or rated in a consistent manner by individuals watching children do the three movement tasks. The second concern was to identify the behavioral manifestations upon which the perception of movement confidence was based. Rater agreement on level of movement confidence would indicate that movement confidence had some stable reality as a construct in the perception of the observers. The identification of behavioral manifestations would provide a general base from which an observational measure of movement confidence could be prepared.

Films were made individually of thirty-six children, aged four, doing three movement tasks selected to minimize skill demands while presenting a perceived but not actual physical harm. The three tasks were (i) falling backward onto a 30-inch-thick foam pad, (ii) jumping from two heights onto a landing mat, and (iii) lifting one arm and/or one leg while standing on the lower bar of uneven parallel bars and holding the upper bar. Various combinations of children and tasks were viewed by nine adults and twenty-seven children, aged ten to twelve. All generalizability coefficients were .9 or higher, indicating high rater agreement within and across groups and tasks, and across occasions (first and second ratings). Children were variable across tasks but adults and children had a high level of agreement within and between their groups.

The rating scale used by the observers was a simple scale ranging from '1' (high) to '3' (low). No formal definition of movement confidence was provided beyond a general description of one who is assured. It was deliberate on our part to use these simple procedures as a sterner test of observer agreement.

Movement confidence appeared to have some reality in the minds of observers in that they agreed with each other, even when using a global definition and making a simple rating. As something of a caution, observer recognition of movement confidence does not mean that the participant is or is not confident in a movement situation. The agreement of observer perception and participant perception is a matter to be tested at a later time. However, observers presumably interact with participants based on their observer perceptions. It is important on this basis alone to study observer perceptions of movement confidence.

Adult observers were asked, after having made their initial ratings, to describe what they saw that made them think a child was low or high in movement confidence. Transcriptions of observer descriptions were analyzed to identify behavioral manifestations of movement confidence. Three general categories of behavioral manifestations of movement confidence were identified, indicating changes in performance and behavior that the observer saw as reflecting movement confidence. The three categories of behaviors are identified as movements, tempo, and attention, as presented in Figure 6. Observer comments for each category were divided into behaviors which are part of two phases: preparation to move and the movement attempt. For example, approaching the side of the pool would be preparation for entering the water and the movement attempt would be whatever occurs while attempting the head-first dive to enter the water.

Observers apparently had an expected range of behaviors for each movement situation such that behaviors outside the expected range were interpreted as signs of low or high levels of movement confidence. Observers described low levels of movement confidence primarily in terms of protective movements and unnecessary movements. Movements indicating lack of confidence were noted both while preparing for the movement to be performed and when attempting

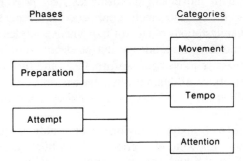

FIGURE 6   Categories of behavioral manifestations of movement confidence as a part of two movement phases

the movement. Twisting, turning, shuffling feet, and reaching for support were preparatory movements identified as indicating lack of confidence. Movement attempts sometimes were varied or incomplete as if to protect the performer (e.g. flexing at the waist to sit down rather than falling straight back). Tempo of movements was described as lack of confidence when the child was going too slow or too fast or not moving at all. Variation in attention also was described as indicating lack of confidence, primarily in terms of visual focus, such as looking excessively at the instructor, apparatus or body parts.

A considerable portion of the descriptors provided by the adult observers was negative rather than positive, which supports our earlier statement that effects of positive levels of movement confidence are more difficult to observe and predict. Also, many of the observer descriptors were indicative of a lower level of achievement of movement outcomes. Children were described as sitting down rather than falling straight back, stepping down rather than jumping off, and bending their body but not letting go of the bar. Movement skill was not a demand in these movement situations, at least not at a high level. But it seems that a high level of physical harm was perceived as probable and the minimal demand for movement skill often was not achieved. This finding fits the general notion that high level of perceived potential harm ($MS_H$) will have a negative impact upon performance.

Many of the observer descriptors were not related to movement perfor- mance, rather they were behaviors indicating a lack of assurance while not necessarily related to poor movement performance. Shuffling feet, reaching for support, hesitation, and looking excessively at the instructor were seen as signs that children were not confident, but some of these children were able to perform adequately. It is important that behavioral signs of this sort be dis- tinguished from poor movement performance, recognizing that poor movement performance often results in such behavioral signs (e.g. sitting down instead of falling straight back). The point is that behavioral signs or manifestations not directly a part of poor movement performance may provide an observable, external criterion of lack of movement confidence. A simple scaling might be: (i) no behavioral manifestations of lack of movement confidence; (ii) behavioral manifestations of movement confidence but no decrease in movement perfor- mance; (iii) a decrease in movement performance; and (iv) not continuing the movement to completion. Additional observations and thought are needed to examine this possibility of providing an external criterion of movement con- fidence.

Another way to think about behavioral manifestations of movement con- fidence is the amount and kind of support an individual needs or seeks during participation (Griffin and Keogh, in press). Change in support conditions is a way for the mover and others to manipulate the demands of a movement situation. A child can ride a bicycle with 'no hands' to increase movement demands or use the brakes to go slower, thus lowering movement demands. A parent can hold the bicycle upright for a start or let the child cope with starting the bicycle. Need for support might be a useful, general indicator of confidence. Does the child 'let go' or use the brakes? Does the child seek the support of others? Depending on the question, support can be an independent variable when manipulating support conditions or a dependent variable when observing movement response in terms of the amount and kind of support a mover seeks and uses.

## DEVELOPMENT OF MOVEMENT CONFIDENCE AND MOVEMENT SKILL

The relationship of movement confidence and movement skill throughout the developing years should be similar to the general predictions provided in our model, noting again that outcomes are limited to movement skill and moving sensations. A lower level of movement confidence for a young child likely will lead to poor movement performance, relative to what the young child should be able to do, and the same should be true for older children and adults. Absolute levels will be different and relationships within elements of movement confidence, attention, and performance may change but the overall effect should be the same.

The important developmental issue is the long-term impact of immediate events which become part of an ongoing sequence. The negative and positive participation spirals noted in the involvement cycle are generally what might be expected as a long-term sequence of events and effects. We will place our more immediate and situational view of movement confidence into a long-term, quite speculative perspective of the developmental of movement confidence and movement skill. We will begin with a simple, two-level view of movement skill development. The development of MOVSENSE and MOVCOMP, as the basic components of movement confidence, will be considered separately. The concluding paragraphs will be an effort to bring all pieces of the discussion into a general developmental perspective.

Movement skill development can be characterized as gaining control of movement-for-self and movement-with-others (Keogh, 1978). Infants and young children must first achieve control of their own movements in terms of basic postural control, locomotion, and manipulation before they can move in relation to other persons and objects. Sitting upright, walking, and holding a ball are at a first level of control, indicating that children are establishing control of their own body. Sitting on a moving bicycle, walking in step with a friend, and catching a ball are at a second level of control in that movements are made in relation to external force-time-space requirements. Movement-for-self involves attending to internal information whereas attention in movement-with-others is more externally directed. Infants and young children will be attending to internal sensations of moving. Older children will be attending more to external information, generating additional information and making related decisions.

The development of MOVSENSE seems intuitively to be a critical factor in early movement skill development. Early experiences of being moved by others, which is what happens in the early months of life, should have a profound effect on a child's perceptions of moving. As an infant experiences new movements, sensations of moving will be evaluated as enjoyed or not enjoyed and as involving or not involving physical harm. MOVSENSE is viewed as a reasonably simple set of perceptions and a simple developmental process. MOVSENSE likely is well established and reasonably stable for specific situations after a few years of life. The direct importance of MOVSENSE probably is the effect on early movement skill development with a compounding effect in subsequent participations. A beginning walker likely will persist if the pain of the constant falling is not perceived as too unpleasant, whereas a child more aware of movement-related pain may decide to sit it out for a while.

The development of MOVCOMP is a more difficult and complex issue. An important developmental consideration is that younger children may not have the same perceptions as adults of skill and ability. Preschool and primary grade children perceive effort as sufficient to produce an achievement, thus not recognizing ability except perhaps that ability is perceived as effort (Harter, in press; Nicholls, 1978). Nicholls reported that primary grade children could not identify their ability level in reading in relation to classmates whereas older children were quite accurate in self-ratings of reading ability. Harter (in press) found that effort rather than ability was perceived by younger children. Harter (1975) also found that younger children were satisfied with effort to produce an effect (marbles dropping) whereas older children were not satisfied unless the task was solved or mastered. Younger children might be pleased to get in the water and try to swim; older children likely would be more aware of and value how well they swam.

Infants and young children also are not likely to recognize ability in the sense that we think of adults evaluating their ability to perform the requisite skills in a movement situation. Perhaps adult perceptions of ability develop from early attempts to be effective. White (1959) proposed that effectance or competence motivation is a striving of individuals to have an effect on their environment. Stott (1961) independently came to a similar view based on systematic observations of his young child. Many early movements may be to produce an effect or a change in the environment, as illustrated by banging pots to make noises. Young children soon come to know that their movements can produce an effect in general terms. As children develop, they become involved in more complex situations which require skill or ability beyond just being involved and doing. the sound must now be of a certain character and quality which requires precise control of the bow on the strings. Competence may begin with simple, personal observations of having an effect, progress to recognizing that amount of effort is important, and culminate in perceptions of ability.

Another consideration in development of MOVCOMP is that movement situations become more complex as a child becomes more competent. A child who puts on the brakes when learning to ride a bicycle, may pedal faster and do wheelies when more proficient. The child seeks more complicated outcomes and others in the environment expect more as the child becomes older. This means that the personal evaluation process to determine MOVCOMP in a particular movement situation will be more complex.

A general developmental perspective can be summarized beginning with infants and young children who are developing control of movement-for-self. MOVSENSE probably develops to a fairly full degree during these years with a major impact on movement skill development. MOVCOMP probably is not functional during these years as we generally think of competence and ability but is more a simple sense of effectance or recognizing that one's movements have an effect in the environment. Movement-with-others, as the important movement problem for children in preschool and elementary-school years, is a complex development involving greater information-processing demands and more complicated personal-evaluation processes. MOVCOMP becomes more than effectance and effort to establish complex notions of ability, thus adding to the complexities of this level of movement skill development. MOVSENSE now is a simple additive factor in the movement confidence equation without changing greatly in character or intensity, except in relation to MOVCOMP.

If we consider development as the full range of life, development of young adults and beyond likely will be diversified within a group and intensified within an individual. A third level of movement skill development exists in that individuals may pursue a limited number of movement skills to a higher personal level of skill, assuming that there is a large amount of participation time. MOVSENSE may now become paramount for some as the outcome to be achieved. Runners may seek 'a high' or state of moving sensation that seems to be a physiological response to exercise. Individuals presumably avoid moving sensations that are neutral or negative. MOVCOMP can be positive if individuals select movement situations appropriate to their skills. However, individuals often choose to compete which raises the demand level and complicates matters.

## SUMMARY

A working model was presented to describe movement confidence as both a consequence and a mediator. The model was limited in this presentation to movement situations in which outcomes and demands are related to movement achievements and moving sensations. The model provides a general structure which can later be expanded to include personal-social aspects of participation choice and persistence. Predictions within the model were limited to negative aspects of movement confidence, both as a consequence and a mediator.

A formal definition of movement confidence is expressed in the equation: $C + (MS_E - MS_H) = MC$. A personal (performer) evaluation of self in relation to demands of a movement situation produces a sense of movement competence (MOVCOMP) and expectations of sensory experiences related to moving (MOVSENSE). The level of MOVSENSE (MS) is based on the level of anticipated personal enjoyment of the expected moving sensations ($MS_E$) and the potential physical harm ($MS_H$). The general sense of the equation is that MOVCOMP (C) is modified by MOVSENSE ($MS = MS_E - MS_H$) to produce a state of movement confidence (MC) for a particular situation. Level of movement confidence can be altered most quickly and markedly by changing important aspects of the movement situation demands that lead to changes in $C$, $MS_E$ and $MS_H$.

Movement confidence functions as a mediator in the processing of information related to movement performance. The level of movement confidence will have an influence upon information-processing operations in terms of contributing directly to attention load and direction, thus indirectly to the achievement of desired movement outcomes. The general effect is to change attention in terms of amount to be processed and what is processed, or what is not processed. Movement confidence, attention load and direction, and movement performance are proposed as having a neutral relationship which becomes negative at critical points. When level of movement confidence decreases below a critical negative level, attention load will be increased and attention will be narrowed, possibly misdirected, thus leading to a lowering of performance level.

The evaluation and clarification of this working model of movement confidence requires the testing of our general predictions, which immediately poses the problem of measuring the three elements of the equation ($C$, $MS_E$ and $MS_H$) and establishing a separate, criterion measure of movement confidence (MC). Several ways of manipulating situation demands were discussed as possible approaches to measuring the three elements of the equation. Behaviors which are a normal part of a movement situation were suggested as possible indicators of movement confidence, thus might be used as behavioral manifestations of movement confidence to provide a criterion measure. A particularly important indicator might be the amount and kind of support an individual needs and seeks during participation.

The relationship of movement confidence and movement skill throughout the developing years should be similar to the general predictions in the model.

Absolute levels will be different and relationships within elements of movement confidence, attention and performance may change but the overall effect should be the same. MOVSENSE probably develops to a fairly full degree during early years with a major impact on the development of control of movement-for-self. MOVCOMP probably develops in a more complicated manner beginning with a simple sense of effectance and effort, and progressing to complex perceptions of ability within which personal skill is recognized. Increased processing demands and more complicated personal-evaluation processes are characteristic of later development, and are important in the interaction of MOVCOMP and development of control of movement-with-others. The larger impact of movement confidence in the development of movement skill is in determining the direction of the spiral of the movement involvement cycle. The practical concern is to maintain a positive spiral: more likely to seek and choose participation and to perform and behave in ways that are satisfying to the individual.

## NOTE

1. Preparation of this chapter was supported in part by grants from the Bureau of Education for the Handicapped (OEG00770997), Biomedical Research Support Grant (USPHS-RR07009) and the Research Council, Faculty Development Fund and School of Health, Physical Education and Recreation of the University of Nebraska-Lincoln. We are most appreciative of the critical comments and suggestions of Dorothy Allen, Richard Maybee, Glyn Roberts, Tara Scanlan and Robin Woods who reviewed earlier drafts of this chapter.

## REFERENCES

Atkinson, J. W. (1964). *An Introduction to Motivation*, Princeton, NJ: Van Nostrand.

Bain, L. L. (1979). Perceived characteristics of selected movement activities, *Research Quarterly*, **50**, 565–573.

Bandura, A. (1977). Self-efficacy: Toward a unifying theory of behavioral change, *Psychological Review*, **84**, 191–215.

Caskey, S. R. (1973). Influence of group and individual success-failure experiences in a throwing task of movement concept and level of aspiration of children in grades three, four and five, unpublished doctoral dissertation, Purdue University.

Coelho, G. V., Hamburg, D. A., and Adams, J. E. (eds.) (1974). *Coping and Adaptation*, New York: Basic Books.

Connolly, K., and Bruner, J. (eds.) (1974). *The Growth of Competence*, New York: Academic Press.

Deci, E. L. (1975). *Intrinsic Motivation*, New York: Plenum Press.

Feltz, D. L., Landers, D. M., and Raeder, U. (1979). Enhancing self-efficacy in high-avoidance motor tasks: A comparison of modeling techniques, *Journal of Sport Psychology*, **1**, 112–122.

Griffin, N. S., and Keogh, J. F. (in press). Movement confidence and effective movement behavior in adapted physical education, *Motor Skills: Theory into Practice*.

Griffin, N. S., Keogh, J. F., and Spector, R. (1979). Behavioral manifestations of movement confidence, paper presented at the meeting of the North American Society for Psychology of Sport and Physical Activity, Trois Rivières, Canada, June 1980.

Griffin, N. S., Keogh, J. F., and Spector, R. (in press). Observer perceptions of movement confidence, *Research Quarterly for Exercise and Sport*.

Harter, S. (1975). Developmental differences in the manifestation of mastery motivation on problem-solving tasks, *Child Development*, **46**, 370–378.

Harter, S. (1978). Effectance motivation reconsidered, *Human Development*, **21**, 34–64.

Harter, S. (in press). A model of intrinsic mastery motivation in children: Individual differences and developmental change, *Minnesota Symposium on Child Psychology* (Vol. 14), Hillsdale, NJ: Lawrence Erlbaum.

Keogh, J. F. (1978). Movement outcomes as conceptual guidelines in the perceptual-motor maze, *Journal of Special Education*, **12**, 321–329.

Keogh, J. F. (1981). A movement development framework and a perceptual-cognitive perspective, in G. Brooks (ed.), *Perspectives on the Academic Discipline of Physical Education*, Champaign, Ill.: Human Kinetics.

Keogh, J. F., Griffin, N. S., and Spector, R. (in press). Observer perceptions of movement confidence, *Research Quarterly for Exercise and Sport*.

Lewis, S. (1974). A comparison of behavior therapy techniques in the reduction of fearful avoidance behavior, *Behavior Therapy*, **5**, 648–655.

Marteniuk, R. G. (1976). *Information Processing in Motor Skills*, New York: Holt, Rinehart & Winston.

Maul, T., and Thomas, J. R. (1975). Self-concept and participation in children's gymnastics, *Perceptual and Motor Skills*, **41**, 701–702.

Nicholls, J. C. (1978). The development of the concepts of effort and ability, perception of academic attainment, and the understanding that difficult tasks require more ability, *Child Development*, **49**, 800–814.

Shavelson, R. J., Hubner, J. J., and Stanton, G. C. (1976). Self-concept: Validation of construct interpretations, *Review of Educational Research*, **46**, 407–441.

Stott, D. H. (1961). An empirical approach to motivation based on the behavior of a young child, *Journal of Child Psychology and Psychiatry*, **2**, 97–117.

Tanner, P. W. (1969). The relationship of selected measures of body image and movement concept to two types of programs of physical education in primary grades, unpublished doctoral dissertation, Ohio State University.

Weiner, B. (1974). *Achievement Motivation and Attribution Theory*, Morristown, NJ: General Learning Press.

White, B. L. (1978). *Experience and Environment* (Vol. 2), Englewood Cliffs, NJ: Prentice-Hall.

White, R. (1959). Motivation reconsidered: The concept of competence, *Psychological Review*, **66**, 297–323.

# PART III

## Timing Behavior in Development

One would receive little argument from the contributors to this volume that timing is a key issue in the development of motor skill. One has only to watch a two-year-old child attempting to catch a ball to be persuaded of this fact. But we know little about how timing may develop. Not only is there a need for more developmental research on this topic but also for a conceptual sharpening of what it means to time a movement. Recent human ethological research by Esther Thelen suggests rather strongly that the organism possesses a high degree of *intrinsic* temporal organization at a very young age. Thus the kicking pattern of a one-month-old displays the same temporal pattern of flexion and extension as the gait of a mature adult (Thelen *et al.*, in press).[1] But movements occur in both space and time: motor organization has to accommodate changing environmental demands. Wade reports the beginnings of a set of studies on what is traditionally defined as motion prediction or coincident timing. Some differences in timing behavior occur across age but, as he himself recognizes, the results are not yet sufficiently clear to force a single interpretation. Wade promotes the Gibsonian perspective (see also Chapter 1) that information in the environment directly specifies the temporal details of activity and, that this specification is scaled to the dimensionality of the child. There is much that is promissory here but the direction promoted by Wade is a challenging one.

Christopher Wickens takes an entirely different tack on the problem. What mechanisms underlie the human's capability to do two things at once? This is a far-reaching topic in psychology and requires that one use the term 'skill' in its most global sense with due recognition given to perceptual and cognitive limitations. Wickens has spent a fair portion of his time pondering upon this problem and developing the methodology to study it – sufficiently so as to identify four quite distinct processes all dealing with the deployment of attentional resources. The developmental data that might differentiate Wickens' carefully drawn hypotheses are sparse to say the least and we can only hope that someone will take up the gauntlet soon.

237

## NOTE

1. Thelen, E., Bradshaw, G., and Ward, J. A. (in press). Spontaneous kicking in month-old infants: Manifestation of a central locomotor program. *Behavioral and Neural Biology*.

The Development of Movement Control and Co-ordination
Edited by J. A. S. Kelso and J. E. Clark
© 1982, John Wiley & Sons, Ltd

CHAPTER 8

# Timing Behavior in Children[1]

MICHAEL G. WADE

## INTRODUCTION

There is probably universal acceptance among scientists interested in the production and control of movement that timing or a time-sense is crucial for skilled action. Yet in spite of this, the issue of chronometry as it relates to motor skills has received few serious attempts at its resolution. This criticism applies to both general models of motor skill learning (Adams, 1971; Schmidt, 1975); and models conceived for the developing organism (Connolly, 1970; Bruner, 1973). As Ashton (1976) observed, the 'sub-routine hypothesis' advanced by Connolly pays little attention to the temporal relationship between the subroutines as they are combined into skilled activity. Lashley's (1951) contention regarding serial order in skilled behavior left unanswered the question of 'how' that serial order occurs. The assumption is that it is sequentially linear and has a location somewhere within the central nervous system (CNS). For example, Schmidt's (1975) attempt to understand how the temporal configuration of the desired movement is organized is by reference to a blueprint termed 'schema' located somewhere in the nervous system. In addition to the blueprint, Schmidt's theory further entails a specification of 'initial conditions' within the nervous system. The problem with Schmidt's theory is that it does not apply directly to the issue of how timing arises. This theory *presumes* an already existing theory of schema timing.

Let us consider the two prominent theoretical positions about timing behavior as expressed in motor learning theory. One theory implicates a central, or open-loop, role for the timing of skilled behavior (Lashley, 1951; Schmidt, 1975). The other theory implicates a peripheral or closed-loop view of timing (Adams, 1971). Although these two theories are invariably discussed as opposing viewpoints, they do in fact both share a common style of control, namely that of error-controlled servomechanisms. Such models imply that sensory and motor nerves are logically independent, separated by an error-correcting device. The underlying assumption entails an explicit reference signal for each goal-directed activity. In addition to optimizing motor output each reference signal requires an explicit correction-determining device. Problems with such a solution quickly ensue when a collection of servo-mechanisms is organized in a hierarchical manner. Such a solution has not been proposed unreasonably in attempts to resolve the problem of fine-grain variables such as muscle fibers acting in reference to a more abstract coarse-grain variable such as an animal's activity. It has been argued elsewhere (Fowler and Turvey, 1978; Kugler and Turvey, 1979) that such a solution may prove to be formally intractable.

Both central and peripheral theories describe the role of timing but do not explain it. Nowhere, for example, does Schmidt's (1975) theory account for how the ordering of the sequence of 'initial conditions' could have come about. In a similar vein there is clear evidence that deafferented subjects, both animal preparations (Taub and Berman, 1968) and humans (Lashley, 1917), can learn motor skills without the aid of feedback from the periphery, thus questioning the peripheralist viewpoint. Criticism of the above theories should in no way detract from their contribution to motor skills research. Suffice to say that if a timer does in fact exist, an explanation, rather than a description, must be forthcoming in a theory that implicates it in motor skill behavior.

The notion of an internal pace-maker is not new and some evidence for such a mechanism exists from studies of the sucking behavior of newborn infants (Wolf, 1967, 1968a). The view here is that such behavior is under some form of central control and that this is a precursor of the timing system that controls the motor behavior of older children and adults. Wolf argued further (1968b) that under stress this complex rhythm may break down, producing stereotyped activity in the young infant. There is little evidence of this in the motor skills literature, suggesting again that it has engendered a low level of interest. Some indirect evidence for this breakdown may be found in the recent work of Shapiro (1977) who investigated the effects of speed-stressing a particular movement and traced the breakdown of the time-sharing relationship between the subcomponents of the movement to a point where the speed requirement was such that the total movement sequence 'broke down.' Shapiro viewed this as the limit of the motor program. If this is so then the qualitative performance level of such motor programs may be directly due to the integrity of such an internal timing system.

The environmental milieu in which the motor skill is emitted also has an important influence on timing, particularly with respect to the anticipation of events. Such activities are concerned with objects moving around in space, and requiring a response with respect to a change in speed or position. Little is known about the control exerted by the exogenous temporal system. What are the features in the environment that permit such control? Coincidence anticipation clearly involves practice and certainly conventionally we think of the subject making decisions with respect to the kinematic parameters (time, distance, acceleration, displacement) of the object. This second issue, the exogenous temporal influences on skill, is the central focus of this chapter.

The interpretation of possible exogenous timing centers for motor behavior is open to both a conventional and an ecological interpretation. This latter view is essentially a perspective reflected in the writings and teachings of the late James Gibson (1966), and expounded by Turvey, Shaw, and Mace (1978) and coworkers Fowler and Turvey (1978), Fitch and Turvey (1977), Kugler, Kelso, and Turvey (1980) who make the point that in order to best understand motor behavior, man cannot be viewed outside the environmental context in which he resides. Fundamental to this interpretation is the notion that our actions and perceptions are body-scaled.

The central idea behind body-scaled information is that objects which are perceived by the animal are defined relative to the animal's capacity for activity. Objects are distinguished not on geometrical dimensions but on activity-related dimensions. The use of the term information is owing to Gibson (1966) and not Shannon. Conventionally information is a measure of uncertainty (Shannon and Weaver, 1949), but Gibson's use of the term defines information as the correspondence between environmental properties as they relate to the animal and the energy medium (e.g. light) as patterned by those properties. Thus the metrics of activity within the environment are not related to some abstract and animal-independent scale (such as feet, inches, feet per second, or pounds-weight) but are environmentally and animal-referential. An object passing across the visual field is not perceived as travelling at so many feet per second, at least at the first-order level. Rather questions are asked of the moving object as it relates to the organism such as: 'Can I reach it?'; 'Can I catch it?'; 'When will it hit me?' In other words the organism within the environment asks 'time to contact' questions of the moving object.

The conventional view of the problem has perhaps been best expressed by Poulton (1957) who has proposed a three stage model:

(1) Primarily a pursuit-tracking task in which the eye follows the target for the purposes of acquiring the necessary perceptual information about motion characteristics.
(2) Prediction of the location of the site at which contact will be made and the necessary decisions regarding the time of arrival of the target at that site.
(3) Organization of the appropriate response along with the necessary reorientation of body segments. Latency in the CNS caused by this body reorientation causes delay between stages (1) and (3).

The idea is that the organism acquires a knowledge about the object's velocity and this is then coded internally. Recent evidence for this viewpoint has been provided by Rosenbaum (1975) whose experiments suggest that velocity is directly perceived by adult subjects. One criticism of Rosenbaum's data however is that he utilized relatively slow velocities (18.76 cm/sec; 42.9 cm/sec) which might not prove to be very sensitive discriminants. Rosenbaum's use of faster velocities appears constrained possibly by the capabilities of his experimental apparatus.

The three stages of Poulton's (1957) model require solutions which are unwieldy. Exact solutions to the problem posed in the various stages of the model would take longer than real time to complete, whether they are attainable via memory search or some form of algorithmic procedure. Solutions which are soluble in principle are too time-consuming to be of practical value. Kugler and Turvey (1979) have argued that this type of problem might fall into the class of N-P complete (cf. Lewis and Papdimetrious, 1978 for an elegant account of N-P complete problems).

The velocity of the target obviously plays a role in the accuracy of the response, and here again the literature is sparse. Some work exists on motion-prediction tasks where velocities were varied. For example, Gerhard (1959) used target speeds between 4.23 cm/sec and 0.8 cm/sec, and Ellingstad (1967) used velocities between 4 cm/sec and 0.2 cm/sec. These speeds are relatively slow and easy to reproduce in the laboratory but have little correspondence to typical velocities that are experienced in the environment. This is particularly true for children and the variety of motor activities in which they engage that require anticipatory timing behavior. The more recent Rosenbaum paper (1975) examined the perception and extrapolation of velocity and accleration. Rosenbaum's data and conclusions show perception of velocity to be *direct* and incorporate both concrete and abstract characteristics of the motion seen. But again, as noted above, he used rather slow velocities in his experiments.

Data on children's timing behavior are limited. Kay (1970) recorded ball-catching by children of different ages and produced a topological description that showed evidence of the development of anticipatory behavior. This was shown primarily by the positioning of the hands prior to catching the approaching ball. Children two- and five-years-old showed little anticipatory behavior, whereas fifteen-year-olds were 'co-ordinated and unhurried' in catching the ball.

A paper by Alderson and Whiting (1974), using college students (but alluding to its developmental implications!), showed that the additive effects of prediction distance (target obscured) and stimulus velocity showed a linear relationship between prediction time and errors. Further, their data showed that a range effect about modal prediction time may be operating to explain why both fast and slow target speeds produce large errors.

Two experiments are presented here which explore changes in the performance of young children on a coincident timing task. The data from Experiment 1 have been reported more fully elsewhere (Wade, 1980), Experiment 2 reports new data.

## EXPERIMENT 1

The apparatus used is described more fully elsewhere (Wade, 1980).

The task required the subject to strike a target (a cartoon figure) moving from right to left, by rolling an aluminum 'donut' down a trackway (a steel rod) such that it struck the figure coincident with it reaching the end of the trackway. Subjects performed under three conditions of target speed: 152.4 cm/sec (5 ft/sec); 91.4 cm/sec (3 ft/sec); 30.5 cm/sec (1 ft/sec). The apparatus was similar to a 'shooting gallery' found in amusement parks across the nation but with the difference that, instead of a gun, the subject generated a ballistic response to hit the target. The trackway comprised a moving belt approximately 153 cm long. the cartoon targets were attached to the belt with 'velcro.' A variable speed motor appropriately adjusted propelled the targets at the selected velocities.

The subjects were familiarized with the apparatus and the task objective. Each subject was positioned directly in line with the coincidence point, and knowledge of results (KR), either 'hit' or 'miss,' was given immediately after each trial. Each subject, according to his or her assigned condition, performed 90 trials, 30 trials for each of the three velocity conditions. The order of the speed presentation was counterbalanced.

To preclude a biassing in the results (error scores) the data were analyzed in terms of errors of distance rather than errors of time. If the errors were recorded on a time scale, the different target velocities would preclude large errors for the high-velocity condition.

Subjects for the first experiment were 41 boys and girls (22 male and 19 female) divided into three age groups: 7–9 years, 9–11 years, and 12–14 years.

### Results and Discussion

The data (Figure 1A) illustrate the age by condition interaction for variable error. Generally the youngest group of subjects were the most variable, and the slowest target velocity produced relatively higher error scores than the medium-to-fast velocities. Although three data points 'do not a U function make' there is a suggestion here of the effect first noted by Alderson and Whiting (1974), with both the fast and slow target velocities producing the large errors. The question is, why?

A conventional interpretation of such data might explore two issues: first that the requirement both to perceptually determine the speed of the target and generate a movement response may be counterproductive, with the 'movement'

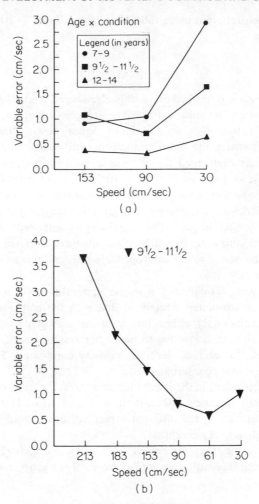

FIGURE 1    Variable error scores for Age by
Target velocity information. (A) Experiment 1
(Reproduced by kind permission of *J. Pub.
Assoc.*, Santa Barbara, CA); (B) Experiment 2

requirement interfering with the perceptual activity. Secondly it may be that
some kind of conventional 'look-ahead' model may be poorly developed in
young children. The conventional information-processing approach might well
explain the first issue along the following lines. For the child, whose
information-processing capacities are not equal to those of the adult, the

requirement to make both a velocity decision at the perceptual level, and in addition, generate an appropriate well-organized motor response may introduce a lag in the CNS that produces errors in coincident anticipation stemming directly from information overload. For the second, a poorly developed 'look-ahead' model may be the result of the child's limited experience in solving motion-prediction problems.

I have discussed elsewhere (Wade, 1976) the role of experience as a factor in becoming sensitive to different aspects of information. A much larger question to be dealt with, however, is whether or not conventional interpretations of such issues as timing errors serve to advance our knowledge of the developing organism's motor behavior (cf. Fowler and Turvey, 1978; Kugler and Turvey, 1979; Kugler, Kelso, and Turvey, 1980). The essential problem with an information-processing model, as computer analogs of skill representation, is that all the constraints are exclusively with reference to the processing system, with little or no consideration of environmental constraints. Quite simply, it is in a sense poor logic to set up an 'in the head' model that must be constrained to represent a system that seems unconstrained yet stable. Criticism of such a hierarchical model of control recently has been offered (Fowler and Turvey, 1978; Kugler and Turvey, 1979). They argue that the task of organizing the system at its lower levels cannot realistically be controlled by an all-powerful executor at the cortical level. In contrast the ecological position attempts to move away from such intermediate representations of timing behavior. An ecological interpretation of the present data described in Experiment 1 might go as follows.

The child's limited interaction with his/her environment, as a function of his/her time spent in that environment, leads to a limited set of perceptual distinctions regarding objects moving around in that environment. As noted above, a child understands best the movement of objects that relate to his/her own body size. Thus velocities in the environment are best understood when they are compatible with the child's dynamics. There are no absolute values for different velocities, rather they are always system-referential (cf. Kugler, Kelso, and Turvey, this volume, for a discussion of 'system-scaled variables'). What is fast or slow 'to the child' is unqualified in the nature of the perceptual event. Outside that frame of reference errors become larger. Concurrent with this view is the recognition that at no time does the child perceive the velocity of moving objects in terms of some standard metric of time, distance, or velocity.

As the child develops, its functional relationships with the environment change with time (see Kugler, Kelso, and Turvey, this volume). The data reported in Experiment 1 used only three target velocities (30.5 cm/sec; 91.4 cm/sec; and 152.4 cm/sec). To test further for the suggested range effect in children's errors in coincident timing a wider range of target speeds was used with another group of similarly aged children.

## EXPERIMENT 2

The apparatus was the same as described in the first experiment except that the target velocity was scaled up to six velocities: 213 cm/sec (7 ft/sec); 183 cm/sec (6 ft/sec); 152.4 cm/sec (5 ft/sec); 90.4 cm/sec (3 ft/sec); 61 cm/sec (2 ft/sec); and 30.5 cm/sec (1 ft/sec).

Experimental procedures were again essentially the same with subject performing on six velocity conditions in a counterbalanced order. There were 30 trials for each velocity presentation. Data was collected on nine children ranging in age from 7–12 years.

**Results and Discussion**

The data for variable error scores are illustrated in Figure 1B. Again the presence of the hypothesized 'U' function was not apparent, although the elements of such a curve are present. Errors decreased from the highest velocity of 213 cm/sec (7 ft/sec) and appear minimal for subjects at the 61 cm/sec (2 ft/sec) velocity. Errors then begin to increase at speeds slower than 61 cm/sec (2 ft/sec). The failure to demonstrate strongly a uniform 'U' function at the slower velocities may be a result of a biassing effect generated by the fact that the subjects viewed the target continuously, producing different levels of information at different velocities. Admittedly the data are not totally persuasive of the point I am trying to make, however they do serve as an empirical first step.

## GENERAL DISCUSSION AND CONCLUSIONS

The intent of this chapter was to present some data on children's timing behavior at different developmental levels. The data suggest that as children get older (7 years to 14 years) their performance gets less variable, and they appear to experience problems with motion prediction outside a particular range of target speeds. In a sense the data presented pose more questions than they answer, and some discussion of them is in order.

First let us consider the question as to whether or not 'timing' is really a tangible issue in a valid theory of motor skill. Certainly it appears to be an important element in skill expression and further there is considerable evidence that our 'timing' improves as we develop from childhood to adulthood. The question is whether timing is an element in the motor skill story or merely a by-product of an increasingly efficient action system. The argument goes beyond the search for the location of the 'timer' (Ashton, 1976) to whether or not 'time' is a variable with a dimension. Gibsonites such as Lee (1980) and Turvey (1977) argue that it is not.

Up to this point when we have talked about timing in motor skills there have seemingly been two issues that have needed to be addressed – the temporal components that: (i) influence decisions regarding response formulation, and (ii) guide response execution.

It seems pretty clear that the former (i) rather than the latter (ii) is the major issue here. Namely the temporal aspects that are evident in the subject's interaction with the environment. Such interactions generate questions with respect both to the selection and the initiation of the response. Subsumed under this issue is the problem of motion prediction as it relates to what we have traditionally referred to as coincidence anticipation.

The latter issue (ii), namely response execution, relates more to the internal functioning of the joint-muscle system. Whether we rely on 'initial conditions' (Schmidt, 1975) or the more recent 'mass spring' analogy (e.g. Schmidt, 1980) there seems to be essentially a constancy in the time-sharing activity of the limb movement involved in the performance. I alluded to this in my remarks about the Shapiro (1977) paper above where the temporal components of the movement are robust across quite broad, speed-stressed boundaries. Appropriate timing in this context may well be an inherent quality of the dynamics of purposeful joint-muscle activity.

There can be no doubt that the developing child is sensitive to visual information about moving objects and related 'time to collision' problems. Such sensitivity has been observed in extremely young (sixteen weeks) infants (Yonus et al., 1977). For the young child performing motor skills that require the resolution of 'time to collision' problems, the location of any errors produced has different interpretations between those who rely on a conventional view of the organism possessing a knowledge of velocity ($V = d/t$), and an internal coding mechanism for producing accurate motion prediction (Alderson, 1972; Alderson and Whiting, 1974), to those (Fowler and Turvey, 1978; Fitch and Turvey, 1977; Turvey, Shaw, and Mace, 1978; Kugler, Kelso, and Turvey, 1980) who take a direct realist view of perception and action. The conventional view (Poulton, 1957; Adams, 1971; Schmidt, 1975) has been outlined above. The alternative, ecological realism (Shaw, Turvey, and Mace, in press; Shaw and Turvey, in press) reflects the notion that it is a function of an animal's 'encounter' with its environment. It is the time-varying pattern or optic flow field that is the normal stimulus for vision (Lee, 1980) and produces the information to control activities.

Let us return briefly to the data presented above (Figure 1). The young children exhibit some difficulty with both fast and slow velocities. The difficulties may be due to a lack of sensitivity of the visual system to a class of 'time to collision' problems outside the child's econiche. The child's environmental experience serves to constrain activity with reference to classes of motion problems requiring coincident behavior.

At this point no single interpretation (conventional or otherwise) can be considered correct. There are, however, recent data which suggest that the proposed direct relationship between perception and action holds a more fruitful avenue of investigation. Lee's (1980) data on the diving behavior of the gannet (Sula Bassana) presents a mathematical argument that the spatio-temporal information necessary for successful entry into the water is derived from 'time to contact' rather than distance away. The bird's final wing-folding prior to entry seems to rely more on visual information picked up *during* the dive, rather than on an *a priori* computation of how long it will take to reach the water from its hovering altitude. 'Time to collision' data presented recently by Todd (1981) also demonstrate that the human visual system rapidly and accurately detects an object's boundaries (The Figure-Ground Problem) directly and without any 'search' time. Todd argues that current computer technology cannot solve such a problem without some 'search' time, thus rendering its validity in such situations as impractical.

The reliance on intermediary mechanisms seems not to be the way the organism solves motion-related problems. Our traditional view of timing mechanisms has relied almost entirely on the notion that a 'timing receptor' and a logically independent concept of time be present somewhere in the central nervous system. It is via this mechanism that we co-ordinate our actions. The fact that such a mechanism is subject to failure (i.e. solvable in real time) for the solution of 'time to collision' or 'time to contact' problems argues for an information base whose time vocabulary is more commensurate with the task and not independent of the task. The information for the solution of such problems is derived directly from the visual information available in the animal's encounter with its environment. As Lee, (1980) notes: 'The time derivative of the 'time-to-contact' optic variable ... is a dimensionless quantity. Nonetheless the dimensionless optic variable affords information for controlling space-time activity.'

What can be said by way of summary? Data have been presented which are suggestive of some kind of range effect in terms of accuracy of coincidence anticipation in children. Both a 'conventional' and an 'ecological' interpretation of the data have been presented. Certainly it can be said that the child changes its sensitivity to information over time. Physical growth changes, and increasing sensitivity, account for much of this improvement. Does 'timing ability' change in the same vein? From a conventional viewpoint the location of the 'timer' has yet to be determined beyond the broad cyclical nature of most biological systems. This really does not get us very far because we can record periodicity from the cellular to the cosmological level. The most parsimonious view at this point in time is perhaps that timing *per se* does not develop in and of itself but is a concomitant feature of the dynamics of muscular action in the context of environmental constraints. Hubbard (1960) seems to imply this when he says: 'The control lies in aiming the stroke and providing the right combination of forces to initiate it, like aiming and firing a rifle' (p. 32). It seems that to understand fully the production of skilled movement we must analyze the dynamics of movement rather than the kinematics. This would seem a particularly good idea for studying timing behavior, for the kinematic level of analysis velocity (distance/time) is not perceived as such (Runeson, 1974) by the human visual system.

We might view timing as a property of relative perspectives. One perspective (exogenous) views only the environmental events with its various contingency schedules. A second view (endogenous) is concerned only with the organism and its various contingencies. The ecological view, however, argues for a view of timing in which the proper system for analysis is the animal/environment synergy whereby a compatibility is sought which is sensitive both to the environmental rhythms of timing and to the animal's evolving design which is the complement.

## REFERENCES

Adams, J. A. (1971). Closed-loop theory of motor learning, *Journal of Motor Behavior*, **3**, 111–150.

Alderson, G. J. K. (1972). Variables affecting the perception of velocity in sports situations, in H. T. A. Whiting (ed.), *Readings in Sport Psychology*, London: Henry Kimpton.

Alderson, G. J. K., and Whiting, H. T. A. (1974). Prediction of linear motion, *Human Factors*, **16**, 495–502.

Ashton, R. (1976). Aspects of timing in child development, *Child Development*, **47**, 622–626.

Bruner, J. S. (1973). Organization of early skilled action, *Child Development*, **44**, 1–11.

Connolly, K. J. (1970). Response speed, temporal sequencing and information processing in children, in K. J. Connolly (ed.), *Mechanisms of Motor Skill Development*, London: Academic Press.

Ellingstad, V. S. (1967). Velocity estimation for briefly displayed targets, *Perceptual and Motor Skills*, **24**, 943–947.

Fitch, H. L., and Turvey, M. T. (1977). On the control of activity: some remarks from an ecological point of view, in D. M. Landers and R. W. Christina (eds.), *Psychology of Motor Behavior and Sport*, Champaign, Ill.: Human Kinetics.

Fowler, C., and Turvey, M. T. (1978). Skill acquisition: An event approach with special reference to searching for the optimum of a function of several variables, in G. Stelmach (ed.), *Information Processing in Motor Control and Learning*, New York: Academic Press.

Gerhard, D. J. (1959). The judgment of velocity and prediction of motion, *Erognomics*, **2**, 287–304.

Gibson, J. J. (1958). Visually controlled locomotion and visual orientation, *British Journal of Psychology*, **49**, 182–194.

Gibson, J. J. (1966). *The Senses Considered as Perceptual Systems*, Boston: Houghton Mifflin.

Hubbard, A. W. (1960). Homokinetics: Muscular function in human movement, in W. R. Johnson, (ed.), *Science and Medicine in Exercise and Sport*, New York, Harper, pp. 7–39.

Kay, H. (1969). The development of motor skills from birth to adolescence, in E. A. Bilodeau (ed.), *Principles of Skill Acquisition*, New York: Academic Press.

Kay, H. (1970). Analyzing motor skill performance, in J. J. Connolly (ed.), *Mechanisms of Motor Skill Development*, London: Academic Press.

Kugler, P. N., Kelso, J. A. S., and Turvey, M. T. (1980). On the concept of coordinative structures as dissipative structures: I. Theoretical lines of convergence, in G. E. Stelmach and J. Requin (eds.), *Tutorials in Motor Behavior*, Amsterdam: North-Holland.

Kugler, P. N. and Turvey, M. T. (1979). Continuing commentary, *The Behavioral and Brain Sciences*, **2**, 305–312.

Lashley, K. S. (1917). The accuracy of movement in the absence of excitation from the moving organ, *American Journal of Physiology*, **43**, 169–194.

Lashley, K. S. (1951). The problem of serial order in behavior, in L. A. Jeffress (ed.), *Cerebral Mechanisms in Behavior*, New York: Wiley.

Lee, D. N. (1980). Visuo-motor coordination in space-time, in G. E. Stelmach and J. Requin (eds.), *Tutorials in Motor Behavior*, Amsterdam: North Holland.

Lewis, H. R., and Papdimetrious, C. H. (1978). The efficiency of algorithms, *Scientific American*, **238**, 96–109.

Poulton, E. C. (1957). On prediction in skilled movements, *Psychological Bulletin*, **54**, 467–478.

Rosenbaum, D. A. (1975). Perception and extrapolation of velocity and acceleration, *Journal of Experimental Psychology & Human Perception and Performance*, **1**, 395–403.

Runeson, S. (1974). Constant velocity – not perceived as such, *Psychological Research*, **37**, 3–23.

Schmidt, R. A. (1975). A schema theory of discrete motor skill learning, *Psychological Review*, **82**, 225–260.

Schmidt, R. A. (1980). On the theoretical status of time in motor program representations, in G. E. Stelmach and J. Requin (eds.), *Tutorials in Motor Behavior*, Amsterdam: North-Holland.

Shannon, C. E., and Weaver, W. (1949). *The Mathematical Theory of Communication*, Urbana, Ill.: University of Illinois Press.

Shapiro, D. C. (1977). A preliminary attempt to determine the duration of a motor program, in D. M. Landers and R. W. Christina (eds.), *Psychology of Motor Behavior and Sport*, Urbana, Ill.: Human Kinetics.

Shaw, R. E., Turvey, M. T., and Mace, W. (in press). Ecological psychology: Consequences of a commitment to realism, in W. Weimer and D. Palermo (eds.), *Cognition and Symbolic Processes II*, Hillsdale, NJ: Lawrence Erlbaum.

Shaw, R. E., and Turvey, M. T. (in press). Coalitions as models for ecosystems: A realist perspective on perceptual organization, in M. Kubovy and J. Pomerantz, (eds.), *Perceptual Organization*, Hillsdale, NJ: Lawrence Erlbaum.

Taub, E., and Berman, J. (1968). Movement and learning in the absence of sensory feedback, in S. J. Freedman (ed.), *The Neurophysiology of Spatially Oriented Behavior*, Homewood, Ill.: Dorsey.

Todd, J. T. (1981). Visual information about moving objects, *Journal of Experimental Psychology & Human Perception and Performance*, **7**, 795–810.

Turvey, M. T. (1977). Preliminaries to a theory of action with reference to vision, in Shaw, R. and Bransford, J. (eds.), *Perceiving, Acting and Knowing: Towards an Ecological Psychology*, Hillsdale, NJ, Lawrence Erlbaum.

Turvey, M. T., Shaw, R. E., and Mace, W. (1978). Issues in the theory of action: Degrees of freedom, coordinative structures and coalitions, in J. Requin (ed.) *Attention and Performance VII*, Hillsdale, NJ, Lawrence Erlbaum.

Wade, M. G. (1976). Developmental motor learning, in J. Keogh and R. S. Hutton (eds.), *Exercise Science and Sport Reviews* (Vol. IV), Santa Barbara, CA: Journal Publishing Affiliates.

Wade, M. G. (1980). Coincidence anticipation of young normal and handicapped children, *Journal of Motor Behavior*, **12**, 103–112.

Wolf, P. H. (1967). The role of biological rhythms in early psychological development, *Bull. of the Meninger Clinic*, **13**, 197–218.

Wolf, P. H. (1968a). The serial organization of sucking in the young infant, *Pediatrics*, **42**, 943–956.

Wolf, P. H. (1968b). Stereotypic behavior and development, *Canadian Psychologist*, **9**, 474–484.

Yonas, A., Bechtold, A. G., Frankel, D., Gordon, F. R., McRoberts, G., Norcia, A., and Sternfels, S. (1977). Development of sensitivity to information for impending collision, *Perception & Psychophysics*, **21** (2), 97–104.

## NOTE

1. Preparation of this chapter was supported by NICHHD Program Project Grant No. HD05951 and State of Illinois Department of Mental Health and Developmental Disabilities Grant No. 704–01, awarded to the author. Peter Kugler is acknowledged for his critical comments on earlier drafts of this chapter.

The Development of Movement Control and Co-ordination
Edited by J. A. S. Kelso and J. E. Clark
© 1982, John Wiley & Sons, Ltd

CHAPTER 9

---

# The Development of Time-sharing Skills

---

CHRISTOPHER D. WICKENS AND DENISE C. R. BENEL

## ABSTRACT

This paper discusses the mechanisms by which time-sharing efficiency improves with age. Drawing upon literature from skill learning and individual differences studies, four possible sources of dual-task improvement may be identified once artifacts related to measurement-scale properties are accounted for. These consist of single-task automation, expanding processing resources, greater structural separation of resources, and improved deployment of resources. Paradigms and techniques for operationally distinguishing between these mechanisms are discussed. A review of developmental investigations reveals few studies that unambiguously argue for an improvement in time-sharing skills. Furthermore, little affirmative evidence is available to suggest that either expanding capacity or increased resource differentiation underlies any ontogenetic changes in dual-task performance efficiency. Instead, automation appears to play a major role, while the time-sharing 'skill' component underlying developmental changes appears to be related to the characteristics of attention switching, allocation and stimulus sampling, referred to collectively as attention-deployment skills.

## OVERVIEW

The ability to time-share, to divide attention between concurrent activities or information sources, is a critical element in the acquisition of perceptual motor skills (Klein, 1976). For example, a major component in the development of motor skills is represented by the hierarchical combination of separate 'basic' motor programs (reach, grasp, etc.) into more complex integrated patterns of action. While late in practice it is safe to assert that this integration has generated a new motor program and the original components have become automated; during the early stages of learning performance clearly entails the division of processing resources or attention between the component sub-programs. Limitation of these resources in early stages is clearly revealed by the awkwardness of performance. If the skill is one performed under conditions of environmental uncertainty, so that processing needs to be divided between perceptual encoding and response co-ordination, then the division of attention itself may represent a critical component of the skill and not simply a limitation whose role is evident only during the early phases of skill integration. Lastly the learning process often entails the division of attention between performance of the skill itself (execution of the appropriate motor commands) and concurrent processing of visual or auditory information related to task instructions or external feedback. The ability to do this will bear critically upon the speed and efficiency with which the skill can be mastered.

The assertion that time-sharing ability increases with age is supported by a modest number of experimental investigations (e.g. Birch, 1971; Lipps-Birch, 1976; Hiscock and Kinsbourne, 1978), as well as by informal observations that the young child must concentrate to a much greater extent than the adult when performing one of a pair of concurrent activities at the expense of performance on the other. This paper will address the possible mechanisms that underlie this increase in time-sharing efficiency with age.

To provide a framework for addressing the developmental time-sharing issue, data and theory will be drawn from two additional domains of experimental inquiry. (i) Research that has addressed the acquisition of time-sharing skills – the increased levels of dual-task performance observed across practice with adult subjects (e.g. Bahrick and Shelley, 1958; Damos and Wickens, 1980; Gopher and North, 1977; Kalsbeek and Sykes, 1967; Schneider and Shiffrin, 1977). (ii) Investigations of individual differences in time-sharing ability (e.g. McQueen, 1917; Jennings and Chiles, 1977; Sverko, 1977; Hawkins, Rodriguez, and Reicher, 1979; Wickens, Mountford, and Schreiner, 1981). Both lines of inquiry have in common with each other and with the developmental area the goal of establishing why dual-task performance is more efficient in one circumstance (level of development, level of training, or a given individual) than in another. Given the relative paucity of developmental investigations on time-sharing, it is anticipated that the skill learning and individual differences research described can provide a framework for formulating future lines of developmental inquiry.


## BASELINE ARTIFACTS: THE MEASUREMENT-SCALE PROBLEM

To observe that dual-task performance is better in one condition than in another does not of course warrant the conclusion that a time-sharing skill or ability differentiates these two conditions. If, for example, an improvement in dual-task performance is paralleled by an equivalent change in the single-task level of both tasks, then the change in the former need not be attributed to time-sharing skills – only to improved single-task performance. Therefore the investigator needs to establish the presence of a greater difference between single- and dual-task performance (dual-task decrement) in one condition than in another (Figure 1a). We shall refer to this decrement difference as the 'critical interaction.' As Lipps-Birch (1976) has noted, however, even when the critical interaction is observed caution must be employed to insure that the underlying measurement scale upon which these decrements are assessed is a linear one, so that decrements of equal size have the same implication in terms of degree of interference at all absolute levels of the scale. If the scale is not linear, as might be suggested by a highly skewed distribution of data, then a scale transformation to its linear representation might eliminate a difference in two decrements that were measured from different single-task baselines (Figure 1b).

The time-sharing investigations of Lipps-Birch (1976, 1978) illustrate this potential source of artifact. Her six-, ten- and thirteen-year-old subjects performed a tracking task concurrently with an auditory same-different judgement task, and the critical interaction was observed. However, suspicious that baseline difference in single-task performance between the two groups might account for the different time-sharing decrements, Lipps-Birch (1978) replicated some aspects of the first study in a second investigation. In the replication, the younger subjects received extensive single-task training on both tasks so that their single-task performance was equivalent to that of the older group. After equating baseline performance in this fashion, the developmental difference in time-sharing decrement vanished.

Lane (1979) has criticized the approach taken by Lipps-Birch on the grounds that providing different levels of single-task practice between groups may render them incomparable, as different strategies might be applied by each

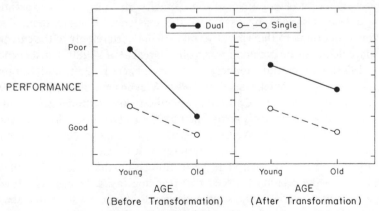

FIGURE 1    Elimination of the 'critical interaction' between taskload and age, with data transformation

as a function of the training difference. Nevertheless, Lipps-Birch's study clearly demonstrates that caution must be applied when different single-task baselines are compared, and the critical interaction is not a strong one.

A recommended course of action when baseline differences exist, is to insure that the critical interaction obtains even when an extreme (but plausible) transformation of the measurement scale is employed in a direction that would tend to equate the dual-task decrements across groups (e.g. a log transformation of the data in Figure 1a). Suc an approach was taken by Damos and Wickens (1980) in supporting their argument that time-sharing skills had developed as task pairs were practiced concurrently.

An alternative approach, if task-load conditions are manipulated within subjects, is to test within each group, if decrements correlate with baseline performance. If this correlation is negligible, then greater assurance is provided that baseline differences do not account for the critical interaction.

## A STRUCTURE-SPECIFIC RESOURCE MODEL OF DUAL-TASK PERFORMANCE

To provide a theoretical framework for considering the relation between four possible mechanisms of improved dual-task performance, it is important to describe briefly the original formulation and a subsequent elaboration of the capacity or resource concept of attention. An underlying assumption of this conception is that the human possesses some limited capacity reservoir of processing resources that may be mobilized and deployed to tasks as required by their difficulty or desired level of performance (e.g. Kahneman, 1973; Knowles, 1963; Moray, 1967). Time-sharing decrements occur when the joint demand for resources of concurrent tasks exceeds the supply available for adequate performance on either or both.

However, recent elaborations of the capacity view argue that experimental data are best described by assuming the existence of more than a single reservoir. According to this view, two tasks will interfere only to the extent that they share demands on common reservoirs (Isreal et al., 1980; Kinsbourne and Hicks, 1978; Navon and Gopher, 1979; Roediger, Knight, and Kantowitz, 1977; Sanders, 1979; Wickens, 1979, 1980; Wickens and Kessel, 1979, 1980).

A simplified version of the structure-specific resource model is illustrated in Figure 2. Here resource pools are defined by three conventionally distinguished stages of processing (e.g. Welford, 1976). If two tasks demand commond resources, as in case I on the left, interference will result and increases in the difficulty of one task will derogate performance on the other. This might be exemplified by the relation between two tracking tasks. In case II, However, there is minimal overlap of resource demands. Such might define the task structure of reading silently while holding a cup of coffee while a passenger in an aircraft. As the difficulty of the passage increases, demanding greater resources, performance on the coffee cup 'task' will be little impaired.

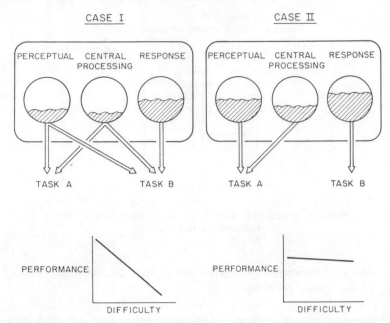

FIGURE 2  A simplified representation of stage-defined processing resources. Case I: Common resource demands of two tasks. Case II: Separate resource demands

Experimental evidence reviewed elsewhere (Wickens, 1980) suggests that the three-stage model of Figure 2 may be elaborated to define separate resource reservoirs by modalities of processing within stages (auditory-visual perception, vocal-manual response), and cerebral hemispheres of processing (verbal versus spatial processing). Furthermore, evidence suggests the existance of just two stage-defined pools, perception and central processing competing for common resources. This elaboration is portrayed in Figure 3.

Employing the structure-specific resource framework as a descriptive model for adult time-sharing performance, differences in the time-sharing performance of children might be attributed to any of the following four factors:

(1) *Automation* reflects a smaller demand of tasks for resources from reservoirs of a constant fixed capacity.

(2) *Expanded capacity* reflects a greater capacity available within each reservoir.

(3) *Increasing functional separation* of resource pools would be manifest if the separate resource reservoirs characteristic of adult processing, depicted in Figures 2 and 3, emerge with development from a structure of undifferentiated capacity.

(4) *Improved deployment of resources* is manifest when the same fixed quantitiy and structure of resources is better and more optimally

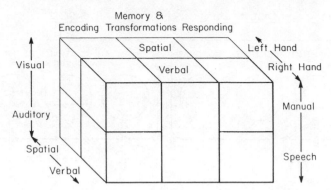

FIGURE 3   The structure of processing resources defined by stages of processing, modalities of processing, and cerebral hemispheres of processing

allocated between tasks, given the constraints imposed by task and environmental variables.

Of these four potential sources of improvement in dual-task performance it should be noted that only the latter three may be legitimately labeled time-sharing skills, since automation represents a characteristic of the specific task, as performed by the learner, and not a more general change in processing efficiency. Each of these sources will be considered in turn and efforts will be made to identify mechanisms for operationally distinguishing between them.

## SOURCES OF IMPROVEMENT IN DUAL-TASK PERFORMANCE

### Automation

Norman and Bobrow (1975) have characterized the *performance-resource function* as that relationship between the hypothetical processing resources invested in a task and the level of performance obtained. Automation can be said to occur if across practice, or development, the maximum performance on a task remains unchanged, but the quantity of resources required to obtain that maximum is diminished. In this case, more 'residual' resources remain available for the performance of concurrent activities, and an apparent improvement in dual-task efficiency will result. To cite one example, a child who has only recently learned to tie her shoes and a well-practiced adult may both perform the task at the same rate. Yet the adult can perform the task better while engaged in a concurrent task, not because of superior time-sharing skills, but simply because of the greater automation, and thereby shift to lower levels of control of the motor commands necessary for shoe-tying.

It should be noted that the phenomenon of automation is not restricted to tasks involving substantial levels of motor control (Posner and Keele, 1969; Keele, 1968), but has manifestations in perceptual phenomena (Schneider and Shiffrin, 1977; LaBerge, 1973a; Lansman, 1978) and in tasks requiring heavy information-transmission loads from stimulus to response (Pew, 1974; Bahrick and Shelley, 1958; Kalsbeek and Sykes, 1967).

## Expanding Resources

The concept of expanding resources – that a task places constant demands on a greater pool of resources – is in theory quite distinct from the view that a task places smaller demands on a constant pool of resources (automation). However, both imply that more residual capacity will be available for concurrent tasks, and therefore that dual-task efficiency will improve. Operationally these two conceptions prove to be somewhat difficult to distinguish, particularly within the developmental framework.

In attempting to dissociate experimentally automation from expanding resources it is important to bear in mind that automation is a phenomenon that may be associated purely with single-task practice. It may be argued, in fact, that automation should develop more rapidly under single-task training than under dual. This characteristic makes automation a relatively easy source to isolate in the area of skill learning when seeking evidence for time-sharing skills. One may predict that if two groups are compared after transfer to a dual-task condition, one group which was trained exclusively under a single-task regime (e.g. alternating trials on the component tasks), and the other under concurrent conditions, any superiority of the dual-training group over the single would, of necessity, be related to time-sharing skills acquired during the dual-task regime, since automation would form at least as well in the single-task regime (Damos and Wickens, 1980).

When isolating automation as a source of dual-task performance differences in the individual differences domain, a different characteristic of automation may be exploited: since automation is defined to be a property only of the specific automated task as performed by the individual and does *not* reflect a more general characteristic of his or her processing efficiency, its contribution should be isolated exclusively to task pairs that share a common component task (the automated one). Therefore automation should *not* be responsible if a general factor of dual-task efficiency emerges that transcends a number of qualitatively different dual-task combinations. Unfortunately, the experimental literature has provided scant evidence for the existence of such an 'A' factor in time-sharing, analogous to the 'g' factor of intelligence proposed by Spearman, (1904); (Jennings and Chiles, 1977; McQueen, 1917; Sverko, 1977; Wickens, Mountford, and Schreiner, 1981). At best, these investigations have isolated only time-sharing factors specific to a given dual-task combination.

In the training paradigm, the task-specific property of automation would imply that its contribution to superior dual-task performance should *not* transfer to a qualitatively different dual-task pair. Damos and Wickens (1980), for example, provided subjects with dual-task training on two discrete tasks (digit categorization by physical size and value, and running short-term memory of digits), and then transferred the group to a dual-axis tracking task. The positive transfer observed to this qualitatively different task pair, relative to a control group who had received only extensive single-task practice, indicated development of a time-sharing skill since automation of the classification and memory tasks would have provided little benefit to the subsequent tracking tasks.

Unfortunately, it appears that neither of the defining properties of automation can be properly exploited adequately to define its role in ontogenetic development and thereby provide affirmative or negative evidence for expanding capacity. This is because any changes with age in capacity are probably invariably confounded with changes in automation. It must be assumed that older children as a group simply have received greater practice on all of the task components to which they might be exposed in a laboratory setting.

Therefore, given an apparently insoluble confounding of automation and expanding resources when developmental changes in time-sharing are exhibited, it is apparent that research focus must be directed to affirmative signs of developmental changes in time-sharing behavior. These affirmative indications are exhibited in the two remaining sources of dual task improvement: resource differentiation and resource allocation.

**Functional Differentiation of Resource Reservoirs**

Figure 3 portrays a conceptual representation of the structure of adult processing resources. A potential source of improvement in time-sharing performance would be exhibited if the differentiated resources of Figure 3 emerged from an 'undifferentiated capacity' structure. Wickens (1980) has argued that the critical experimental results necessary to establish the presence of separate processing structures characteristic of adult performance is the *structural alteration effect* or SAE. If two tasks are time-shared, and the processing structure of one is altered in such a way that its processing demands are unchanged (e.g. a change from visual to auditory presentation), then a resulting change in dual-task efficiency (the SAE) indicates that the different structures relied upon separate resource reservoirs. When separate, as opposed to common, reservoirs are required, time-sharing efficiency increases.

As an example of an SAE, Wickens (1980) required subjects to perform a manual tracking task concurrently with a running memory mental arithmetic task (consecutive differencing of digits). When the modality of presentation of the digit employed for the arithmetic task was shifted from visual (the common modality with tracking) to auditory, improved time-sharing efficiency was observed. When the digit response modality was altered from manual (common with tracking) to verbal, a further improvement resulted. Similar SAEs have been reported with shifts in input modality (Treisman and Davies, 1973; Brooks, 1970), cerebral hemispheres of processing (Kinsbourne and Hicks, 1978), and verbal versus manual response modalities (McLeod, 1977; Harris, Owens, and North, 1978). With regard to the developmental issue, the critical evidence to be sought to suggest increasing resource differentiation with age is a corresponding increase in the *magnitude* of SAEs with age.

**Attention Deployment Skills**

It is conceivable that a major developmental difference in time-sharing may be reflected in how the resources available for task performance are deployed, rather than in their absolute availability or their structural composition. An analogy can be drawn to developmental research on memory. It is argued in this context that a major source of developmental change is not so much the absolute capacity of the memory system, but in the appropriate selection of mnemonic strategies such as rehearsal or encoding by semantic relatedness (Hagan, Jongward, and Kail, 1975). These strategies Flavell, Friedrichs, and Hoyt (1970) have labeled as 'meta memory.'

In seeking developmental changes in resource deployment, two approaches may be adopted. One may examine changes in time-sharing strategies as they are manifest through careful microanalysis of dual-task performance; alternatively it is possible to identify allocation and deployment skills that are known to be of use in efficient time-sharing performance and then determine the degree to which these deployment skills emerge with development.

*Modeling the Microstructure of Time-sharing*

When time-sharing studies require the full processing of two streams of information (e.g. stimuli, transformations, and responses are associated with both tasks) then considerable insight concerning the strategies employed in dual-task performance can be gained through time-series, correlational, and information theory analysis. These can reveal the patterning and contingencies existing between stimuli and responses, and allow inferences to be drawn concerning the qualitative characteristics of the underlying processing mechanisms.

One example of this kind of analysis is provided by an investigation of the acquisition and transfer of time-sharing skills by Damos and Wickens (1980). When subjects time-shared performance on two tracking tasks, the investigators employed time-series analysis between the perceived error and control response signals to identify the extent of parallel processing or independence between the two tasks or, conversely, the extent of 'cross-talk' between them. A parallel processing strategy was observed to emerge with practice. Further analyses of these data also indicated systematic changes in the times at which subjects chose to exert control on one task and the contingencies of these responses upon the error state of the other task.

In a different condition, subjects time-shared two discrete tasks, a running memory, digit-cancellation task and a categorical classification task. Both were associated with visual stimulus displays and manual responses. Damos and Wickens were able to dichotomize subjects into two categories according to their response strategies: those that processed the two tasks in parallel (executed simultaneous responses to both), and those that performed them in a serial fashion. In the parallel group, by comparing the latency of the simultaneous response in the dual-task condition, with the sum of the latencies of the two tasks performed singly, they were able to estimate the amount of overlap in processing. For the serial-processing group, a similar differencing procedure allowed them to estimate the time taken to switch attention from one task to the other. Both of these estimates were observed to change systematically with dual-task practice.

In a related approach with two discrete tasks, Fisher (1975) described time-sharing performance according to a criterion model. In this model the parameter posited to be critical to time-sharing efficiency was the time criterion set by the subject for switching from one task to the other, rather than continuing through with the response programmed on the task at hand. Different criterion settings will lead to different performance measures on both tasks, and Fisher argues that there exists an optimum criterion value to maximize dual-task efficiency. In both the analyses of Damos and Wickens and of Fisher, the nature of the response pattern adopted by the subject indicates the presence of more or less optimal strategies of attention deployment. Thus age differences in the patterning of responses between tasks as reflected by model parameters should be carefully examined in developmental investigations to reveal the existence of such trends where evidence may not be provided by global analyses of performance decrements.

An alternative approach to assessing attention deployment skills is to search more directly for the availability and utilization of capabilities and strategies that are known to facilitate dual-task performance. Three such capabilities can be briefly described: *attention switching*, reflecting the hardware limitation of the resource deployment process; *resource allocation* and *information sampling*, the latter two both reflecting the software properties of an executive resource management system (Moray and Fitter, 1973; Moray, 1976, 1978).

*Attention Switching*

A number of paradigms have been employed to measure attention switching times between perceptual channels or concurrent mental operations in adult subjects, and time constants associated with specific paradigms have been fairly well validated (e.g. LaBerge, 1973ab, 1969; Kristofferson, 1967; Hawkins, Church, and deLemos, 1978). Furthermore, data from Damos and Wickens (1980) and Hawkins, Church, and deLemos (1978) suggested that switching speed represents a potential source of improved time-sharing skill. Major differences in these times with age, or in the efficiency with which a switch might be 'called,' could readily account for an important source of variance in developmental time-sharing abilities.

### Resource Allocation by Priorities

The ability to allocate resources in proportion to priorities imposed by task instructions or internal goals underlies many instances of successful dual-task performance. Navon and Gopher (1979) have shown by theoretical analysis that for a given dual-task combination, one particular policy of resource distribution between tasks yields optimal performance. Given the characteristics of the underlying performance-resource function, a subject who overemphasizes one task may produce only a minimal performance gain on that task while affecting a disproportionate loss in performance of the other, thereby producing a derogation of overall time-sharing efficiency.

Several investigations have demonstrated that adults can effectively allocate resources between tasks according to experimenter-defined priorities (e.g. North and Gopher, 1976; Navon and Gopher, 1980; Sperling and Melchner, 1978; Wickens and Gopher, 1977), and monetary payoffs (Shulman and Briggs, 1971; Kahneman, 1970). Brickner and Gopher (1981) observed that time-sharing efficiency of subjects was greatly facilitated if they had received prior training on differential resource allocation. This allocation policy appears to be far less optimal when task demands are continually fluctuating within a trial (Wickens and Tsang, 1979). In young children it is possible that the allocation policy is considerably more rigid or adheres less closely to optimum policies.

### Information Sampling

The ability to sample different information sources in the environment, in direct proportion to their information content (Senders, 1964), and/or the expected value of sampling (or cost of ignoring: Sheridan and Tulga, 1978) is a skill in which adult subjects are observed to perform nearly optimally according to normative models of information theory and cueing theory (e.g. Carbonell, 1966; Sheridan and Ferrell, 1974; Moray, 1976, 1978). The presence of such sampling strategies implies that the subject possesses an internal model of the environment that represents the statistical characteristics of input sources. Differences in the fidelity of the model across age could easily produce large variance in time-sharing performance manifest with any task combinations which are dependent upon the processing of uncertain environmental information.

## DEVELOPMENTAL EVIDENCE

Considering the apparent importance of differences between adults' and children's dual-task performance in understanding developmental changes in perceptual, cognitive, and motor skills, it is surprising that such a small number of developmental studies have been conducted that allow these differences to be considered within the theoretical framework presented above. The following section will consider these investigations and their implications for developmental time-sharing differences.

### Affirmative Evidence for the Critical Interaction

Clearly the presence of different time-sharing skills in adults must, at a minimum, be supported by the appearance of the critical interaction between task load and age, preferably in such a form that it cannot be accounted for by baseline differences, as was the case of Lipps' (1976, 1978) data described earlier. Perhaps the strongest evidence of this interaction has been provided by Hiscock and Kinsbourne (1978). Their three- to twelve-year-old subjects performed a finger-tapping task with the right and left hands, either in a control condition or concurrently with verbal activity (reciting nursery rhymes or animal names). A time-sharing decrement in tapping performance was observed at all ages and was quantified as a ratio measure of single- to dual-task tapping rate. More importantly, this ratio score decreased with age, suggesting improved time-sharing. To guard against a baseline artifact the investigators also established that the decrement score did not correlate with single-task tapping rate.

Stratton (1977) required subjects aged seven and eleven to perform a rhythmic arm-swinging task under single-task conditions and concurrently with a simple reaction-time task. Temporal error was the performance measure employed on the rhythmic task. Stratton observed that the dual-task decrement in rhythmic temporal error was reliably larger for the younger group. Despite differences in single-task baseline, it appears that this difference in decrement is great enough to withstand transformations of the data.

Evidence for changes in time-sharing decrements with age is also provided by comparing the results of a study by Birch (1971) with children (aged three to six) with similar conditions in an investigation by Schvaneveldt (1969) with adults. In both studies subjects were required to respond to a single stimulus with either a manual response, a vocal response, or a combined vocal-manual response pattern. In Birch's study only a single stimulus was ever presented, while Schvaneveldt associated the manual and vocal responses with the spatial location and value respectively of a digit stimulus. Birch noted reliable delays in the combined condition as compared to the two single-response controls, while Schvaneveldt, in the simpler conditions more comparable to those employed by Birch, observed no increase in response time. Since no decrement at all was obtained by adults, baseline differences do not represent a problem because any transformation would still generate zero decrement for adults and a nonzero value for children.

An investigation by Piazza (1977) provides equivocal evidence concerning developmental differences, and again illustrates the measurement-scale problem. Like Hiscock and Kinsbourne, Piazza required children of different ages (three, four and five) to perform tapping concurrently with either verbal activity or humming. No interaction between task loading and age was reported with tapping rate as the dependent variable. However, if a reciprocal measure of intertap interval is employed, thereby using time as the dependent variable, a very large interaction with age is evident. The difference in tap intervals between single and dual conditions is quite small for the five-year-olds relative to the two younger groups.

Unfortunately, neither in the investigations of Hiscock and Kinsbourne, nor in those of Stratton or Piazza can an automation explanation be ruled out since a microanalysis of the data was not undertaken. In fact, in a prior study by Kinsbourne and McMurray (1973), the authors argue that automation of tapping may account for differences in tapping-verbal interference between adults and children. Birch (1971), however, did perform a microanalysis and reports trends in his data that suggest the emergence of time-sharing response strategies. The youngest subjects tended to exhibit direct competition (nonsimultaneity) in the release of the bimodal response, whereas the older ones showed a greater tendency toward co-ordination, both responses being released in synchrony, albeit delayed from the unimodel response conditions. As noted above, the bimodal responses of Schvaneveldt's adult subjects were not delayed. In addition, in the comparable conditions there was evidence for neither competition nor co-ordination (synchrony) of the manual and vocal responses, but for complete independence. Collectively then, the investigations of Birch and of Schvaneveldt argue for age-dependent increases in independence, or channel capacity of the output stage of processing.

**Negative Evidence**

Negative evidence for decrement changes with age appears to be as strong as the positive evidence. As indicated, Piazza's data is equivocal. In a developmental investigation of time-sharing memory, Lane (1979) required children of two ages (nine and thirteen), and adults simultaneously to maintain visual and verbal items in memory for later recall. The memory load (number of items) for each subject was adjusted adaptively, so that approximately constant single-task performance was achieved across all age groups. (The younger subjects were thereby required to retain a smaller number of items in memory.) Under dual-task conditions, all age groups again demonstrated equivalent levels of recall. That is, the magnitude of the decrement was equal across age groups when single-task baselines were equated. Therefore the results paralleled the observation of Lipps-Birch (1978). In contrast to Lipps-Birch, however, the equation of baselines was accomplished through differential adjustments of task difficulty rather than differing amounts of single-task practice.

Holden (1974) reports an investigation that does not strictly involve a dual-task paradigm, but does reflect upon the availability of resources between different stages of processing. In this experiment, subjects were required to enumerate the number of events in a rapid stimulus train. Events occurred either entirely within one modality of alternated between the auditory, visual, and tactile modalities. In the two enumeration conditions compared, subjects either covertly counted the number of events, or executed a manual tap, following each event. The added motor requirement of tapping was observed to produce a decrement in enumeration performance (e.g. the sum total of taps in the tap condition was in greater error from the number of events, than the accuracy of counts in the count condition). Of major importance was the observation that the decrement in enumeration accuracy from counting to tapping, imposed by adding the response requirement, was no greater in younger than older children. In terms of a ratio of tap to count errors, this decrement was in fact greater for the older children.

An additional source of negative evidence for developmental time-sharing differences is provided by two developmental investigations of divided auditory attention in a dichotic listening task (Hiscock and Kinsbourne, 1977; Geffen and Sexton, 1978). Both studies demonstrated an improvement with age in selective or focused attention (the ability to withhold processing or nonrelevant information), an observation substantiated by other developmental research (e.g. Doyle, 1973; Hagan and Hale, 1973). However, neither study indicated any improvement with age in the ability of subjects to process in parallel the two independent sources of auditory information (a decrement score between a divided and focused attention condition).

## Sources of Developmental Time-sharing Differences

### Structural Alteration Effects

The evidence then for decreasing time-sharing decrements with increasing age is decidedly mixed. Where such evidence exists, automation explanations cannot be easily discounted since, with the exception of Birch's (1971) study, microprocessing analysis has not been undertaken in potentially crucial experiments. In the search for evidence of development in time-sharing skills it is appropriate therefore to examine evidence supportive either of increasing functional separation of resources or of independent development of attention-deployment skills.

The thrust of evidence for developmental differences in the former category is again more negative than positive. As described above, support would be provided if structural alteration effects are observed to be greater in adults than children. Such results would indicate the greater functional separation of resources upon which the compared structures depend in adults. The investigations described above by Hiscock and Kinsbourne (1978) and Piazza (1977) both addressed this issue. Processing structures (controlling hemispheres) were altered by requiring left- versus right-handed tapping and, in Piazza's investigation, either a verbal (left-hemispheric) or humming (right-hemispheric) oral task.

In both experiments structural alteration effects were observed. However, in neither case was an interaction noted such that the advantage of employing separate versus common hemispheres was greater for older than younger subjects. In fact, Piazza's results indicated the opposite effect. *Greater* lateralized interference was observed for the younger subjects. In support of this finding Kinsbourne and McMurray (1975) report that lateralized tapping-verbal interference effects (SAEs) are observed with children, but not with adults.

Structural alteration effects with input modalities were investigated in Stratton's (1977) investigation of simultaneous performance of a rhythmic arm-swinging and a reaction-time task. The stimuli to be processed in the latter task could be delivered in either the auditory or visual modality, while the rhythmic task required timing of motor movements with auditory stimuli from a metronome. In comparing results of seven- and eleven-year-old subjects Stratton noted, as described above, a greater decrement for the younger group, but SAEs were absent. That is, no interaction in the size of this decrement was observed between reaction-time stimulus modality and age.

Finally, considering resource pools defined by stages of processing rather than by modalities or hemispheres, an interpretation of Holden's (1974) results on enumeration performance provides further negative evidence for increased differentiation. According to this interpretation the requirement to tap, rather than simply count, produced a performance decrement because of the necessary mobilization of extra processes associated with the manual response. If younger children's performance drew resources from a less differentiated pool (e.g. the stage-defined pools of Figures and 2 and 3 were less distinct), the decrement of the added response requirement should have been greater for this group. In fact, as noted above, it was less.

*Attention Deployment*

Drawing an analogy from the metamemory literature, it is likely that the search for developmental differences in time-sharing should be directed toward differences in deployment. Here again, within the framework provided above, experimental evidence is scant, but is more affirmative than negative. Concerning the hardware component of switching speed, Holden's (1974) data may be cited again. The greater enumeration error (in both the tap and count conditions) observed in the inter- as opposed to the intramodality conditions is argued by Holden to result from a failure to switch attention rapidly enough between modalities in the former condition. As a consequence events are sometimes missed by the time attention has switched to the next modality and enumeration is consistently underestimated. This intra-inter-modality decrement was greater for the younger children, consistent with the view that switching speed for this group was slower than for the older.

Developmental differences in the 'software' component of priority allocation was directly addressed in Lane's (1979) time-sharing memory investigation described above. Recall conditions were compared in which the experimenter-defined priorities (and payoffs) emphasized either the auditory or the visual material. Lane's adult subjects and older children showed differential recall performance on the two modalities that reflected these priorities. However, the youngest subjects failed to do so. In a related investigation, Hale *et al.* (1978) showed that the ability of children to allocate attention between two attributes (color and shape) of a stimulus according to priorities improved reliably from the ages of five to twelve.

With regard to developmental differences in information sampling, the numerous demonstrations and observations that young children are more distractable, and more likely to attend to irrelevant sources of stimulus information in concept learning, dichotic listening, incidental learning, and memory paradigms are certainly pertinent (e.g. Doyle, 1973; Hagan and Hale, 1973). Absent however are careful quantitative analyses of the conformity or departure of children from optimal sampling strategies in paradigms involving multiple channels of relevant information. However, extrapolation from the developmental data on distraction and irrelevant information processing suggests that systematic age differences in these strategies should be manifest and presumably these can account for large portions of developmental variance in time-sharing efficiency. Data should be collected here that parallel the research efforts of Moray (1976), Sheridan and Tulga (1978), Senders (1964), and Carbonnell (1966).

## SUMMARY

It is apparent that the available evidence for developmental differences in time-sharing behavior is scarce. The studies that provide appropriate data are few in number. Furthermore, much of the data of those investigations can be accounted for by alternative and more parsimonious explanations in terms of automation and measurement-scale artifacts. The former, in particular, renders the concept of expanding capacity with age nearly impossible to validate. The strongest experimental support seems to suggest that differences lie in resource deployment policies rather than in the availability or structure of those resources, but much more experimental data is called for before answers can be conclusive.

## REFERENCES

Bahrick, H. P., and Shelly, C. (1958). Timesharing as an index of automatization, *Journal of Experimental Psychology*, **56**, 288–293.

Birch, D. (1971). Evidence for competition and coordination between vocal and manual responses in preschool children, *Journal of Experimental Child Psychology*, **12**, 10–26.

Brickner, M. and Gopher, D. (1981). Improving time-sharing performance by enhancing voluntary control of processing resources. Technion Israeli Institute of Technology Technical Report AFOSE-77-3131C., 24.

Brooks, L. (1970). An extension of the conflict between reading and visualization, *Quarterly Journal of Experimental Psychology*, **22**, 91–96.

Carbonell, J. R. (1966). A cueing model of many instrument visual sampling, *IEEE Transactions and Human Factors and Electronics*, HEF-7, No. 4.

Damos, D., and Wickens, C. (1980). The identification and transfer of timesharing skills, *Acta Psychologica. Acta Psychologica*, **6**, 564–577.

Doyle, A. (1973). Listening to distraction: A developmental study of selective attention, *Journal of Experimental Child Psychology*, **15**, 100–115.

Fisher, S. (1975). The microstructure of dual task interaction, 2, *Perception*, **4**, 459–474.

Flavell, J. H., Friedrichs, A. G., and Hoyt, J. D. (1970). Developmental changes in memorization processes, *Cognitive Psychology*, **1**, 324–340.

Geffen, G., and Sexton, M. (1978). The development of auditory strategies of attention, *Developmental Psychology*, **14**, 11–17.

Gopher, D., and North, R. (1977). Manipulating the conditions of training in time-sharing performances, *Human Factors*, **19**, 583–593.

Hagen, J., Jongeward, R., and Kail, R. (1973). In H. Reese (ed.), *Advances in Child Development and Behavior* (1973). (Vol. 10), New York: Academic Press.

Hagen, J. W., and Hale, G. A. (1973). The development of attention in children, in Pick, A. D. (ed.), *Minnesota Symposia on Child Psychology* (Vol. 7), Minneapolis: University of Minnesota Press.

Hale, G. A., Taweel, S. S., Green, R. Z., and Flaugher, J. (1978). Effects of instruction on children's attention to stimulus components, *Developmental Psychology*, **14**, 494–506.

Harris, S., Owens, J., North, R. (1978). A system for the assessment of human performance of concurrent verbal and manual control tasks, *Behavior Research Methods and Instrumentation*, **10**, 329–333.

Harris, S., and Wickens, C. D. (1979). Interaction of processing structures and task difficulty in a dual-task paradigm, Navy Aeromedical Research Laboratory Technical Report.

Hawkins, H., Church, M., and deLemos, S. (1978). Time-sharing is not a unitary ability, University of Oregon Center for Cognitive and Perceptual Research, ONR Technical Report No. 2, June.

Hawkins, H., Church, M., and deLemos, S. (1978). Time-sharing is not a unitary ability, University of Oregon Center for Cognitive and Perceptual Research, ONR Technical Report No. 2, June.

Hawkins, H. L., Rodriguez, E., and Reicher, G. M. (1979). Is time-sharing a general ability? University of Oregon Center for Cognitive and Perceptual Research, ONR Technical Report No. 3, June.

Hiscock, J., and Kinsbourne, M. (1977). Selective listening assymetry in preschool children, *Developmental Psychology*, 12, 217–224.

Hiscock, J., and Kinsbourne, M. (1978). Ontogeny of Cerebral Dominance: Evidence from time-sharing asymmetry in children, *Developmental Psychology*, 14, 321–329.

Holden, E. (1974). Enumeration vs. tracking during unimodal and multi-modal sequential information processing in normals and retardates, *Developmental Psychology*, 10, 667–671.

Isreal, J., Chesney, G., Wickens, C., and Donchin, E. (1980). P-300 and tracking difficulty: Evidence for multiple resources in dual task performance, *Psychophysiology*, 17, 259–273.

Jennings, A., and Chiles, D. (1977). An investigation of time-sharing ability as a factor in complex performance, *Human Factors*, 19, 535–548.

Kahneman, D. (1970). Remarks on attention control, *Acta Psychologica*, 33, 118–131.

Kahneman, D. (1973). *Attention and Effort*, Englewood Cliffs, NJ: Lawrence Erlbaum.

Kalsbeek, J. W. H., and Sykes, R. N. (1967). Objective measurement of mental load, in A. F. Sanders (ed.), *Attention and Performance III*, Amsterdam: North Holland, pp. 253–261.

Keele, S. W. (1968). Movement control in skilled motor performance, *Psychological Bulletin*, 70, 387–403.

Kinsbourne, M., and Hicks, R. (1978). Functional Cerebral Space, in J. Requin (ed.), *Attention and Performance VII*, Hillsdale, NJ: Lawrence Erlbaum.

Kinsbourne, M., and McMurray, J. (1973). Effect of cerebral dominance of time-sharing between speaking and tapping by preschool children, *Child Development*, 46, 240–242.

Klein, R. M. (1976). Attention and movement, in G. E. Stelmach (ed.), *Motor Control: Issues and Trends*, New York: Academic Press.

Knowles, W. B. (1963). Operator loading tasks, *Human Factors*, 5, 155–161.

Kristofferson, A. B. (1967). Attention and psychophysical time, *Acta Psychologica*, 27, 93–100.

LaBerge, D. (1973a). Attention and the measurement of perceptual learning, *Memory and Cognition*, 1, 268–276.

LaBerge, D. (1973b). Identification of two components of the time to switch attention: A test of serial and a parallel model of attention, in S. Kornblum (ed.), *Attention and Performance IV*, New York: Academic Press.

Lane, David. (1979). Developmental changes in attention-deployment skills, *Journal of Experimental Child Psychology*, 28, 16–29.

Lansman, M. (1978). An attentional approach to individual differences in immediate memory, ONR Technical Report, University of Washington, June.

Lipps-Birch, L. (1976). Age trends in children's time-sharing performance, *Journal of Experimental Child Psychology*, 22, 331–345.

Lipps-Birch, L. (1978). Baseline difference, attention, and age differences in time-sharing performance, *Journal of Experimental Child Psychology*, 25, 505–513.

McLeod, P. (1977). A dual-task response modality effect: Support for multiprocessor models of attention, *Quarterly Journal of Experimental Psychology*, 29, 651–667.

McQueen, E. N. (1917). The distribution of attention, *British Journal of Psychology*. Monograph Supplements, Vol. II, Cambridge.

Moray, N. (1967). Where is capacity limited? A survey and a model, *Acta Psychologica*, 27, 84–92.

Moray, N. (1976). Attention Control and Sampling Behavior, in Sheridan and Johansson (eds.), *Monitoring and Supervisory Control*, New York, Plenum Press.

Moray, N. (1978). Strategies in Sampling and Control, in G. Underwood (ed.), *Strategies of Information Processing*, New York: Academic Press.

Moray, N., and Fitter, M. (1973). A theory and the measurement of attention, in S. Kornblum (ed.), *Attention and Performance IV*, New York: Academic Press.

Navon, D., and Gopher, D. (1979). On the economy of the human processing system. Psychological Review, 86, 217–255.

Navon, D., and Gopher, D. (1980). Interpretations of task difficulty in terms of resources, in R. Nickerson (ed.), *Attention and Performance VIII*, Englewood Cliffs, NJ: Lawrence Erlbaum.

Norman, D. A., and Bobrow, D. J. (1975). On data-limited and resource-limited processes, *Cognitive Psychology*, 7, 44–64.

North, R. A., and Gopher, D. (1976). Measures of attention as predictors of flight performance, *Human Factors*, 18, 1–14.

Pew, R. W. (1974). Levels of analysis in motor control, *Brain Research*, 71, 393–400.

Piazza, D. (1977). Cerebral lateralization in young children as measured by dichotic listening and finger tapping tasks, *Neuropsychologia*, 15, 417–425.

Posner, M. I., and Keele, S. W. (1969). Attention demands of movements, *Proceedings of the Seventeenth Congress of Applied Psychology*, Amsterdam: Zeitlinger.

Roediger, H. I., Knight, J. L., and Kantowitz, B. H. (1977). Inferring decay in short term memory: The issue of capacity, *Memory and Cognition*, 5, 167–176.

Sanders, A. (1979). Some remarks on mental load, in N. Moray (ed.), *Mental Workload: Its Theory and Measurement*, New York: Plenum Press.

Schneider, W. and Shiffrin, R. M. (1977). Controlled and automatic human information processing: I. Detection, search, and attention, *Psychological Review*, 84, 1–66.

Schvaneveldt, R. W. (1969). Effects of complexity in simultaneous reaction time tasks, *Journal of Experimental Psychology*, 81, 289–296.

Senders, J. (1964). The human operator as monitor and controller of multi-degree of freedom systems, *IEEE Transactions on Human Factors in Electronics*, HFE-5, 2–5, September.

Sheridan, T., and Ferrell, W. (1974). *Man-Machine Systems: Information, Control, and Decision Models of Human Performance*, Cambridge, Mass., MIT Press.

Sheridan, T. B., and Tulga, M. K. (1978). A model for dynamic allocation of human attention among multiple tasks, Fourteenth Annual Conference on Manual Control, University of Southern California (Los Angeles), April.

Shulman, H. G., and Briggs, G. G. (1971). Studies of performances in complex aircrew tasks, Ohio State University, Research Foundation. Air Force Project 2718, Final Report.

Spearman, C. (1904). 'Generalized Intelligence' objectively determined and measured, *American Journal of Psychology*, 15, 201–293.

Sperling, G., and Melchner, M. (1978). Visual search, visual attention and the attention operating characteristic, in J. Requin (ed.), *Attention and Performance VII*, New York: Lawrence Erlbaum.

Stratton, R. (1977). Development of attention in motor task performance of children, doctoral dissertation, Florida State University.

Sverko, B. (1977). Individual differences in time-sharing performance, Technical Report ARL-77-4/AFOSR-77-4, Aviation Research Laboratory, January.

Triesman, A. M., and Davies, A. (1973). Divided attention to ear and eye, in S. Kornblum (ed.), *Attention and Performance IV*, New York: Academic Press.

Welford, A. T. (1975). *Skilled Performance*, Glenview, Ill.: Scott Foresman.

Wickens, C. D. (1979). Measures of workload, stress and secondary tasks, in N. Moray (ed.), *Human Workload: Its theory and measurement*, New York: Plenum Press, 77–99.

Wickens, C. D. (1980). The structure of processing resources, in R. Nickerson (ed.), *Attention and Performance VIII*, Englewood Cliffs, NJ: Lawrence Erlbaum.

Wickens, C. D., and Gopher, D. (1977). Control theory measures of tracking as indices of attention allocation strategies, *Human Factors*, **19**, 349–366.

Wickens, C. D., and Kessel, C. (1979). The effect of participatory mode and task workload on the detection of dynamic system failures, *IEEE Transactions on System Man and Cybernetics*, **13**, 24–31.

Wickens, C. D., and Kessel, C. (1980). The processing resource demands of failure detection in dynamic systems, *Journal of Experimental Psychology: Human Perception and Performance*, **6**, 654–577.

Wickens, C. D., Mountford, S. J., and Schreiner, W. (1981). Multiple resources, task-hemispheric integrity, and individual differences in time-sharing, *Human Factors*, **23**, 211–229.

Wickens, C., and Tsang, P. (1979). Attention allocation in dynamic environments, Paper presented at the 15th Annual Conference on Manual Control, Wright State University, March.

# PART IV:

# From Description to Explanation: An Emerging View

We are reminded as we arrive at this final section that for all developmental scientists regardless of theoretical orientation the fundamental issue remains the same, namely, to understand the nature of developmental change. In both the Roberton essay as well as the Seefeldt and Haubenstricker chapter we find a basic commitment to explaining developmental change in motor skill. Although the research reported in both chapters is descriptive in approach, we think the reader will agree that the research is far from a mere charting of the motor milestones so frequent in the 1920s and 1930s (see for example Shirley, 1931). Rather, those scientists who have chosen to describe motor skill change across the lifespan have provided us with invaluable evidence regarding the developing system's control and co-ordination of segmental actions necessary to any theory of motor skill development. Seefeldt and Haubenstricker, for example, report on their extensive work on the biomechanical analysis of the so-called fundamental motor skills. Their approach has been one of studying the natural development of these actions with a view toward the eventual determination of their stages of development. In a similar vein, Roberton takes up the issue of stage theory, arguing for its primacy in developmental theory and more pointedly for the need to understand stages of motor development. She and her colleagues have sought to identify the putative invariant and universal sequence of motor development which stage theory might predict. Along the way, their research has given rise to a component analysis of motor co-ordination which may well provide the future basis for identifying elemental units of behavior that may transfer across tasks.

Interestingly this cross-task approach is also emerging in the field of ethology where the focus is shifting to what Fentress (1976) has called *relational dynamics*, namely an understanding of which behaviors share common features. For example, the pecking behavior of chickens while eating and fighting is likely to be much less similar than pecking and *kicking* behavior

while fighting. The fundamental issue here is that the components are related —
across tasks — to the extent that they share common functions. In motor
development this might mean that spinal-pelvic rotation will codevelop to a
greater degree in functionally similar tasks, such as forceful projection of a ball
in throwing and striking, than in tasks (such as throwing a ball for distance and
throwing a ball for accuracy) which share the same physical form but are
functionally dissimilar.

Finally, the section includes two integrative papers, one by Rarick and the
other by Smoll, which attempt to bring some order to the diversity and sometimes polarity found in the descriptive and process-oriented approaches to
research in motor development. However, as we look across the essays of this
volume it would seem that though there is diversity of approach, ultimately we
are all seeking to understand the same thing, namely the developmental
principles of movement control and co-ordination.

The Development of Movement Control and Co-ordination
Edited by J. A. S. Kelso and J. E. Clark
© 1982, John Wiley & Sons, Ltd

CHAPTER 10

# Descriptive Research and Process-oriented Explanations of the Motor Development of Children

G. Lawrence Rarick

The purpose of this symposium was to bring together investigators whose research in motor behavior has been essentially descriptive and those whose research has been process-oriented with the view of building a conceptual framework for the study of motor development. The rationale for the foregoing was based on the premise that motor development research has in the past operated primarily at a descriptive level with much of the work oriented to charting the course of development with an emphasis on stage-dependent theories such as those proposed by Gesell (1946) and McGraw (1941), the thrust of such research being primarily on 'when' as opposed to the more analytical question of 'how.' A perusal of the early literature on motor development does indeed support the contention that research in this area has been largely descriptive.

The extent to which this earlier research has contributed to our understanding of human motor development is debatable as is the question of the methodological approaches that future research should take in order to provide explanations of the processes underlying this aspect of human development. This would seem to be particularly important in view of the growing awareness expressed by some developmental psychologists (Piaget, 1952; Bruner, 1970; Connolly, 1970) and such educators and therapists as Ayres (1975), Frostig and Maslow (1973), and Kephart (1960) of the impact of motor experiences early in life on cognitive development. Similarly, it would be hoped that a symposium such as this might serve as a much needed source of information for practitioners involved in teaching motor skills to developmentally young as well as to disabled children. The foregoing are indeed worthy goals, for while research may have as its primary mission the advancement of knowledge, sight must not be lost of the need for applied research which shows promise of having immediate beneficial effects on humanity.

Bridging the gap between description and explanation is indeed a worthy focus for a symposium such as this, for research which does not go beyond assessment and description has limited scientific value. One might ask if descriptive research is, in fact, limited solely to description, or if, when properly used, it may be an effective tool, and in some instances the only one, that can be used in providing information from which plausible explanations may come. For example, one can point to the theories and explanations regarding the origin and evolution of the universe and the accurate predictions of astronomical events that have come from mathematical calculations based on descriptive data. Similarly, inferences about the lifestyles and cultures of early man have come from anthropological and archeological studies using essentially descriptive methods.

It would be less than accurate to conclude that well-planned descriptive studies are not appropriate in providing information useful in explaining natural phenomena. On the other hand, few would question that much descriptive research is poorly designed, global in nature, and does not address itself to explicit questions. Controlled experimentation, where appropriate, is clearly our most effective research tool. Its value in providing meaningful explanations, however, depends on the insight and design capability of the researcher. Sight should not be lost of the fact that controlled experimental research involves elements of description, for the kinds of measurements that are used and the type of data collected are essentially descriptive. Explanations are not easy to come by and many approaches are useful in providing insights into the processes of nature.

The remainder of this paper will consider the nature of human development, its neurological foundations, some descriptive approaches that have been used in studying motor development, process-oriented research, and lastly some comments on what can be done to bridge the gap between description and explanation.

## NATURE OF HUMAN DEVELOPMENT

Within the confines of the topic it would seem appropriate to comment first on the nature of human development and its neurological foundations and some of the contributions that descriptive research has made to our understanding of the development of motor functions in humans.

Development, by its nature, is characterized by change. Thus, any attempt to study this phenomenon, whether it be done in a free and natural environment or under well-controlled experimental conditions, must make repeated observations on the same individuals over specified periods of time. This is not a difficult task for those studying animal behavior, but it poses major problems with humans, particularly when one wishes to manipulate experimental variables and study their long-range impact. It is therefore not surprising that much of our information on human motor development has come from cross-sectional descriptive studies. Exceptions to this are the longitudinal investigations on infants by such early researchers as Gesell (1946), McGraw (1942), and Shirley (1931); and the research on school-age children by Espenschade (1940), Jones (1949), Clarke (1971), and Rarick and Smoll (1967).

Most of the early research on motor development of infants and young children was mainly descriptive, using observational and cinematographic techniques. These studies provided age-related data on the acquisition of a wide range of motor skills although some gave attention to the biomechanical aspects of human movement. Sight should not be lost of the fact that both Gesell and Thompson (1929; 1941) and McGraw (1935), as well as others, employed co-twin techniques in studying the impact of early training upon the trend of motor development. The findings of the latter pointed to the significance of instrinsic developmental factors as prime determinants of motor behavior in early life. The action of these inherent forces constitutes a biological maturation which governs the expanding motoric capabilities of the infant and young child. As such they exert a major influence on the time and sequence of such motor events as creeping, crawling, standing, and walking.

It was evident to these early researchers (McGraw, 1941; Tilney and Kubie, 1931) that the course of early motor development is preset, as evidenced by the gradual decline in subcortical movements resulting from the onset of cortical inhibitory influences, followed by the emergence of cortical control of generalized motoric responses appearing in essentially a cephalo-caudal direction. One might legitimately ask 'what did these early investigations tell us about processes *per se*?' Perhaps very little, but they did provide considerable insight into the significance of innate factors in shaping the course of early motor development, a concept that has over the years had a marked influence on child-rearing practices.


## NEUROLOGICAL FOUNDATIONS OF MOTOR DEVELOPMENT

The neurological foundations for many of the so-called natural movements such as walking, running, and jumping are held by many to have phyletic origins. Such movements have been observed during prenatal life and have been routinely noted during the first few days of postnatal life (Peiper, 1929). These are reasonably well-co-ordinated movements controlled at this time by subcortical centers, gradually coming under the control of the motor area of the cerebral cortex as the child matures.

It has been recognized for some time that in eliciting a body movement muscles work in groups, seldom acting alone. Movements involving one or more joints are strikingly similar from person to person and hence the term movement pattern has been used to describe them. Movement patterns once acquired are for the most part executed with little if any conscious direction. Herrick (1931) labeled such movements as 'acquired automatisms,' for once initiated the movements continue automatically, although the specific muscle groups controlling the act can, in whole or in part, be consciously controlled. The central control mechanism lies in the motor area of the cortex, although other areas of the central nervous system serve to modulate and control the movements.

The development and refinement of complex movement patterns as young children grow are readily observable phenomena and have been subjected to considerable scientific investigation. The research of Hellebrandt et al. (1961) on the development of broad jumping behavior in early childhood is noteworthy. The impact of practice on this maturing motoric capability is nicely illustrated in Figure 1 which shows the transition from the relatively infantile jumping form at thirty-seven months of age to the relatively mature jumping behavior six months later, a behavior that was not elicited with practice at the earlier age. The conclusion reached by these investigators was that 'jumping is a phylogenetic acquisition which unfolds progressively "pari passu" with the growth and development of mechanisms capable of mobilizing the mechanical forces required' (Hellebrandt et al., 1961).

Patterned movements are characterized by an ordered and properly timed sequence of subroutines which, when viewed in total, give the movement its quality or form. Each movement subroutine is dependent upon those that precede it and the degree to which the subroutines are synchronized in their time-force relationships is the basis for skillful, well-co-ordinated movements. The significance of the body's feedback mechanisms in serving as modulating control systems (servomechanisms) in the many motor activities of daily life involving relatively slow controlled movements is self-evident. However, it has been known for some time that rapid movements of a ballistic character are carried out with such speed that once the movement is initiated the feedback control mechanisms do not have time to affect the course of the movement (Hubbard and Seng, 1954; Stetson and McDill 1923). In such cases the error-detecting mechanisms monitoring such movement must play their role in succeeding movements (Schmidt, 1975). That the subroutines of complex rapid (ballistic) movements operate without conscious direction once the act is under way is generally recognized. How these mechanisms function in the learning and development of motor skills should be of major concern to motor and behavioral researchers.

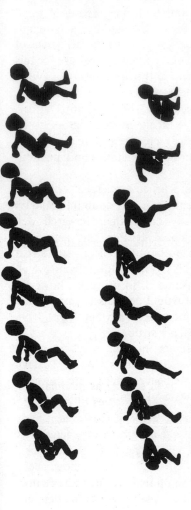

*Row 1.* John performing the standing broad jump at 37 months of age. *Row 2,* full-blown "winging" at 41 months. The poise is that of a bird in soaring flight.

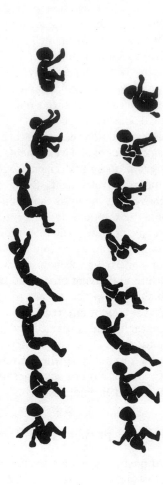

Transition from infantile to more mature arm positioning during a jump from a two footed take-off by John at 43 months of age. The first attempt to bring the arms forward during the propulsive phase of the jump was disastrous. The second was successful.

FIGURE 1   Transition from infantile to relatively mature form in the standing broad jump (from Hellebrandt *et al.*, 1961)

## CINEMATOGRAPHY AS A DESCRIPTIVE RESEARCH TOOL

Among the research tools available for the study of human movement cinematography has proved to be one of the most effective. It is essentially a descriptive technique providing a pictorial frame-by-frame record of rapid movements, one which can be repeatedly used for both qualitative and quantitative analysis. As such it is an ideal method for studying the biomechanics of motor development. Unfortunately, it has not enjoyed widespread use for this purpose. Cross-sectional studies of age differences in throwing behavior (Wild, 1938), jumping performance (Roy, 1971; Hellebrandt et al., 1961; Glassow, Halverson, and Rarick, 1965), and running behavior (Beck, 1966; Dittmer, 1962) have materially advanced our knowledge of age-related factors in the biomechanical execution of these skills. In this sense reasonable levels of performance expectations can serve as guides for both qualitative and quantitative aspects of motor skill development.

Some might propose that cinematography is a process-oriented tool in the study of motor development. Such a contention is of doubtful validity, although movement analysis specialists usually carry their research well beyond mere description. It is a process-oriented tool in the sense that cinematography provides valuable information on biomechanical factors that are important in the execution of motor skills, information from which processes or underlying mechanisms may be deduced. In no sense, however, does it measure underlying processes. In fact, it would perhaps be appropriate to ask at this point if processes per se are ever measured – products, yes, from which processes may be inferred – but processes, per se no.

Cinematography has provided valuable insights into the ways in which complex motor skills are executed, and enlightened inferences have been drawn concerning the mechanisms which control the sequence, timing, and power of component parts of motoric acts, particularly when electromyography is used in conjunction with cinematography.

## PROCESS-ORIENTED RESEARCH

In the recent past considerable attention has been directed to the role of information processing, proprioceptive feedback, knowledge of results, and closed- and open-loop systems in motor performance. In any study of behavioral constructs such as these the investigator is dealing with abstractions that lend themselves to study only in indirect ways. The conditions of the experiment, the circumstances under which the subject performs, the nature of the motor response itself, and the measurements that are taken determine the plausibility of the inferences that can be drawn regarding processes or mechanisms co-ordinating the act. What happens may be measured, but the 'how' and the 'why' can only be inferred.

It might be enlightening to review briefly a process-oriented experiment conducted by Connolly (1970) as reported in *Mechanisms of motor skill development*, one of the few studies described in detail therein. This experiment used a card-sorting task for its data base, one in which the subjects (children, adolescents, and young adults) were asked to sort a pack of 24 cards and place each card one by one in a tray which matched the color design of the card that was sorted (turned over). The color designs of the cards for each of the four tasks and the corresponding trays in which the cards were to be placed differed for each task so the load of information the child had to handle varied materially according to the task. The respective tasks involved 2, 4, 6, and 8 choices corresponding according to the investigator to 1, 2, 2.585, and 3 bits of information.

The time required to complete the task was the criterion measure. Since the task involved both movement and decision time, measurements were also taken on the time it took each child to place the same number of blank cards into unmarked trays using for this task 2, 4, 6, and 8 trays, respectively. The latter was defined as movement time and the difference between total time and movement time as decision time.

The results clearly pointed to well-defined and systematic age differences in decision time with the slope of the regression line for the younger children differing materially from that of the older children with the increasing number of choices (see Figure 2). The movement time, while differing systematically with age, did not differ within age regardless of the number of choices (see Figure 3). The author concludes that 'the information-processing abilities are an important limiting factor in the sequencing of the subunits which go to make up basic motor skills.' Note that the investigator has previously pointed out that within age level the number of choices had no bearing on movement time. What then is the writer's basis for saying that information load of the kind used here was a limiting factor in the *execution* of this kind of movement? What was differentially affected within each age group was the time required to select the proper tray, not the time required to execute the movement. One might then legitimately question what in fact was measured. The *time* required to complete a prescribed task under defined conditions was measured – but was a motor process *per se* measured?

The comments on the foregoing do not mean to imply that well-designed experimental research may not lead to plausible explanations of the processes that govern defined aspects of motor behavior and motor learning. One might question, however, whether such an experiment as the one just cited sheds much light on the processes underlying the motor development of children. True, many motor skills that children acquire necessitate decision-making, such as how much force to apply or the proper timing of sequential movements, but these relate essentially to the movement aspect of the task and thus have a true motoric orientation.

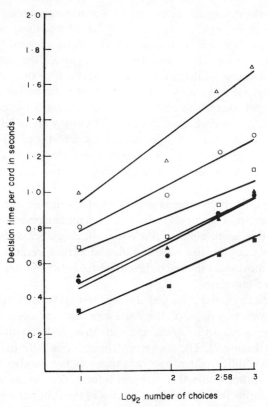

FIGURE 2    Linear regression lines of the form
$Y = A + b \log_2 X$ fitted to choice time data ($\Delta$, 6
years; $\bigcirc$, 8 years; $\square$, 10 years; $\blacktriangle$, 12 years; $\bullet$, 14
years; $\blacksquare$, adult) (from Connolly, 1970)

Vision has long been recognized as a significant factor in motor development and as such its impact on gross motor behavior is worthy of study in humans. One of our graduate students at Berkeley has recently completed an investigation on an aspect of the motor behavior of blind children which might by some be considered to be process-oriented. The investigation (Gipsman, 1979) was designed to identify factors which affect the performance and learning of a novel balance task by blind children. Totally blind, blindfolded, legally blind, sighted, and sighted blindfolded boys and girls in two age levels, eight to ten years and twelve to fourteen years, were tested using the stabilometer as the novel experimental task (Bachman, 1961). The sample included forty-eight subjects equally divided into eight groups according to visual categories and age levels. Two stabilometer tasks were used with all subjects, one in which the

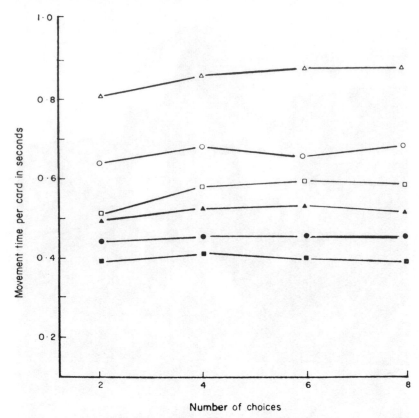

FIGURE 3    Movement time as function of number of response locations for the various age groups (Δ, 6 years; O, 8 years; □, 10 years; ▲, 12 years; ●, 14 years; ■, adult) (from Connolly, 1970)

body was oriented at right angles to the stabilometer plane of rotation (Figure 4), the other with the body parallel to it (Figure 5). Ten trials of twenty seconds each with thirty seconds rest between trials were given on each task. This procedure was repeated one month later to test for retention.

In addition to the above, a specially designed test was employed with all subjects blindfolded to assess their sensitivity to the vertical position. The equipment for this included a chair mounted on the stabilometer platform, in which the subject sat, and which through a subject-controlled power source movement of the platform could be regulated through a range of ten degrees from the vertical (Figure 6). The task required that the subject, while seated in the chair, should regulate the movement of the board through the range of motion, stopping when, in the subject's judgement, the vertical position had been reached.

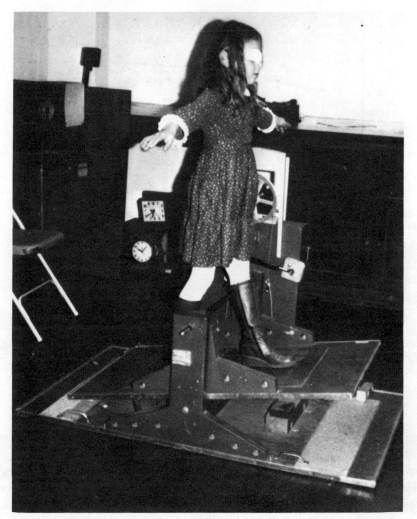

FIGURE 4    Body position for stabilometer test: body alignment parallel to axis
of rotation

The results were as hypothesized in that stabilometer performance on both
tasks was best for the sighted, and was significantly better for the totally blind
than for the legally blind or for the sighted blindfolded groups at both age
levels. The hierarchy from the best to the poorest performance proceeded from
sighted, to totally blind, to legally blind, to sighted blindfolded. Learning
occurred in all groups, the older blind subjects on the average showing more
learning than the younger. However, the findings indicated that with the

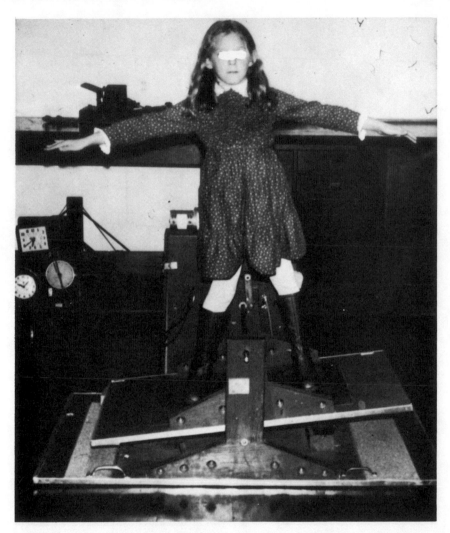

FIGURE 5    Body position for stabilometer test: body alignment perpendicular to axis
of rotation

sighted there was an adolescent balance lag even when the performance scores
were adjusted for differences in height and weight. This lag was not apparent
for either the totally blind or the legally blind groups when similar adjustments
in body dimension were made. The investigator (Gipsman, 1979) proposed that
the blind adolescent may be more effective in using proprioceptive feedback
during this developmental period, a time when additional demands are made on
this mechanism.

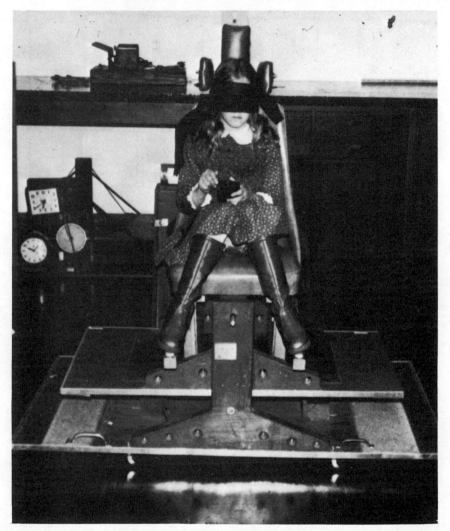

FIGURE 6   Subject seated in preparation for the test of sensitivity to the upright
position

It is worth noting that there were no significant differences between the blind
and the blindfolded sighted children on the test for sensitivity to the vertical
position. Nor did the scores on this test have any substantial correlations with
performance scores on either of the stabilometer tasks for the sighted, legally
blind, or the totally blind children. The reason for this seeming inconsistency is
not at this point entirely clear. It would seem reasonable to believe, however,

that the rapid and sudden movements of the board in the stabilometer tasks would evoke materially stronger sensory input from the joint receptors and from the vestibular system than would result from the slow and passive tilting of the seated subject during the vertical sensitivity test. Hence, it is perhaps not surprising that the performance relationships between these tasks were not high.

While this study was cross-sectional in its immediate approach, it has longitudinal overtones, for these totally blind and legally blind children had been completely or partially deprived of sight from birth; hence, the impact of visual loss early in life on this skill could in this sense be developmentally assessed. Based on these findings it would seem that complete deprivation of sight from birth is not incompatible with the development of an age-related equilibrium adjustment capability, one that in a task of this kind resulted in better performance in the blind than occurred in the fully sighted with vision occluded.

The sparsity of published process-oriented research of a developmental nature on the motor behavior of children is not meant to imply that we have no insight into age or maturity factors that affect the development of motor skills in the childhood years. We do know that with advancing age children's levels of performance in most motoric skills gradually become more adultlike. For example, cinematographic observations on such a basic skill as running show that with advancing age children increase both the frequency and length of the stride while decreasing the relative rise in the center of gravity per strike (Beck, 1966; Dittmer, 1962; Fortney, 1964). While the increases in stride length and frequency that accompany greater running speed are in part a function of increasing muscular power, the role of co-ordinated movements of the arms and trunk in maintaining balance and assisting in the forward thrust of the body is clearly significant in accounting for age-performance changes in this skill. Yet such information provides us with little basic information on neurological and developmental processes *per se*. It does, however, give us some insight into how the human body accommodates itself to the requirements of the task of locomotion. It would seem apparent that analyses of age changes in the movement patterns of this skill and such other basic skills as jumping and throwing provide important insights into developmental trends. Research of the above kind, while essentially descriptive, is an important means of understanding some of the critical factors responsible for the changes in motor performance that occur with advancing age.

One of the most promising process-oriented concepts that has both developmental and practical implications is Schmidt's Schema Theory of Discrete Motor Learning (1975). In essence this theory proposes that through many different motoric experiences one establishes a set of rules or a strategy for solving a broad range of motor problems. The theory, for example, suggests that variable practice which requires variable response specifications results in the development of a motor schema which facilitates transfer to a similar but not previously attempted task. While the validity of this theory has yet to be established, evidence is accumulating that it may well have credence with children. For example, Kelso and Norman (1978) reported that variable practice on a simple novel motor task by young children (two years, eleven months to four years) resulted in greater transfer to an unpracticed task of the same response class than occurred following constant practice. Similar findings were reported recently by Moxley (1979), using a complex gross motor task with older children, aged six to eight. Schmidt (1975) (see also Shapiro and Schmidt, this volume) believes that the theory holds promise for the teaching of motor skills to children by reaffirming the intuitions of those in movement education that the instructional emphasis with children should be placed on the development of a variety of movement patterns thus leading to the establishment of a generalized motor schema.

Other recent research such as the investigation by Shapiro (1977) of the importance of knowledge of results in skill acquisition in four-year-old children is a promising direction for future studies. Although the findings relative to errors on a linear positioning task were in no sense conclusive they pointed to the need for providing children with rather specific feedback information in motor learning situations rather than depending primarily on verbal cues.

Another study of a process-oriented nature that has some developmental implications is one by Dorfman (1977) on the anticipatory timing of boys and girls aged six to nineteen. The task required subjects to co-ordinate the interception of dots on a cathode ray oscilloscope by use of a manual slide control. As was expected, the errors declined with advancing chronological age reaching an asymptote at fourteen to fifteen years. Dorfman made no attempt to speculate on the processes at work other than to say that the complexity of the task was such that its successful execution required the synchronous action of many control mechanisms, most of which were beyond the response capabilities of young children. This was in many ways a well-designed study, but one in which the data provided limited insight into the probable mechanisms at work.

As mentioned earlier most of the process-oriented research has dealt with slow precision-type movements, motions of a nonballistic type. Evidence that an error-detecting mechanism is operating during the learning of a ballistic skill has been provided by the research of Schmidt and White (1972). Support for this is based on the finding of these investigators that with repeated trials of a ballistic movement the subjects developed a strong error-detecting mechanism as indicated by the increasing within subject correlation between actual errors and subjectively evaluated errors and the decreasing difference in magnitude of the two errors during the course of learning. The experiment used solely young adults so there are as yet no data on the developmental nature of this phenomenon.

It is clear from the foregoing that those involved in process-oriented motoric research have directed only limited attention to children. Other than the research cited here and the investigations of Whiting and Cockerill (1972) on the development of a ballistic skill with and without vision, very little age-related process-oriented research has been published.

## BRIDGING THE GAP BETWEEN DESCRIPTIVE AND PROCESS-ORIENTED RESEARCH

The literature is filled with data on age changes in motor responses ranging from reaction-time data to test results on measures of strength and fine and gross motor co-ordination. All point to improvements in performance as defined by various performance scores. Although we have information on biomechanical changes and changes in body size that accompany age gains in performance scores we have very little scientific information on the processes that are responsible for these improvements.

The differences between descriptive research and process-oriented research of an experimental nature need no further comment here except to point out once again that both depend upon data usually quantified in the form of one or more numerical values. The difference in part relates to what the values or scores assess and the inferences that can be drawn from the scores. There would seem to be little question that well-thought-out experimental process-oriented investigations will move us closer to an understanding of the body's mechanisms and how they work than will result from the usual types of descriptive studies. But one should not assume that just because an investigation is well-designed, processes *per se* are being measured.

If we are serious about providing information on the processes that affect the development of motor skills in normal and handicapped children, the research base must be broadened to include well-designed descriptive studies (bio-mechanical and factor analytical) and process-oriented studies on children of a variety of ages including preschoolers, and where possible to make provision for repeated observations on the same children over extensive periods of time. At present the process-oriented research has, with few exceptions, been centered on college age populations, an understandable situation in view of the logistical problems encountered in experimental research with children.

Lastly, it would perhaps be wise to consider modification of the types of tasks usually employed in process-oriented research. Often relatively slow precision tasks are used which may provide valuable insights into the factors affecting these tasks under specific task conditions, but one might question the relevance of these findings to tasks with a sports orientation. Perhaps – given the high degree of skill specificity – we need to pay more attention to examining the processes that underlie the basic motor abilities that children need for the development of a broad range of sports skills.

## REFERENCES

Ayres, A. J. (1975). Sensorimotor foundations of academic ability, in W. M. Cruickshank and Hallahan, D. P. (eds.), *Perceptual and Learning Disabilities in Children* (Vol. 2), Syracuse: Syracuse University Press.

Bachman, J. C. (1961). Specificity vs. generality in learning and performing two large muscle motor tasks, *Research Quarterly*, **32**, 3–11.

Beck, M. C. (1966). The path of the center of gravity during running in boys grades one to six, unpublished doctoral dissertation, University of Wisconsin, Madison.

Bruner, J. S. (1970). The growth and structure of skill, in K. Connolly (ed.), *Mechanisms of Motor Skill Development*, New York: Academic Press.

Clarke, H. H. (1971). *Physical and Motor Tests in the Medford Boys' Growth Study*, Englewood Cliffs, NJ: Prentice-Hall.

Connolly, K. (ed.) (1970). *Mechanisms of Motor Skill Development*, New York: Academic Press.

Connolly, K. (1970). Response speed, temporal sequencing, and information processing in children, in K. Connolly (ed.), *Mechanisms of Motor Skill Development*, New York: Academic Press.

Dittmer, J. (1962). A kinematic analysis of the development of the running pattern of grade school girls and certain factors which distinguish good and poor performance at the observed ages, unpublished master's thesis, University of Wisconsin, Madison.

Dorfman, P. W. (1977). Timing and anticipation: A developmental perspective, *Journal of Motor Behavior*, **9**, 67–79.

Espenschade, A. (1940). Motor performance in adolescence including the study of relationships with measures of physical growth and maturity, *Monographs of the Society for Research in Child Development*, **5**, 1–126.

Fortney, V. (1964). Trends and traits in the action of the swinging leg in running, unpublished master's thesis, University of Wisconsin, Madison.

Frostig, M., and Maslow, P. (1973). *Learning Problems in the Classroom*, New York: Grune and Stratton.

Gesell, A. (1946). The ontogenesis of infant behavior, in L. Carmichael (ed.), *Manual of Child Psychology*, New York: Wiley.

Gesell, A., and Thompson, H. (1929). Learning and growth in identical infant twins: An experimental study by the method of co-twin control, *Genetic Psychology Monograph*, **6**, 1–124.

Gesell, A., and Thompson, H. (1941). Twins T and C from infancy to adolescence. A biogenic study of individual differences by co-twin control, *Genetic Psychology Monograph*, **24**, 3–121.

Gipsman, S. C. (1979). Factors affecting performance and learning of blind and sighted children on a balance task, unpublished doctoral dissertation, University of California, Berkeley.

Glassow, R. B., Halverson, L. E., and Rarick, G. L. (1965). Improvement of motor development and physical fitness in elementary school children, Co-operative research project No. 696, University of Wisconsin, Madison.

Hellebrandt, F. A., Rarick, G. L., Glassow, R. B., and Carns, M. L. (1961).

Physiological analysis of basic motor skills, *American Journal of Physical Medicine*, **40**, 14–25.

Herrick, D. J. (1931). *An Introduction to Neurology* (5th edn.), Philadelphia: W. B. Saunders.

Hubbard, A. W. (1960). Homokinetics: Muscular function in human movement. In W. R. Johnson (ed.), *Science and Medicine in Exercise and Sports*. New York: Harper & Row.

Hubbard, A. W., and Seng, C. N. (1954). Visual movements of batters, *Research Quarterly*, **25**, 42–57. (See also (1955), Rebuttal to comments on 'Visual movements of batters', *Research Quarterly*, **26**, 366–368.)

Jones, H. (1949). *Motor Performance and Growth*, Berkeley: University of California Press.

Kelso, J. A. S., and Norman, P. E. (1978). Motor schema formation in children, *Developmental Psychology*, **14**, 153–156.

Kephart, N. C. (1960). *The Slow Learner in the Classroom*, Columbus, Ohio: Bobs Merrill.

McGraw, M. B. (1935). *Growth: A Study of Johnny and Jimmy*, New York: Appleton-Century.

McGraw, M. B. (1941). Development of neuro-muscular mechanism as reflected in the crawling and creeping behavior of the human infant, *Journal of Genetic Psychology*, **58**, 83–111.

McGraw, M. B. (1942). *The Neuro-Muscular Maturation of the Human Infant*, New York: Columbia University Press.

Moxley, S. E. (1979). Schema: The variability of practice hypothesis, *Journal of Motor Behavior*, **11**, 65–70.

Peiper, A. (1929). Die schreitbewegungen der neugeborenen, *Monats Zeitschrift fur Kinderheilkunde*, **45**, 444–448.

Piaget, J. (1952). *The Origins of Intelligence in Children* (2nd edn.) New York: International Universities Press.

Rarick, G. L., and Smoll, F. L. (1967). Stability of growth in strength and motor performance from childhood to adolescence, *Human Biology*, **39**, 295–306.

Roy, B. G. (1971). Kinematics and kinetics of the standing long jump in seven-, ten-, thirteen-, and sixteen-year-old boys, unpublished doctoral dissertation, University of Wisconsin, Madison.

Schmidt, R. A. (1975). A schema theory of discrete motor skill learning, *Psychological Review*, **82**, 225–260.

Schmidt, R. A., and White, J. L. (1972). Evidence of an error detection mechanism in motor skills: A test of Adams' Closed-Loop Theory, *Journal of Motor Behavior*, **4**, 143–153.

Shapiro, D. C. (1977). Knowledge of results and motor learning in preschool children, *Research Quarterly*, **48**, 154–158.

Shirley, M. M. (1931). *The First Two Years: A Study of Twenty-Five Babies: Vol. 1, Postural and Locomotor Development*, Minneapolis: University of Minnesota Press.

Stetson, R. H., and McDill, J. A. (1923). Mechanisms of the different types of movement, *Psychology Monographs*, **32**, 18–40.

Tilney, F., and Kubie, F. S. (1931). Behavior and its relation to the development of the brain, *Bulletin of the Neurological Institute*, **1**, 229–313.

Whiting, H. T. A., and Cockerill, I. M. (1972). The development of a simple ballistic skill with and without visual control, *Journal of Motor Behavior*, **4**, 155–162.

Wild, M. R. (1938). The behavior of throwing and some observations concerning its course of development in children, *Research Quarterly*, **9**, 20–24.

The Development of Movement Control and Co-ordination
Edited by J. A. S. Kelso and J. E Clark
© 1982, John Wiley & Sons, Ltd

CHAPTER 11

# Describing 'Stages' within and across Motor Tasks

MARY ANN ROBERTON

## THE DESCRIPTIVE APPROACH

In his landmark book, *The Study of Behavioral Development* (1973), Joachim Wohlwill lists the 'interesting' questions that developmentalists should be asking. He also explores possible methodologies that could be used to answer those questions. The book is organized around five tasks which Wohlwill feels are involved in the study of developmental change. Briefly, these are:

(1) discovery and synthesis of developmental dimensions – that is, determining what behavioral phenomena change regularly over time and how one might measure that change;
(2) descriptive study of 'ages changes' along the developmental dimension chosen;
(3) study of the interpatterning of changes along two or more developmental dimensions;
(4) study of the determinants of development;
(5) study of individual differences in development.

Description within Wohlwill's framework is placed not as the first task of the developmentalist, but as the second. Description is not to be a willy-nilly collection of miscellaneous facts about behavior at some point in the lifespan. Rather, it should be a systematic study of longitudinal changes in behavior that occur along some carefully selected, developmental dimension. Further, Wohlwill suggests that several steps should take place *within* the descriptive process. If the data collected are quantitative, these steps consist of (i) determining the presence and direction of developmental change; (ii) determining the shape of the developmental function; and (iii) specifying the mathematical parameters of the developmental curve. If the collected data are qualitative,

293

questions about the form of the developmental function are replaced by the specification of the sequence in which behaviors appear, together with a study of how invariant this sequence is within individual children.

When the task of description is pictured in this light, it is very clear that the bulk of literature in motor development carries little descriptive information of this kind. How many developmental functions exist for how many dimensions? Those few graphs one can even visualize are from mixed longitudinal or cross-sectional data (Espenschade and Eckert, 1980). The qualitative 'stage' sequences being popularized in new motor development texts and scales are also from cross-sectional studies. No published longitudinal validation attempts have been made on those sequences.

For these reasons the research course my associates and I have chosen begins at level 2 in Wohlwill's paradigm. We are trying to study developmental functions, particularly qualitative sequences generated longitudinally, to see how individuals' movements change over time. Secondly, we are interested in the longitudinal interplay across these functions and sequences, a question ultimately relating to the possibility of stages in motor development but also of interest for its own sake. This question would be classified as level 3 in Wohlwill's paradigm. Once we understand some of these sequences and their interrelationships, *then* we will move to Wohlwill's level 4 by asking about the processes which underlie a *particular* developmental function.

## STAGE THEORY

We have tried to approach descriptive work within the framework of developmental theory so that data gathering is directed by theory and then the theory is modified by the data obtained. The theoretical framework that has guided our work may be called 'classical stage theory.' It has provided the framework for Piaget's (1976) stages of cognitive development and Kohlberg's (1963) stages of moral development. While receiving criticism in recent years (Brainerd, 1978), the heuristic value of stage theory cannot be denied. Hundreds of studies have been performed in the cognitive realm alone, trying to refute or support Piaget's stages. As a result, we have learned a great deal about the course of cognitive development. Kohlberg's announcement of stages of moral reasoning set off a new renascence within the study of moral development as researchers hurried to, again, support or refute his claims. That stage theory would be natural to study in motor development should be readily apparent. Often cognitive psychologists illustrate 'what stages are' with motor examples. Indeed, many of us reared in the descriptive tradition of motor development grew up using the term 'stage' as a natural part of our descriptive vocabulary. Our forerunners in motor development, such as Burnside (1927), Shirley (1931), Ames (1937), Wild (1937), and Gesell (1946), all seemed to believe in a universal, invariant sequence of motor skill development, a stage sequence which represented observed, qualitative transformations in response selection.

The remainder of this paper will review some recent studies in which we have used the predictions of stage theory to test the validity of hypothesized developmental sequences within the overarm throw for force. The paper will close with a presentation of methodology being piloted for an across-task approach to the question of motor stages. In between will be sprinkled some serendipitous findings about motor development methods and models.

## DEVELOPMENTAL STEPS WITHIN THE OVERARM THROW

While there are several stage criteria which can be derived from classical stage theory (Pinard and Laurendeau, 1969; Inhelder, 1971), we chose to work with two: the notions of a universal sequence and of an invariant sequence; that is, do *all* children (universality) go through the same stages in the *same order* (invariance)? We chose to work with the overarm throw for force because Wild's (1937) 'stages' had always been rather well accepted for that skill. Although the literature contained several additions to those stages, no one had actually questioned her original assumption that stages did, indeed, exist in the throw. From our observations of movement, it also seemed that if universal, invariant sequences did exist for any motor tasks, they would most likely appear in all-out, force-production tasks occurring within a 'closed' environment. The closed environment, in this case, is one in which visual cues to the performer are unmoving within each trial and constant from trial to trial (Gentile *et al.*, 1975).

The model of stage development that is associated with classical stage theory is a stage-by-stage, 'staircase' graph. This graph would be hypothetically generated by every child as he developed over time by moving from stage to stage in the order predicted. Using this model as a reference, we can compare it to each child's longitudinal graph to test the assumptions of invariance and universality for a particular hypothesized sequence. This approach is known as an idiographic or case-by-case search for the 'negative instance,' for the one child who takes the sequence out of order or does some movement not allowable within the sequence. This is the approach taken with fifty-four youngsters who were filmed performing the overarm throw for force during kindergarten, first grade, and second grade (Roberton, 1978a). We had hypothesized three developmental sequences: one for the action of the pelvis-spine, one for the action of the forearm, and one for the action of the humerus in the throw. We found that every child who showed development over the three years went through at least some of the hypothesized sequence for the humerus and forearm in the order predicted. This result was not true for the pelvic-spinal categories. Several children skipped categories as they developed over time. Thus, two of the three sequences received good longitudinal support in the sample studied. The only problem was that a three-year study was clearly not long enough: few children went through an entire sequence in that length of time, and one-third of the sample showed no development at all over the three years in the three components studied.

## Prelongitudinal Screening

At this point, a digression may be useful in order to share two offshoots of this three-year longitudinal study. The first by-product is a prelongitudinal screening procedure which seems to hold promise for those interested in testing the universal invariance of developmental sequences (Roberton, 1977). The children who were filmed actually performed ten trials of the overarm throw each year. We reasoned that the children's across-trial stage classifications should reveal something about the invariance of the developmental sequence. For instance, if children were really 'in' a particular stage, they ought to show that stage regularly across the ten trials. We arbitrarily said at least 50 percent of their trials ought to be in their modal stage category; otherwise, they would be too variable to be considered 'in a stage.' Secondly, if any of the children's trials varied away from that modal category, they should vary only to adjacent stages in the hypothesized sequence, if the sequence were invariant. If a child was showing only step 1 and then 'jumped' to step 3 somewhere in the ten trials, this would be a nonadjacent ordering. If children could skip stages at *one point* in time, we reasoned they would be likely to do so *across time*. Therefore, any sequence which had one child showing less than 50 percent stability or one child showing nonadjacent trial variation was probably not a universal, invariant sequence.

To test the validity of this prelongitudinal screening, we calculated for each year of the three-year study the presence of 50 percent stability in each child and looked for nonadjacent, across-trial orderings (Roberton, 1978a). For the humerus and forearm, the screening each year held up: no child ever had less than five trials in his modal category, and no child varied to a nonadjacent ordering across the yearly ten trials. These two components, humerus and forearm, were also the two which eventually held up longitudinally. The action of the pelvis-spine did not hold up to the across-trials screening. This same component was the one which also did not eventually hold up longitudinally. Thus, when the across-trials screening test supported the categories, so did the longitudinal test. Therefore, it may ultimately be wise for developmental researchers to screen potential invariant developmental sequences across trials at one point in time. If the sequence holds up, then longitudinal test would be the next step toward support or refutation. If it does not hold up, then the researcher may wish to revise the sequence before embarking on the time and expense of longitudinal research. We plan continued investigation of the validity of such prelongitudinal screening procedures.

## A Developmental Model

A second spin-off of the three-year study was a new model for intratask motor development. Most 'stages' of motor tasks had described the whole body configuration, that is, what the arms and the legs and the trunk looked like at the same point in time. By serendipitously choosing to work with only components or parts of the body action, we discovered that development in the different components occurred at different rates within the same child. For instance, over the three years that we studied the throw, only 6 percent of the children moved up one developmental step in *each* of the three components; 20 percent progressed in two components; and 39 percent progressed in only one component (Roberton, 1978a). It seemed very clear that the movement components did not develop in the parallel, lock-step fashion that is suggested by the total body configuration stages of Monica Wild (1937). It would seem that the question of an invariant sequence must, therefore, be confined to the ordering of developmental steps within the body components. We have data now that suggest the component approach is developmentally valid for the hop and skip (Roberton and Halverson, 1977) and, possibly, for the forward roll (Williams, 1980), as well as the throw.

## A Further Longitudinal Test

Before this digression into prelongitudinal screening and component models, we had just discussed finding two components (the action of the humerus and the action of the forearm) whose developmental sequences were still intact after three years of longitudinal testing. The staircase graph had been generated by every child who showed development. However, few children had gone through all the 'stairs' of the graph in the three years, so a longer longitudinal test was needed. Fortunately, the University of Wisconsin-Madison has a small, longitudinal, motor development study of seven children which has been running since 1962, thanks to the perseverance of Lolas Halverson (Halverson, Roberton, and Harper, 1973). Some nine to fourteen years of filmed data were available on the children. The overarm throw for force had been included in most of the filming sessions, yielding 785 trials available for analysis. We proceeded to reduce these data in order to ask the question: over nine to fourteen years did all seven children go through all the developmental steps in the order hypothesized?

The briefest answer to that question is 'sort of' (Roberton and Langendorfer,

1980). The developmental data showed approximations to the classic invariant model that ranged from excellent, particularly for the boys' data, to fair. Given the possibility of measurement error and the paucity of useful data at the youngest ages, classic theorists would feel very comfortable with our results. We felt, however, that a model based on probabilistic notions would better represent our empirical findings. To explain this conclusion, a few graphs from the study may be of interest. They are among the first graphs to show motor sequences generated over long periods of time. Figure 1, for instance, traces the action of the forearm over a period extending from a year and ten months to thirteen years of age in one child as he performed the overarm throw for force. Clearly, this result would make any classic stage theorist ecstatic, for the data mimic the classic model precisely. The staircase graph does exist empirically.

Not all our data were like this, however. Figure 2 is particularly interesting. KE showed a lengthy transitional period before she stabilized at each of the higher developmental steps. Such behavior is allowable under the classic model (Roberton, 1978b) and is an excellent example of the 'equilibration process' (Langer, 1969) in which periods of stability alternate with periods of instability.

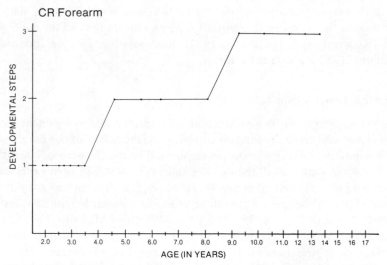

FIGURE 1   'Staircase' development in overarm throw forearm action in child CR (male) from age 1–10 to 13–2 years. Developmental steps are (i) no forearm lag; (ii) partial forearm lag; and (iii) full forearm lag. (See Roberton, 1978a for complete category descriptions.) Reprinted with permission from Roberton, M. A., and Langendorfer, S., Testing motor development sequences across 9–14 years, in K. Newell, G. Roberts, W. Halliwell, and C. Nadeau (Eds.), *Psychology of Motor Behavior and Sport – 1979*, Champaign, Ill.: Human Kinetics, 1980

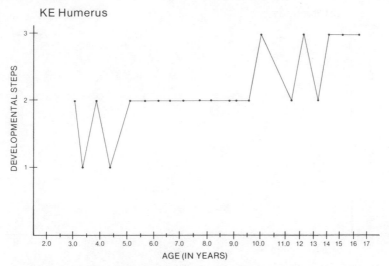

FIGURE 2    Step-to-step development in overarm throw humerus action in child KE (female) from age 3-0 to 16-3 years. Several years of transition occurred before reaching each higher level. Developmental steps are (i) humerus oblique; (ii) humerus aligned but independent; and (iii) humerus lags. (See Roberton, 1978a for complete category descriptions.) Reprinted with permission from Roberton, M. A., and Langendorfer, S., Testing motor development sequences across 9–14 years, in K. Newell, G. Roberts, W. Halliwell, and C. Nadeau (eds.), *Psychology of Motor Behavior and Sport – 1979*, Champaign, Ill.: Human Kinetics, 1980

To developmentalists, these transitional periods should be more interesting to study than the stable 'stage' periods. Both from the perspective of developmental dialectics (Riegel, 1976) and from a process perspective, it would seem that a subject in transition would have something 'interesting' happening endogenously and/or exogenously that should be identified. Once we learn more about developmental sequences, we may be able to select as subjects for process-oriented studies those people in transition within particular sequences.

A third graph from the study illustrates an instance of a 'negative case' (Figure 3). This child exhibited the categories out of sequence. After studying several thousand trials of throwing in three separate research projects, we finally had found one person who seemed to show that the sequence for the action of the humerus was not invariant. This is, unfortunately, not as clean a 'negative case' as we would like, for we found trials of the skipped step 2 appearing in previous years; MR simply never exhibited the level modally.

This first 'negative case' could clearly be measurement artifact and needs to be replicated in subsequent study. It caused us, however, to meditate on the

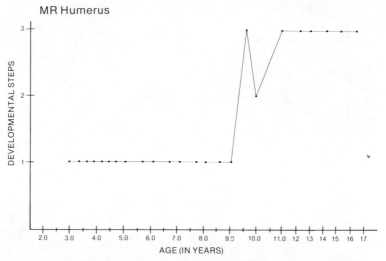

MR Humerus

FIGURE 3   Out-of-sequence development in overarm throw humerus action demonstrated by child MR (female) who 'jumped' from step 1 to step 3. Data represent thirteen years of development. Developmental steps are (i) humerus oblique; (ii) humerus aligned but independent; and (iii) humerus lags. (See Roberton, 1978a for complete category descriptions.) Reprinted with permission from Roberton, M. A., and Langendorfer, S., Testing motor development sequences across 9–14 years, in K. Newell, G. Roberts, W. Halliwell, and C. Nadeau (Eds.), *Psychology of Motor Behavior and Sport – 1979*, Champaign, Ill.: Human Kinetics, 1980

meaning of these data describing the action of the humerus – data which had shown so much order and regularity in numbers of children, yet which now suggested that deviations were possible. As a result, we began to consider an alternative stage model. This model has been mentioned in the theoretical, developmental literature (Feldman and Toulmin, 1976; Wohlwill, 1973) but rarely used with real data. We call it a population or probability stage model (Figure 4). Instead of the staircase graph for each individual, which assigned probabilities of 0 to nonadjacent categories, this model assigns a probability value to the possibility of *any* stage occurring at *any* time. The probability of showing a nonadjacent stage would always be low in the population but still possible for a given individual. In the classic model, the probability of non-adjacency is always 0 for both the population and the individual.

In Figure 4 we have graphed the occurrence of all developmental steps observed at a given age for the boys in the longitudinal study, regardless of whether the steps were exhibited modally. The graph nicely shows the orderly rise and fall of the three stages across the sample. The frequencies on the graph

## Humerus

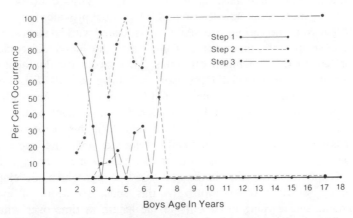

FIGURE 4 Observed occurrence of developmental steps in overarm throw humerus action across three boys studied longitudinally. Graph gives good support for the developmental nature of the three hypothesized steps as a 'population model.' Developmental steps are (i) humerus oblique; (ii) humerus aligned but independent; and (iii) humerus lags. (See Roberton, 1978a for complete category descriptions.) Reprinted with permission from Roberton, M. A., and Langendorfer, S., Testing motor development sequences across 9–14 years, in K. Newell, G. Roberts, W. Halliwell, and C. Nadeau (eds.), *Psychology of Motor Behavior and Sport – 1979*, Champaign, Ill.: Human Kinetics, 1980

give us a 'best guess' as to the probability of observing a given developmental level at a particular age in future samples. As we build up our observations, we should begin to get increasingly accurate estimates. In this figure the boys show a gradual passing away of step 1 and a coming to be of step 2 until each step has a 50–50 percent probability of occurring at the age of three. At the age of four, step 3 has only a 10 percent probability of occurring, but it could occur.

Thus, the notion of a universal, invariant sequence could be considered a legitimate *population notion*, which would be carried out to varying degrees within particular members of the population. The ordered staircase graph (Figure 1) would be one subset of possible probabilities. Indeed, it would seem that most people go through the population stages. The new model, however, allows individual exceptions to occur. This population model thus preserves the ordered regularity with which spatio-temporal transformations seem to occur in motor development. At the same time it provides a flexibility the classic stage model lacked.

At this point it should be stressed that while the probability stage graph uses 'age' along the horizontal axis, the model clearly suggests that, for any individual, development is not age-determined. The model provides only a population 'best guess' of the various probabilities associated with all stages at a given age. The developmental time-course of any particular individual could be far ahead or behind the population estimates. That motor development is 'age-related but not age-determined' (Roberton and Halverson, 1977) is a fact that even the most diehard maturationist would have to concede. Wohlwill (1970) has suggested that age should be considered a dependent rather than an independent variable in developmental research. While his proposal only confuses the issue, it should emphasize to all developmentalists that age acts solely as a 'marker' or 'neutral' variable in their research. 'Time' is an equally-valid, neutral designation for the horizontal axis along which developmental researchers plot their observations. In this sense, students of evolution, development, and learning differ only in the length of time over which they make their observations (Roberton and Halverson, 1977).

The Roberton and Langendorfer (1980) study, then, found that the universality and invariance of developmental sequences for the humerus and forearm action within the forceful overarm throw received moderate support when studied in seven children across nine to fourteen years. However, a possible refutation of invariance was observed in one subject's humeral action. In general, for both components the boys' data were more similar to the classic model than the girls' data. The boys' rate of development was also much faster with shorter transition times between developmental steps. The girls showed an inability to maintain, or failure to achieve, the highest levels of arm action. Boys were less stable at the youngest levels observed. Although more study was needed at the extremes of the age range examined, it may be that a population model of developmental progression would better represent the empirical data than the classic model.

Finally, the data also emphasized the heuristic value of the component model of intratask development. In an earlier study (Roberton, 1977), we had hypothesized from cross-sectional data that early in the course of throwing the pelvic-spinal component would show more developmental progress than the humerus and forearm action. Later both humerus and forearm would show more advanced development than the pelvic-spinal action. Inspection of the longitudinal data for these seven children revealed partial support for this hypothesis among the boys. Their trunk action was initially more advanced than both arm components. When the trunk action stabilized at an intermediate level of block rotation, both humerus and forearm actions changed from the lowest level to an intermediate one. Then, the humerus continued to develop to the most advanced step. Two years later, the forearm and trunk actions reached their advanced levels.

The component model also predicts that individuals may differ in rates of component development. Therefore, the 'profiles' formed by the developmental steps across components at any point in time will also differ over individuals. The longitudinal data substantiated this hypothesis. Each child followed a developmental course with unique rates of change and interaction among the components. At the same time, evidence was found for possible developmental or biomechanical constraints working across the components. A total of sixty-three step combinations or profiles could have occurred randomly across the three components of humeral action, forearm action, and pelvic-spinal action. Only seventeen of these combinations were observed modally in the longitudinal data. Of the seventeen, six were common to a majority of the subjects, but only one was common to all subjects. This observation suggests that components may show diversified sequences of change within a non-random range of profiles. The common 'linkages' (Williams, 1980) across components may be caused by the constraints of biomechanics, neurophysiology, or development itself.

## MOTOR STAGES ACROSS TASKS

Somewhere during the hours of watching films of children throwing, we began puzzling about the fact that cognitive 'stages' generalized across cognitive tasks, while the hypothesized stages we were studying were specific to a task. We then discovered that Flavell and Wohlwill (1969) had suggested that developmental sequences and stage sequences need not be synonymous. Developmental sequences can also be universal and invariant, theoretically, but they only become stage sequences if they reflect 'nodal interrelationships among two or more qualitatively defined variables developing apace' (Wohlwill, 1973, p. 192; Flavell, 1977). The key is that a 'stage' is a multivariate or across-task notion. Its study would come at level 3 in Wohlwill's research paradigm, when one examined the interpatterning of development across several dimensions. Subsequently, we suggested that intratask motor stages would be better called 'steps' because they lacked the criterion of 'structural wholeness,' that is, this concurrent generality across similar tasks (Roberton, 1978b).

We have now begun piloting the methodology for an investigation into motor stages that might generalize across tasks in a fashion analogous to Piaget's cognitive stages. In this model, stage 1 would appear in an individual whether hopping *or* jumping; or whether throwing *or* striking. In some sense we may be talking about the generality-specificity question, or the notion of transfer, couched in terms of the developmental levels of the movements used in the tasks.

Again, we needed a model. What would two tasks 'developing apace' look like if graphed? What interpatterning across them would we accept as evidence for a motor stage common to both? Figure 5 shows our tentative speculation on this problem, stimulated again by Wohlwill (1973). The most simplistic result would be for a given level of the movement to develop in both tasks simultaneously (case A in Figure 5). More than likely, however, we would find some kind of 'horizontal decalage,' as is observed across cognitive tasks (Pinard and Laurendeau, 1969). In these cases the stage manifests itself in one task consistently before it appears in the second task. Cases B and C of Figure 5 show two forms of horizontal decalage, which would still suggest a developmental relationship between the two tasks if the timing of the lag were similar across all children. Case E shows no common stage. Development spurts all the way to conclusion in one task before the other even begins. Case D shows another doubtful relationship.

Thus far, we have data on four children to match against these models. We are trying to compare the rate of development of the pelvic-spinal steps in throwing to those in striking a suspended ball with a forehand drive. We chose the suspended ball in order to 'close' the striking task somewhat, to promote environmental similarity across the two skills. Because the pelvic-spinal sequence is not invariant in the throw, we have some expected jumps in our data. Also we did not consistently film the suspended ball task as the children grew older, causing further gaps in the data. The next graph (Figure 6), however, shows the developmental relationship between the two tasks over a twelve-year period in one child. Interestingly, we get the suggestion of a consistent case B decalage with pelvic-spinal action always advancing in the throw before it advances in the strike. The time lag of the decalage varied from six months to two years. In the data of the other two boys we also got the same 'horizontal crosspiece' created by being at level 4 in both skills, then proceeding to level 5 in throwing first. Because of gaps in the striking data and the long number of years the youngsters stay at level 4 (block rotation), that one decalage is the only replicated part of the staircase sequence so far. The one girl whose data have been reduced suggested a case A relationship. At age four to seven she was in stage 3 on both tasks. She moved simultaneously to level 4 in both tasks and has remained there ever since. If we ultimately get a great variety of these case patterns over a number of children or several 'no relationship' patterns, it would be hard to see how a motor stage could be said to exist across the two tasks.

We clearly have a long way to go to examine properly the codevelopment of similar components across tasks; however, we did want to share our current, albeit primitive, methodology. This inquiry process is the third task of the developmental researcher, according to Wohlwill (1973). Our pilot study will help us sharpen our methods, and then we can decide if the question of motor stages in its broad sense is worth pursuing. Certainly, information about the interpatterning of two developmental sequences would be worthwhile,

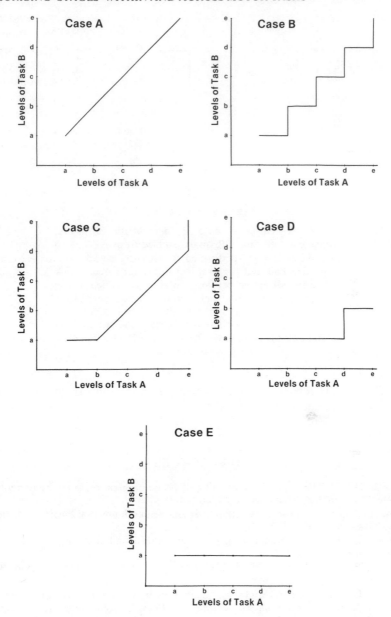

FIGURE 5    Possible models for two developing motor tasks reflecting common stages. Case A shows synchronous development; cases B and C show 'horizontal decalage' in which the stage always manifests itself in one task prior to the other; case D suggests a doubtful developmental relationship between the two tasks; case E shows no common stage across the tasks (after Wohlwill, 1973)

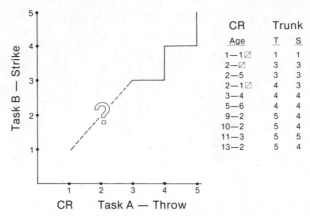

FIGURE 6 Observed case B, across-task horizontal decalage in one child CR (male) studied from age 1-10 to 13-2 years as he performed a sidearm strike of a suspended ball and the overarm throw for force. Trunk (pelvic-spinal) action developmental steps studied across both tasks were (i) no trunk action; (ii) extension of the trunk; (iii) spinal rotation with the pelvis stationary or spinal-then-pelvic rotation; (iv) block rotation; and (v) differentiated rotation. (See Roberton, 1978a for complete category descriptions.)

regardless of the stage question. Ultimately, whether motor stages exist or not will be far less important compared to all we will learn about motor development along the way.

## REFERENCES

Ames, L. (1937). The sequential patterning of prone progression in the human infant, *Genetic Psychology Monographs*, **19**, 409–460.

Brainerd, C. (1978). The stage question in cognitive-developmental theory, *Behavioral and Brain Science*, **1**, 173–214.

Burnside, L. (1927). Coordination in the locomotion of infants, *Genetic Psychology Monographs*, **2**, 283–372.

Espenschade, A., and Eckert, H. (1980). *Motor Development*, Columbus, Ohio: Bobs Merrill.

Feldman, C., and Toulmin, S. (1976). Logic and the theory of mind, in W. Arnold (ed.), *Nebraska Symposium on Motivation – 1975*, Lincoln, Nebraska: University of Nebraska Press.

Flavell, J. (1977). *Cognitive Development*, Englewood Cliffs, NJ: Prentice-Hall.

Flavell, J., and Wohlwill, J. (1969). Formal and functional aspects of cognitive development, in Elkind, D., and Flavell, J. (eds.), *Studies in Cognitive Development*, New York: Oxford University Press.

Gentile, A., Higgins, J., Miller, E., and Rosen, B. (1975). The structure of motor tasks, *Mouvement*, Actes du 7ᵉ symposium en apprentissage psycho-moteur et psychologie du sport, October, pp. 11–28.

Gesell, A. (1946). The ontogenesis of infant behavior, in L. Carmichael (ed.), *Manual of Child Psychology*, New York: Wiley.

Halverson, L., Roberton, M. A., and Harper, C. (1973). Current research in motor development, *Journal of Research and Development in Education*, **6**, 56–70.

Inhelder, B. (1971). Criteria of the stages of mental development, in J. Tanner and B. Inhelder (eds.), *Discussions on Child Development*, New York: International Universities Press.

Kohlberg, L. (1963). The development of children's orientations toward a moral order. I. Sequence in the development of moral thought, *Vita Humana*, **6**, 11–33.

Langer, J. (1969). *Theories of Development*, New York: Holt, Rinehart, & Winston.

Piaget, J. (1976). The attainment of invariants and reversible operations in the development of thinking, in S. Campbell (ed.), *Piaget Sampler*, New York: Wiley.

Pinard, A., and Laurendeau, M. (1969). 'Stage' in Piaget's cognitive-developmental theory: Exegesis of a concept, in D. Elkind and J. Flavell (eds.), *Studies in Cognitive Development*, New York: Oxford University Press.

Riegel, K. (1976). From traits and equilibrium toward developmental dialectics, in W. Arnold (ed.), *Nebraska Symposium on Motivation – 1975*, Lincoln, Nebraska: University of Nebraska Press.

Roberton, M. A. (1977). Stability of stage categorizations across trials: Implications for the 'stage theory' of overarm throw development, *Journal of Human Movement Studies*, **3**, 49–59.

Roberton, M. A. (1978a). Longitudinal evidence for developmental stages in the forceful overarm throw, *Journal of Human Movement Studies*, **4**, 167–175.

Roberton, M. A. (1978b). Stages in motor development, in M. Ridenour (ed.), *Motor Development: Issues and Applications*, Princeton, NJ: Princeton Book Co.

Roberton, M. A., and Halverson, L. E. (1977). The developing child – His changing movement, in B. Logsdon (ed.), *Physical Education for Children: A Focus on the Teaching Process*, Philadelphia: Lea and Febiger.

Roberton, M. A., and Langendorfer, S. (1980). Testing motor development sequences across 9–14 years, in K. Newell, G. Roberts, W. Halliwell, and C. Nadeau (eds.), *Psychology of Motor Behavior and Sport – 1979*, Champaign, Ill.: Human Kinetics.

Shirley, M. (1931). *The First Two Years, a Study of Twenty-five Babies*, Minneapolis: The University of Minnesota Press.

Wild, M. (1937). The behavior pattern of throwing and some observations concerning its course of development in children, unpublished doctoral dissertation, University of Wisconsin-Madison. (See also *Research Quarterly*, 1938, **9**, 20–24.)

Williams, K. (1980). Developmental characteristics of a forward roll, *Research Quarterly for Exercise and Sport*, **51**, 703–713.

Wohlwill, J. (1970). The age variable in psychological research, *Psychological Review*, **77**, 49–64.

Wohlwill, J. (1973). *The Study of Behavioral Development*, New York: Academic Press.

The Development of Movement Control and Co-ordination
Edited by J. A. S. Kelso and J. E. Clark
© 1982, John Wiley & Sons, Ltd

CHAPTER 12

# Patterns, Phases, or Stages: An Analytical Model for the Study of Developmental Movement

VERN SEEFELDT AND JOHN HAUBENSTRICKER

The modern history of motor development dates back to the 1920s and 30s, when physicians and psychologists such as Gesell (1929), Halverson (1931), Shirley (1931) and McGraw (1935) reported the sequential changes that occurred during infancy and early childhood. In this traditional setting, specialists in motor development have been criticized for their reliance on descriptive data in lieu of experimentation, and on their atheoretical attempts to solve developmental problems.

More recently, the subject matter and methodology of motor development have acquired a new dimension, primarily because of the interest shown by investigators who were formerly counted among those in the areas of motor integration, motor control, and motor learning. Much of the recent work in motor development is characterized by an emphasis on the perceptual-cognitive influences of motor skill acquisition; the studies are of short duration and the theories are generally transposed from observations on infra-human beings or college students to children of a specific chronological age. It will be interesting to note whether this 'transfer of theory by age level' will provide solutions to questions about motor skill development.

The question of selecting appropriate research procedures for solutions to existing problems deserves some attention, especially when a large share of this audience is inclined toward basic research. I would like to share with you the thoughts of Gershinowitz (1972) which appeared in *Science*. Gershinowitz suggested that when we seek to use knowledge in the promotion of change, then we must reverse the process that is now commonly used by scientists. His suggested sequence of events for solving problems includes the following: (i) use existing knowledge; (ii) conduct applied research that is specifically designed to answer a practical question; (iii) conduct basic research in the areas that will have the greatest possibilities for practical utility; and (iv) conduct basic research without regard to its practical application.

Gershinowitz went on to explain that the fundamental difference between basic and applied research *is not* in its subject matter, nor in the minds of its practitioners and sponsors, but in its relationship to those who use the knowledge that has been generated. He attributed the efficient transformation of knowledge in physical science and engineering into technology to the techniques and procedures that involve the user, while research in the *life, social,* and *behavioral* sciences has been carried out largely within the isolation of academic institutions, where the communication between scientists and the users of knowledge, and consequently its transfer into action, has been ineffective.

The thoughts of Gershinowitz may be an appropriate commentary on our present status in motor development. We do not wish to suggest that we stop seeking or building theories to explain how motor skills are learned. However, repeated admonitions during the last fifteen years that we do more theorizing have not produced any astonishing results. Perhaps a division of labor, where some theorize, but where others take time to observe the phenomenon in its natural surrounding, would result in information that could eventually be combined in the formulation of theories. Perhaps we lack the basic information to construct useful theories about the phenomenon that we propose to study.

In our laboratory we are committed to the quest for knowledge about how children learn motor skills, primarily for the purpose of using that knowledge to change behavior. Whether this state of mind exists among us because we are constantly reminded of our land grant origin, or whether we have gravitated there because of our interest in applied research, is immaterial. As a consequence of this philosophy, we conduct our three motor developmental programs with the dual purposes of (i) learning what we can about how children move, and (ii) interacting with teachers to dispense the knowledge that we have acquired and to learn from them if our proposed solutions were useful.

The three motor developmental programs that we have conducted for some time are as follows. *Motor Performance Study*: now in its thirteenth year. This longitudinal study involves subjects between the ages of two and twenty years. Measurements of physical growth and motor performance are taken twice each year. Children between the ages of five and fourteen years attend on-campus classes devoted to the teaching of gross motor skills. These classes are held on Saturdays during the school year and daily for five weeks during the summer. *Remedial Motor Program*: now in its tenth year. This program involves the one-to-one instruction of children between four and twelve years of age who have gross motor problems that prevent them from benefitting from large or small group instruction with children who function within the normal range of skill development. *Early Childhood Program*: now in its sixth year, this year-around program enrolls children between the ages of two and six years. The curriculum is devoted to teaching the gross and fine motor skills of childhood. Studies are conducted on the emergence of motor stages with and without instruction.

In 1966 we began viewing movement as a biomechanical phenomenon, through which joint actions could be *identified, ordered,* and *classified.* Through a mixed-longitudinal study that has yielded over 36,000 feet of film on children performing selected fundamental movement skills, we have identified the common patterns and elements of which these skills are comprised. Our work is neither innovative nor unique. The techniques we use were in practice a half-century ago. However, the questions we are asking and the organizational patterns we have described differ from those of the 1920s, 30s and 40s, and may take us a step closer to an explanation of how children learn motor skills.

## HISTORICAL STUDY OF MOVEMENT SKILLS

There is common agreement that the study of motor development involves observation. However, *what* is observed has differed with the investigator. One of the earliest reported sequences of an intraskill sequence was that of prehension (Halverson, 1931). He identified the sequential changes that took place by recording the time when the behavior occurred. Shirley (1931) observed the progression that led to upright locomotion in twenty-five children and described this sixteen-stage process in what we have termed an interskill sequence. Her sequences, and many others that followed, concentrated on the *order* in which the events occurred and not on the *proficiency* with which they were performed. McCaskill and Wellman (1938) identified the common motor acts of infancy and childhood, but departed from the detailed description of qualitative behavior and relied more on the identification, ordering, and quantification of tasks. Godfrey and Kephart (1969) provided a check list of the events that constituted mature performance, and listed as deviations those developmental actions that were ultimately discarded or eliminated from the task when more mature behavior was achieved.

The biomechanical approach that we have used to divide the developmental process into stages, from its most rudimentary to its most mature form, is based on observing the task as it is performed by numerous children across the age span from one to twelve years. The ultimate criterion of 'mature' performance was defined by observing the task as it was performed by highly skilled adult athletes. The shift from one stage to another was characterized by an abrupt change in the positioning of one or more limbs or body segments, in relationship to their previous position in the sequence of joint actions. This change in position within the series of joint rotations always resulted in the potential for the task to be performed more proficiently by permitting one or a combination of the following to occur: (i) permitting a greater range of movement around the force-producing points; (ii) adding more rotating joints to the 'power train'; (iii) permitting greater 'flow' or less interruption of the movement; and (iv) better positioning of the body for a maximum production of force.

An example of how the stages of throwing have been defined according to this observational method is provided in the following description. Most of these characteristics were originally described by Wild in 1938.

*Stage 1*
The throwing motion is essentially posterior-anterior in direction.
The feet usually remain stationary during the throw.
There is little or no trunk rotation in the most rudimentary pattern at this stage but those at the point of transition between stages one and two may evoke a slight trunk rotation in preparation for the throw and extensive hip and trunk rotation in the follow through.
The force of projection of the ball comes primarily from hip flexion, shoulder protraction, and elbow extension.

*Stage 2*
The distinctive feature of this stage is the rotation of the body about an imaginary vertical axis, with the hips, spine, and shoulders rotating as one unit.
The performer may step forward with either an ipsilateral or contralateral pattern, but the arm is brought forward in a transverse plane.
The motion may resemble a sling rather than a throw, due to the extended arm position during the course of the throw.

*Stage 3*
The distinctive characteristic is the ipsilateral arm–leg action.
The ball is placed into a throwing position above the shoulder by a vertical and posterior motion of the arm at the time that the ipsilateral leg is moving forward.
There is little or no rotation of the spine and hips in preparation for the throw.
The follow-through phase includes flexion at the hip joint and some trunk rotation toward the side opposite the throwing hand.

*Stage 4*
The movement is contralateral, with the leg opposite the throwing arm striding forward as the throwing arm is moved in a vertical and posterior direction during the 'wind-up' phase. Thus, the motion of the trunk and arm closely resemble those of stages one and three.
The stride forward with the contralateral leg provides for a wide base of support and greater stability during the force production phase.

*Stage 5*
The shift of weight is entirely to the rear leg, as it pivots in response to the rotating joints above it.
The throwing hand moves in a downward arc and then backward as the opposite leg moves forward.
Concurrently, the hip and spine rotate into position for forceful de-rotation.

As the contralateral foot strikes the surface the hips, spine, and shoulder begin to de-rotate in sequence.

The contralateral leg begins to extend at the knee as the shoulder protracts, the humerus rotates, and the elbow extends, thus providing an equal and opposite reaction to the throwing arm.

The opposite arm also moves forcefully toward the body to assist in the equal and opposite reaction to the throwing arm.

Our stages describe the total body configuration during the performance of a skill. Roberton (1978) has criticized this procedure because she believes that it implies that the segmental actions or components are developing at the same rate. She proposed that tasks be classified according to intratask components, which emphasize the independent description of each component. In her version, stages of development may exist at the component level, but not at the level of total body configuration. We agree that all of the patterns or sub-routines within a stage (as defined by us) do not advance as an indivisible unit. However, we have found sufficient cohesion between certain of these sub-routines so that listing them within a 'stage' appeals to us as the least complicated way to describe a particular developmental task. Our students have also shown a preference for the description by 'total body configuration' when learning to identify the various developmental levels.

Perhaps the most detailed description of an intertask sequence is the one proposed by Milani-Comparetti and Gidoni (1967). Their sequence of achieving the erect posture identifies the body actions and reflexes that must be present and/or extinguished before the next task can be accomplished. Whether this procedure is useful for the classification of movement beyond the age of infancy is not known because work has not progressed beyond this age. However, the work of Kabat (1952), Voss (1967), Knott and Voss (1968), and Shambes and Campbell (1973) suggests that mass movement patterns of proprioceptive neuromuscular facilitation (PNF) can be identified in the motor tasks of infancy and childhood. These mass movement patterns are regarded by some as the substrate for all subsequent motor skills.

In a doctoral dissertation now under way (Evans, 1980), we have found a high degree of agreement between three physical therapists in their identification of the mass movement patterns of the overhand throw, in its five developmental levels as identified by our staff. It was hypothesized that these mass movement patterns would be stable across the five stages of the throw and that the intraphasic modal mass movement pattern would be stable across the five-stage sequence. If the presence or absence of these patterns is associated with movement proficiency, then we have another technique by which we can classify movement. If the hierarchical complexity of the subpatterns corresponds to our sequence of stages, it will provide a model against which to compare our substages.

In our laboratory the classification of fundamental skills into stages has been accomplished for nine tasks, eight of which are shown in Figure 1. This illustration permits us to examine the ages when children are able to perform the tasks that are encompassed within the stages. It also permits us to compare the relative difficulty in achieving the various stages by noting the time-span between their attainment. If one looks at the unusual amount of time between the attainment of stages 3 and 4 in striking, for example, we can surmise that progress, as defined by this system, has been delayed. Either (i) the postural and movement demands for stage 4 are difficult to achieve, or (ii) those required for stage 3 require an unusual amount of time for their mastery, or (iii) the increment in tasks between stages 3 and 4 is too great. The systematic solution to a problem of this type is possible by the following set of procedures, using the five-stage sequence of over-arm throwing as the skill to be analyzed (See Figure 2).

Our study of the developmental sequences for the various skills has revealed that progress can be curtailed for many reasons. We have placed these impedi-

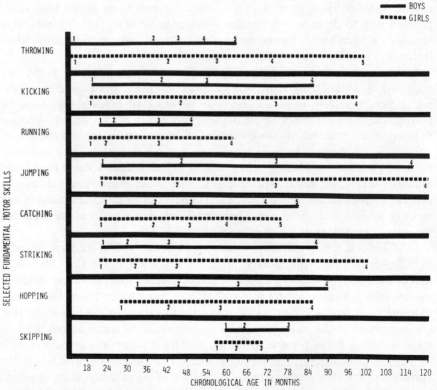

FIGURE 1     Age at which 60 percent of the boys and girls were able to perform a specific developmental level for selected fundamental motor skills

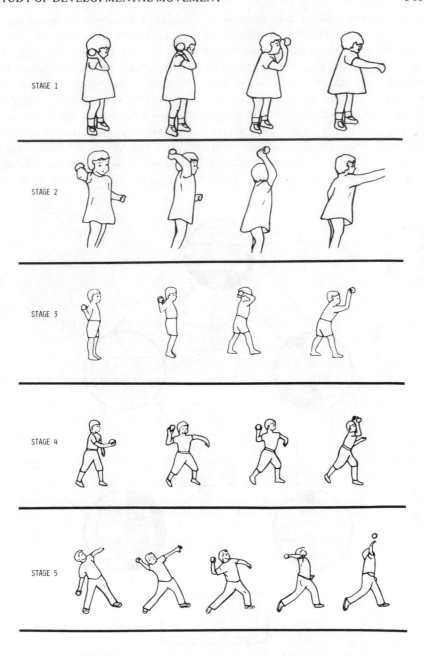

FIGURE 2   Developmental sequence of throwing behavior, redrawn from
Wickstrom

ments to progress into three categories: (i) critical antecedents; (ii) novel situations; and (iii) limiting conditions. A model which describes the inter-relationship of these three categories is provided in Figure 3. The diagram reflects our belief that certain critical antecedents must be attained before the learner can accomplish a novel task. However, the novel task can be accomplished with various degrees of proficiency; thus permitting the learner to move on, even though the task is not performed well. In fact, the influence of limiting conditions on the level of task acquisition is partially responsible for the differences in the proficiency levels between individuals. Children whose motor repertoire is comprised of poorly learned tasks will have difficulty acquiring more demanding tasks within that intratask sequence. To the degree

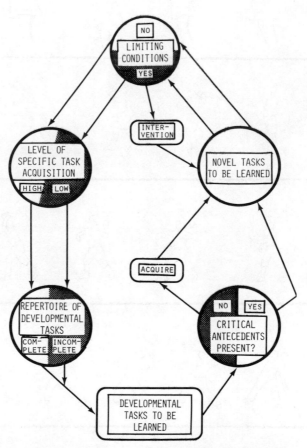

FIGURE 3    Model for the analysis of fundamental motor
skills

| STAGE | CRITICAL ANTECEDENTS | NOVEL SITUATION | LIMITING CONDITION(S) |
|---|---|---|---|
| 1 | ABILITY TO COORDINATE FORCE-FUL EXTENSION OF THE ELBOW AND RELEASE OBJECT AT FULL EXTENSION | INCREASED RANGE OF MOTION THROUGH SHOULDER ELEVATION, SPINAL EXTENSION AND POSTER-IOR MOVEMENT OF THE THROWING ARM | INABILITY TO MOVE THE BASE OF SUPPORT IN CONJUNCTION WITH THE ANTERIOR-POSTERIOR ACTION OF THE TRUNK AND ARM |
| 2 | MOVING BASE OF SUPPORT FOR-WARD WHILE TRUNK IS ROTATING | ROTATION AROUND A LINEAR AXIS; SHIFT OF WEIGHT IN SAME DIRECTION AS ROTATION OF TRUNK | INABILITY TO SEPARATE ROTA-TION OF SPINE AND HIP WHILE MOVING BASE OF SUPPORT |
| 3 | ABILITY TO CONTROL POSTURE OVER BASE OF SUPPORT WHILE MOVING IN AN ANTERIOR-POSTERIOR DIRECTION | SHIFTING WEIGHT AND INITI-ATING OPPOSITION OF MOVEMENT IN AN IPSILATERAL POSITION | INABILITY TO SHIFT THE BODY WEIGHT TO THE CONTRALATERAL SIDE WHILE ROTATING THE TRUNK AND SHOULDER INTO A "WIND-UP" POSITION |
| 4 | ABILITY TO SHIFT WEIGHT TO THE IPSILATERAL SIDE | USING OPPOSITION OF MOVEMENT IN THE UPPER AND LOWER EXTREMITIES | BALANCING AND PIVOTING ON THE SUPPORT LEG WHILE ATTEMPTING OPPOSITION OF MOVEMENT WITH THE UPPER AND LOWER EXTREMITIES |
| 5 | OPPOSITION OF MOVEMENT IN THE UPPER AND LOWER EXTREMITITY | MAINTAINING BALANCE ON THE SUPPORT LEG WHILE ROTATING AND DE-ROTATING A SERIES OF JOINTS IN THE "WIND-UP" AND FORCE PRODUCING PHASES | COORDINATION OF VARIOUS ROTATING JOINTS FOR THE MAXIMUM SUMMATION OF EFFORT |

FIGURE 4    Analysis of the overarm throwing motion, by developmental level

that these tasks are involved in future learning, there will be a reduction in efficiency and effectiveness. Figure 4 illustrates how the five-stage sequence of throwing is acquired by incorporating the components of the model.

Note that the model is presented here only in relation to the biomechanical variables that influence performance. Similar analyses could be made for perceptual-cognitive processes and structural-maturational variables. When all of the requirements for a specific skill have been identified, it is then possible to determine if there are common requirements across skills. Even if there are no pervasive patterns across skills, the analyses that are dictated by the model compel us to identify the specific tasks within a sequence. Thus the environment can be structured in accordance with the learner's capabilities and the demands of the task.

## SUMMARY

The study of motor development has depended upon observational data, designed to provide information about how emerging motor patterns were influenced by maturation, growth, and the social structure. This paper has focused on a systematic method of observing skills and classifying them into stages. This process is then applied to the overarm throw. Current methods of classifying motor sequences are discussed.

## REFERENCES

Evans, R. (1980). Stability and phasic relationships of the mass movement patterns of proprioceptive neuromuscular facilitation across the developmental sequence of the forceful overarm throw in children, unpublished doctoral dissertation, Michigan State University, East Lansing, MI, August.

Gershinowitz, H. (1972). Applied research for the public good – A suggestion, *Science*, **176**, 380–386.

Gesell, A. (1929). Maturation and infant behavior pattern, *Psychological Review*, **36**, 307–319.

Godfrey, B., and Kephart, N. (1969). *Movement Patterns and Motor Education*, New York: Appleton-Century-Crofts.

Halverson, H. M. (1931). An experimental study of prehension in infants by means of systematic cinema records, *Genetic Psychology Monographs*, **10**, 107–386.

Kabat, H. (1952). Studies of neuromuscular dysfunction, XV. The role of central facilitation in restoration of motor function in paralysis, *Archives of Physical and Medical Rehabilitation*, **33**, 521–533.

Knott, M., and Voss, D. E. (1968). *Proprioceptive Neuromuscular Facilitation*, New York: Harper and Row.

McCaskill, C., and Wellman, B. (1938). A study of common motor achievements at the preschool ages, *Child Development*, **9**, 141–150.

McGraw, M. B. (1935). *Growth: A Study of Johnny and Jimmy*, New York: Appleton-Century.

Milani-Comparetti, A. and Gidoni, E. (1967). Routine developmental examination in normal and retarded children, *Developmental Medicine and Child Neurology*, **9**, 631–638.

Roberton, M. (1978). Stages in motor development, in M. Ridenour (ed.), *Motor Development: Issues and applications*. Princeton, NJ: Princeton Book Co.

Schambes, G., and Campbell, S. (1973). Inherent movement patterns in man, *Kinesiology*, **3**, 50–58.

Shirley, M. (1931). *The First Two Years, A Study of Twenty-five Babies*, Minneapolis, The University of Minnesota Press.

Voss, D. (1967). Proprioceptive neuromuscular facilitation: Demonstration with cerebral palsied child, hemiplegic adult, arthritic adult, Parkinsonian adult, *American Journal of Physical Medicine*, **46**, 838–898.

Wickstrom, R. (1977). *Fundamental Motor Patterns*, Philadelphia: Lea and Febiger.

Wild, M. R. (1938). The behavior pattern of throwing and some observations concerning its course of development in children, *Research Quarterly*, **9**, 20–24.

The Development of Movement Control and Co-ordination
Edited by J. A. S. Kelso and J. E. Clark
© 1982, John Wiley & Sons, Ltd

CHAPTER 13

# Developmental Kinesiology: Toward a Subdiscipline Focusing on Motor Development

FRANK L. SMOLL

In a 1964 paper, which was recently elaborated on (Henry, 1978), Henry provided an affirmative answer to the question of whether there is a scholarly field of knowledge concerning human movement. Since then, definition and delineation of the field of study has been the topic of convention sessions, special symposia and, undoubtedly, innumerable faculty meetings. Many articles have dealt with the nature of a human movement discipline (e.g. Eyler, 1967; Kenyon, 1968), the structuring of its hypothetical framework (e.g. Abernathy and Waltz, 1964; Fraleigh, 1967), and the relationships of the discipline with physical education (e.g. Locke, 1977; Norrie, 1977; Park, 1977; Renshaw, 1973). In addition, several books contain chapters on various aspects of the body of knowledge question (e.g. Kroll, 1971; Rivenes, 1978). In a similar vein, attempts have been made at defining discipline-like subfields and clarifying their scope of inquiry (e.g. Kenyon, 1969; Whiting, 1972; Wilberg, 1973; Martens, 1974). Based on the assumption that a conceptual ordering will ultimately enhance systematic extension of knowledge, this paper explores the nature and content of a subdiscipline focusing on the study of motor development.

Most disciplines in the human movement discipline have their origins in a traditional field or fields. During the 1930s and 40s, the study of motor development was included in an emerging area of child development. Today, however, child development researchers primarily address issues relative to the cognitive and affective domains. Given that the study of motor development has been a major concern of students of human movement for some time, it is surprising that this emphasis was omitted from an initial structuring of content areas comprising the body of knowledge (Zeigler and McCristal, 1967). Consideration of this issue is obviously needed and, indeed, long overdue. The discussion that follows is divided into four parts: first, an analysis will be presented of the nature of motor development relative to the concept of development; second, a frame of reference will be developed concerning the human movement discipline; third, the objectives and nature of the subdiscipline labeled *developmental kinesiology* will be examined; and fourth, the content of developmental kinesiology will be delineated.

## THE NATURE OF MOTOR DEVELOPMENT

Motor development may be defined as changes over time in motor behavior that reflect the interaction of the human organism with its environment.[1] The phenomenon is an aspect or subdivision of the total process of development, and as such its salient features may be explored within the context of the developmental concept. In this regard, Harris (1957) identified five ideas commonly included in discussions of development. These ideas will serve as bases for explicating the nature of motor development.

### Organism Conceived as a Living System

Even the most superficial observation reveals that motor development occurs in a very complex dynamic system – the human organism.[2] As a living organism, the human is an open system in which developmental processes evolve out of a high rate of interchange within the system and with the environment in which it exists. Motor development is thus a product of organism-environment interaction and its regulation is subject to an interactional interpretation of the respective roles of heredity and environment.

Concepts of heredity and environment are convenient abstractions or categories of variables that can only theoretically be separated from each other (Ausubel and Sullivan, 1970). Because their interdependency renders them phenomenologically inseparable, this guarantees the bipolar determination of all developmental processes, including motor development. The continuous interaction between heredity and the environment is thus represented by a simple equation: Genotype × Environment = Phenotype. *Genotype* is an individual's genetic endowment or the sum total of all potentialities inherited from one's parents; *phenotype* refers to 'the manifest characteristics of the organism, including anatomical, physiological, and psychological traits' (Montagu, 1963, pp. 389–390) and is always the resultant of the interaction between a certain genotype and a certain environment. Although genes determine potentialities for developing traits and capacities, the predispositions established by genes are never absolute or inevitable in their effects on development. Actualization of inherited potentialities is a function of the relative strength of the genotype and of various environmental factors. Thus we inherit a given genotype which responds in a given way to a given environment, and the result is a given outcome or phenotype.

An important implication of the genetic basis of motor development pertains to a predisposition toward acquiring various levels of skill or proficiency. Hypothetical limits of motor achievement are established by genes, but it is the environment that determines the extent to which the potentialities within these limits are realized. Thus, while the genotype is essentially fixed, it is not a fatalistic or immutable situation. Rather, through the intelligent management of the environment, there is a great deal that can be done about it. In order to make the most of whatever capacities an individual possesses, environmental factors affecting motor development can be manipulated in ways that are most conducive to optimal development.

The uniqueness or individuality of motor development is attributable in part to the bipolar regulation of the process. No two persons are born with the same genotype (identical twins excepted), and it is highly unlikely that two people would be exposed to exactly the same environmental conditions. Furthermore, because of an age trend toward heterogeneity in environmental stimuli, individual differences in motor development tend to become greater with advancing age.

## Time

Time is a natural dimension in which both contemporaneous and developmental phenomena occur. In contemporaneous sciences (e.g. chemistry, physics, physiology) time is of incidental or nominal interest; here scientists are concerned with describing and explaining events and relationships which do not change significantly during the interval in which they are studied. On the other hand, in developmental sciences (e.g. geology, embryology, developmental psychology) *change* as a function of time is the primary phenomenon under investigation (Ausubel and Sullivan, 1970). Thus, with regard to motor development, scientists are interested in determining how and why motor behavior differs (i.e. undergoes changes) from one point in time to another.

The purview of motor development formerly concentrated on changes in motor behavior during infancy and childhood. However, in order to avoid the mistake of ignoring interage networks and other aspects of long-term ontogenetic linkages, emphasis is now placed on exploring the process within the framework of a lifespan concept of development. The lifespan concept emphasizes that developmental change can be pervasive and rapid at all ages (Baltes and Schaie, 1973; Goulet and Baltes, 1970; Nesselroade and Reese, 1973). Motor development is thus viewed as a more or less continuous, lifelong process that begins in utero and persists through adult life (Halverson,

Roberton, and Harper, 1973; Keogh, 1977; Roberton, 1972; Wickstrom, 1975, 1977).

## Change over Time Toward Complexity of Organization

A major aspect of motor development involves an increase in functional complexity, making it possible to perform at progressively higher levels of proficiency. Acquisition of adult standards in *fundamental skills* is central to this process. Fundamental skills (e.g. walking, running, jumping, hopping, throwing, catching, kicking, striking) are the bases or underlying constituents of *complex skills* utilized in game, sport, and dance activities. In essence, complex skills are advanced and refined versions of fundamental skills that have been adapted to the special requirements of particular physical activities.

Development of mature form in fundamental skills (i.e. patterns of performance characteristic of skilled adults) occurs through a sequential progression involving achievement of intermediary developmental (immature) motor patterns. The blueprint for developmental motor patterns is phylogenetically ingrained, and its expression follows an orderly, stage-by-stage sequence with each successive stage representing a higher degree or level. The hierarchical sequence from rudimentary to mature stages is generally viewed, either implicitly or explicitly, as reflecting the gradual maturation of the child. However, in accordance with the bipolar determination paradigm, developmental outcomes are clearly the result of the mediating effects of environmental factors (e.g. stimulation and practice) upon inherent processes. Furthermore, while the developmental sequence of motor events is approximately the same for all children, this does not imply that each separate stage is a prerequisite for the immediately succeeding stage, or that the sequence is absolutely rigid. Omissions and reversals in the process do occur, yet such occurrences do not necessarily result in developmental retardation (Seefeldt, 1970).

Associated with the orderly, predictable pattern of motor development are two well-known trends of developmental direction. The *cephalocaudal* trend is typified by a head-to-foot progression in muscle control and co-ordination, with development in the head and trunk regions of the body preceding development in the lower extremities. According to the *proximodistal* trend, those parts of the body closest to the central axis are brought under control before the peripheral segments. Thus control of large muscle groups near the medial portion of the body is possible before control of body parts near the extremities. Evidences of the cephalocaudal and proximodistal trends are readily observable during infant motor development, particularly in regard to postural-locomotor and reaching–grasping behaviors, respectively. It should be noted, however, that there are some exceptions to these trends; yet they do not negate the validity of the general principles.

In contrast to the generally uniform sequence of motor development, the rate is ontogenetically determined. Consequently, developmental changes in motor behavior are not age-bound. Rather, the ages at which changes take place vary from one child to another. And, as one might expect, this substantially contributes to the individuality of the process.

The preliminary stages of fundamental skills are usually quite well established prior to six years of age. In this regard, Seefeldt (1971) stated that 'the specific nature of these skills and the tremendous amount of time required to gain mastery of them point to the urgency of early practice. If a child does not develop a broad repertoire of fundamental skills prior to first grade, he will probably not find the time to do so thereafter' (p. 21). Although a good foundation must be established, what happens during these early years is only a part of the process. Motor development includes modification and combination of fundamental skills into skills of increasingly greater complexity and precision. The greater complexity of skills used in game, sport, and dance activities is partly attributable to the fact that their development involves integrating and co-ordinating several underlying fundamental skills. Similarly, part of the greater precision accrues as a function of adapting basic skills to the specific requisites of the activity and as a function of incorporating individual stylistic variations into the patterns.

While the present discussion focuses on general characteristics of changes over time in motor behavior, it should be noted that the construct of *organization* is central to the conceptualizations of motor skill development presented by Bruner (1973), Elliott and Connolly (1974), and Keogh (1975). Organization therein refers to the manner in which sequences of movement 'subroutines' are combined to achieve efficient execution or increased control over motor behavior. In this regard, concepts such as sequencing and modularization (Bruner, 1973) and movement consistency and constancy (Keogh, 1975) have been proposed as basic elements of the process. Such models and theoretical formulations have given rise to an orientation toward studying underlying mechanisms of motor behavior in terms of mental operations or information processing. These approaches will receive additional attention in a later section of the paper.

## Comprehension of Parts or Part-systems into Larger Units

It is readily apparent that initial attempts at performing motor tasks are accompanied by excessive and often random bodily movements. As the process of motor development continues along its sequential course, gross awkward movements give way to increasingly discrete movements involving only the appropriate musculature and body segments – a general to a specific progression. If, however, motor development were no more than a process of differentiation and refinement, there would be a tendency for the individual to become a composite of unrelated specifics with little, if any, inclination to function motorically as a unified being. In reality though, the process does entail integration of simpler patterns of earlier years into smoothly functioning patterns of increasing complexity ('wholes' involving the use of many lever systems). Thus, as Rarick (1961) stated, 'in the motor realm, development does involve progressively greater neuro-muscular discreteness and exactness, but at the same time such responses become integrated into smoother and more refined patterns of movement' (p. 24). There is a gradual fusion of new elements with those of established patterns, which contributes to an increasing ability to perform according to adult standards.

### An End-state of Organization Which is Maintained with some Stability

To this point there has been an exclusive focus on aspects of motor development characterized by *progressive* changes as the human organism advances toward maturity. What then is maturity when viewed within the lifespan concept? Bayley (1963) stated that:

> Maturity as a general concept applied to human adults is neither a specific point in time nor a static condition that extends over a span of years, but is rather a complex series of ever-changing processes. There may, however, be long periods of relative stability in a given process or function once that function has reached its full development. (p. 126)

In regard to motor behavior, there are certain genetically determined limits that a person moves toward. However, attainment of adult levels of performance rarely (if ever) represent complete fulfillment of one's developmental potential. Motor development is therefore a purposive or goal-seeking process that progresses toward an individually defined optimal level of skill commensurate with maturity. Yet, while maturity is a relatively stable condition, the status of performance may continue to undergo modification.

When applied to the entire lifespan, maturity becomes a reference against which the processes of progressive change and of aging can be juxtaposed for comparison. Motor development most notably encompasses progressive changes from prenatal origins to maturity, but it also includes changes that occur 'on the other side' of maturity. Specifically, another facet of motor development is the decline in level of performance associated with the aging end of the continuum.

### Addendum

The preceding discussion indicates that motor development is an extremely complex aspect of the total developmental process. As such, it constitutes an important component of the totality of man. However, while achievement of motor competencies is necessary for normal functioning, it should not be assumed that the salience of this process is restricted to the psychomotor domain. Motor development is not only subject to regulation by a variety of endogenous and environmental factors, but likewise it has a profound impact on behaviors and processes that transcend the motor realm. Thus, in order to effect a more comprehensive understanding of motor development, we must be cognizant of its interrelationships with and interdependency on physical, psychological, sociological, and cultural factors as well.

## KINESIOLOGY – A CROSS-DISCIPLINE DEALING WITH HUMAN MOVEMENT

Before discussing the nature and content of the subdiscipline focusing on motor development, it is necessary to clarify my position on some important characteristics of the human movement discipline. This will later serve as a frame of reference for examining issues pertaining to the particular subdiscipline in question. In presenting a rather brief coverage, I have synthesized works that can be consulted for more detailed treatments.

### What is a Discipline?

To begin with, universal agreement does not exist over the definition of a discipline. Of the definitional efforts available, Henry's (1964) formulation concisely captures the essence of a discipline:

> An academic discipline is an organized body of knowledge collectively embraced in a formal course of learning. The acquisition of such knowledge is assumed to be an adequate and worthy objective as such, without any demonstration or requirement of practical application. The content is theoretical and scholarly as distinguished from technical and professional. (p. 7)

Distinguishing between a discipline and a profession is additionally illuminating. The objective of a discipline is to understand some portion of reality. A discipline is thus concerned with describing, explaining, and predicting phenomena in its designated domain for the sake of expanding knowledge alone. A profession, on the other hand, is value-oriented and seeks to improve human welfare by implementing change in some aspects of reality. Consequently, disciplinarians are motivated by curiosity to acquire knowledge *per se*; professionals are altruistically motivated to provide services for the betterment of mankind.

**Is Physical Education a Discipline?**

There has been considerable debate as to whether physical education is a discipline, a profession, or both. Physical education is that aspect of education which seeks to achieve educational objectives through the medium of movement. More precisely, it is a subprofession of the teaching profession that uses specific physical activities to change behavior in the cognitive, affective, and psychomotor domains. Given that a discipline is not synonymous with a profession, it follows that using the term *physical education* to refer to the human movement discipline is no more accurate than equating the practice of medicine with the discipline of biology or the profession of family counseling with the discipline of psychology. In this regard, Kenyon (1969) stated that:

> ... arguing that a given field can be simultaneously a profession and a discipline is little save a logically invalid contradiction of terms. The only solution to this dilemma would be to recognize that, while it is possible for the same phenomenon to serve as the focal point of both a profession and a discipline (subject matter for one, a medium for the other), it is there that the similarity ends. Thus, the expression 'physical education' with its obvious professional connotations is not a suitable label for both the professional *and* disciplinary aspects of human physical activity. (pp. 164–165)

**What Term Should be Used to Designate the Human Movement Discipline?**

Of the numerous labels that have been proposed (e.g. *activity sciences, anthropokinetics, exercise science, homokinetics, kinanthropology*), *kinesiology* is sufficiently descriptive, yet simple, and it is consistent with the generic nomenclature of the other disciplines (Martens, 1974). The term is derived from the Greek *kinein*, meaning 'to move,' and the suffix *-ology*, 'the study of.' Thus, *kinesiology* literally means *the study of movement*. This label is attaining wide acceptance, appearing with increasing frequency in the literature, and has become the name for several discipline-oriented university departments.[3]

**The Nature of Kinesiology**

Kinesiology is the study of human movement with special emphasis on the biophysical and psychosocial parameters which affect it and are influenced by it in the realms of sport, work, play, dance, and exercise (adapted from Department of Kinesiology, University of Washington, 1979). The body of knowledge comprising kinesiology was described by Morford and Lawson (1979) as follows:

> Divided into three segments, the subject matter comprises neuromuscular control and motor learning, biomechanics and exercise physiology and other selected psy-

chological and biological factors and the relation of these factors to human development, the functional status of the individual and his or her ability to engage in movement activities; the historical and contemporary role of athletics, dance, or other forms of physical activity in culture, and in both primitive and advanced societies; the contribution of such activities to the emotional adjustment, aesthetic development and physical condition of the individual. (pp. 36–37)

In view of the above, it is important to note that kinesiology is a *cross-discipline* rather than an *interdisciplinary* field of knowledge. In explaining this distinction, Morford and Lawson (1979) stated that:

whereas the adjective, interdisciplinary, describes the interaction among two or more different disciplines in the form of a communication of ideas to the mutual integration of the fields concerned, the term cross-disciplinary implies the integration and magnification of discrete portions of several disciplines. (p. 34)

Thus, an interdisciplinary framework is characterized by interactional inquiry that lacks emphasis on a communality of focus or concern for integration of the resultant knowledge. Rather, such knowledge is subsumed within a traditional discipline. By contrast, while maintaining a focus of attention on human movement, the cross-disciplinary field of kinesiology integrates and magnifies discrete portions of other disciplines in the physical, biological, and social sciences. Furthermore, because content relative to human movement receives only haphazard and peripheral treatment in the traditional disciplines, it follows that 'a person could be well educated in the traditional disciplines . . ., yet ignorant with respect to comprehensive and integrated knowledge of human motor behavior and capability' (Henry, 1978, p. 14).

### The Relation of Kinesiology to Physical Education

Having thus distinguished between a discipline and a profession, I will now discuss the fundamental question of how kinesiology relates to physical education. It is generally held that a professional field cannot effectively achieve its goal of improving the welfare of humanity without a knowledge base on which to substantiate its practice. Henry (1978) succinctly commented on the dependency nature of the discipline–profession relationship as follows: 'the fundamental knowledge derived from uninhibited basic research is the very life blood of any respectable profession' (p. 25). Because physical education is oriented toward changing behavior through the medium of movement, it may thus be viewed as a field which relies on the application of kinesiological knowledge within an educational context. Kinesiology, then, provides the theoretical underpinnings upon which an effective practice of physical education may be grounded. However, while the body of knowledge has direct relevance for physical education, it bears reiterating that the mission of kinesiology is the scholarly pursuit of knowledge devoid of any requisite of practical application.

## DEVELOPMENTAL KINESIOLOGY – A SUBDISCIPLINE OF KINESIOLOGY

The study of the multifaceted phenomenon of motor development is within the scope of a kinesiology subfield, which I prefer to call *developmental kinesiology*. Developmental kinesiology is the study of the nature and regulation of motor development including the biophysical and psychosocial factors which affect it and are influenced by it.[4]

### Objectives of Developmental Kinesiology

In seeking to expand knowledge, the objectives of developmental kinesiology are threefold. First, it endeavors to *describe* the behavioral manifestations of motor development. In so doing, the principal characteristics (both quantitative and qualitative) of motor behavior at successive developmental levels are described as coherently as possible to permit the abstraction of common trends and of sequential uniformities and differences between individuals. The preliminary descriptive level of analysis is supplemented by the study of reciprocal relationships among motor development and a variety of biophysical and psychosocial variables. Second, developmental kinesiology seeks to *explain* changes over time in motor behavior and their effects on associated behaviors and processes. The explanatory level of analysis involves manipulation of variables in attempting to explain the process of transformation as well as its consequences. Third, developmental kinesiology strives to *predict* the future status of motor development and its effects, which is the final test of scientific explanation.

Developmental kinesiology purports to expand knowledge in its designated domain as an important end in itself without regard for applicability to practical problems. Thus the bulk of fundamental knowledge comprising developmental kinesiology is derived from basic research characterized by value-free inquiry. It should be noted, however, that a portion of the body of knowledge is obtained from applied research which is classified as '. . . a secondary level organization of fundamental knowledge, directed toward specific and immediate practical needs' (Henry, 1978, p. 25). For example, researchers have investigated ways of promoting optimal motor development as well as ways of manipulating motor development to effect enhancement of other aspects of development. Yet, while engaging in applied research, value-free inquiry is exercised in pursuing theoretical and scholarly explanations. In essence, then, such research is guided by theory and adheres to the rigorous requirements of scientific method. It is therefore apparent that the resultant knowledge has a legitimate niche in developmental kinesiology.

## The Nature of Developmental Kinesiology

Having identified the objectives of developmental kinesiology, the nature of the subfield will be examined in terms of three criteria for determining whether a field of study qualifies as a discipline and for distinguishing one discipline from another: a particular focus of attention; a unique body of knowledge; and a particular mode of inquiry (Kenyon, 1968).

### Focus of Attention

There is essentially unanimous agreement that the focus of kinesiological inquiry is on human movement. Similarly, for developmental kinesiology, it is doubtful whether anyone would dispute that motor development is the central phenomenon or particular piece of reality about which understanding is sought. Some may argue, however, that the study of the effects of motor development on other aspects of development is beyond the scope of developmental kinesiology. How may this apparent dilemma be resolved? Kenyon (1968) noted that '... the boundaries of disciplines are indeterminant and usually in flux' (p. 37). Thus, while each discipline has a particular focus of attention, virtually all disciplines overlap in certain areas. It follows that attempting to conceive subdisciplines as mutually exclusive categories is unrealistic and, indeed, a futile pursuit. I contend that exclusion of the study of the effects of motor development from the domain of development kinesiology implies a narrow interpretation of the phenomenon and denies appreciation and concern for its impact as an aspect of the total development of human beings.

### A Unique Body of Knowledge

No other discipline or subdiscipline has claimed motor development as a central focus. It was noted earlier that the study of motor development was originally subsumed within the area of child development. Yet it did not attract the attention of many investigators, nor did it attain prominence in that field. In fact, examination of child development texts and courses reveals a primary concern for cognitive and social development with little, if any, attention given to motor development. On the other hand, the research of numerous students of human movement has produced a growing body of knowledge which uniquely focuses on motor development and its effects. This particular body of knowledge is characterized by the presence of special constructs not found in any other field. To illustrate, conceptual terms such as *motor stage*, *developmental motor pattern*, and *movement processes* are indigenous to developmental kinesiology. Furthermore, this subdiscipline draws upon certain portions of traditional disciplines and subdisciplines. For example, knowledge concerning motor development has accrued from neurophysiological research, and understanding of relationships between physical growth and motor development has emanated from research incorporating concepts and techniques from physical anthropology. Therefore, in creating a unique body of knowledge, developmental kinesiology (like its parent discipline) is characterized by a cross-disciplinary perspective.

*A Particular Mode of Inquiry*

The third criterion refers to the methodology or logic of discovery employed for the creation of knowledge. Kenyon (1968) stated that established disciplines tend to embrace a single mode of inquiry based on one of the following three 'ways of knowing:' empirical operations or reliance on sensory observations for the actual experience of reality; formal operations or the ordering of symbols without resorting to observations of reality; and intuitive or mystical operations involving some inner spontaneous experience or 'revelation.' Developmental kinesiologists have uniformly adopted an empiricist epistemology in further understanding in their domain. Employment of the methods of science has been instrumental in generating a discursive subject matter (i.e. expressed in the form of systematically arranged linguistic statements). This knowledge is capable of public verification and thus fulfills the requisite of potential universal agreement.

**Future Developmental Kinesiology Research**

At this point it seems appropriate to interject some comments on research design and on the relation of empirical and theoretical approaches. Because of the concern for investigating changes over time, both cross-sectional and longitudinal designs have been employed in developmental kinesiology research.[5] Most available information has been derived from cross-sectional studies in which the data reflect differences across successive age groups, or cohort differences. The longitudinal approach, on the other hand, provides data on the same individuals over time, thereby enabling analysis of the true nature of developmental change and gaining insight into the processes which are operating to produce age-linked differences. Therefore, in spite of its inherent difficulties, the longitudinal method has been advocated as the most appropriate approach for answering questions concerning motor development (Halverson, Roberton, and Harper, 1973; Seefeldt, 1974a; Wickstrom, 1977).

It should be noted that some developmentalists maintain that studies which do not use longitudinal methods are not developmental. Bijou (1968) in contrast pointed out that this is far too limited and recommended the application of experimental designs in developmental research. Similarly, with regard to the study of motor development, Roberton (1978) and Seefeldt (1974a) have expressed the need for designing experiments and manipulating variables whose effects are theoretically derivable from analysis of previously studied developmental processes. However, as Bijou (1968) stated, 'which procedure is used in a study depends on the objective of the study, the training and boldness of the investigator, and the situation in which the study is conducted' (p. 424).

The issue of research design is directly related to that of descriptive versus explanatory levels of analysis, which in turn may be viewed as an aspect of the contrast between empirical and theoretical approaches. It is well known that descriptive analysis via normative studies is a logical precursor of explanatory or hypothesis-based research. Before attempting to explain how or why certain changes take place during the course of development, precise information is required regarding the actual changes that do occur. Without an accurate description of the phenomena in question, researchers can '... do little more than speculate about speculations (i.e. about the nature of hypothesized events) instead of testing hypotheses that might explain demonstrably occurring events' (Ausubel and Sullivan, 1970, p. 8). While acknowledging the importance of descriptive data, consideration is equally due to the role of theoretical frameworks in explanatory analyses. Theoretical formulations enable the identification of relevant questions, the answers to which are less likely to contribute miscellaneous facts to what Forscher (1963) referred to as a 'chaotic brickyard.' Theories not only serve as a guide in the collection of normative data, but also provide for the orderly integration and interpretation of empirical evidence. In addition, they lead to structuring of specific explanatory hypotheses that are consistent with generalizations derived from a larger body of empirical findings. In view of this, Ausubel and Sullivan (1970) commented on the interdependency of empirical and theoretical approaches as follows:

> Unrelated to a comprehensive theoretical framework, hypothesis-based research is wasteful and uneconomical; both the data from which it is derived and the findings it yields, considered as ends in themselves, are chaotic and unintelligible. On the other hand, specific explanatory hypotheses as well as larger bodies of theory that are not anchored to and continually corrected by empirical data are dealing with phenomena and problems the very existence of which is purely speculative. (p. 9)

Thus, while it is imperative that developmental kinesiologists continue to move from descriptive to explanatory levels of analysis, the body of knowledge will be most efficiently and meaningfully expanded by a productive combination of empirical and theoretical approaches.

## DELINEATING THE CONTENT OF DEVELOPMENTAL KINESIOLOGY

The diversity of the body of knowledge comprising developmental kinesiology is in part a reflection of the multifaceted nature of motor development. In order to delineate the content of the subdiscipline, consideration will be given to a variety of topics to which researchers have directed their attention and to the methodological approaches which they have employed. The discussion does not constitute either a summary of knowledge or a critique of the research. Rather, the intent is to provide an overview of traditional issues and research approaches as well as some current investigatory lines. For this purpose, the subject matter has been divided into four categories: overt motor behavior; endogenous determinants of motor development; environmental factors influencing motor development; and the psychological impact of motor development.[6]

### Overt Motor Behavior

The vast majority of developmental kinesiology research has involved studies in which the motor behavior of children was observed and chronicled, thereby providing descriptive or normative accounts of change over time. In mapping the course of motor development, basically two kinds of data have been generated. *Movement product* data represent achievement of performance scores in specific motor skills, such as speed of running, distance of throwing, and height or distance of jumping. While this information is useful, the end result of a motor act tells little about its manner of execution. On the other hand, *movement process* data indicate how motor skills are performed, or more precisely, they reflect the mechanical actions of constituent motor patterns which are integrated in a space–time–force context. These data have been utilized to describe qualitative changes which take place as mature form is acquired in fundamental skills.

### Movement Process-oriented Research

Classic studies of motor development were concerned with descriptions of stages and timetables for attainment of postural, locomotor, and prehensile control (Ames, 1937; Bayley, 1935; Burnside, 1927; Gesell, 1946; Halverson, 1931; McGraw, 1941; Shirley, 1931). Utilization of more advanced cinematographic techniques enabled Wild (1938) and Hellebrandt *et al.* (1961) to identify and describe characteristic developmental patterns for overarm throwing and jumping skills, respectively. Biomechanical approaches incorporating both kinetic and kinematic analyses (e.g. Clouse, 1959; Dittmer,

1962; Garrett and Widule, 1971; Roy, Youm, and Roberts, 1973) and electromyographic techniques (Okamoto, 1973) have also been applied to the study of children's motor behaviors. At the University of Wisconsin's Motor Development and Child Study Center, movement process-oriented research has been conducted on the overarm throw (Halverson and Roberton, 1966), vertical jumping (Poe, 1976), sidearm striking (Halverson and Roberton, 1966; Harper and Struna, 1973), and punting (Halverson and Roberton, 1966; Poe, 1973). In addition, descriptions of intraskill sequences for throwing, catching, horizontal jumping, and running have emanated from the Motor Performance Study at Michigan State University (Seefeldt, Reuschlein, and Vogel, 1972). In order to effect a fuller understanding of motor development, the study groups at Wisconsin and Michigan State have included analyses of interskill progressions as well as intraskill sequences. At this time, the most comprehensive synthesis of information on fundamental skill development is contained in Wickstrom's second edition of *Fundamental Motor Patterns* (1977).

A current investigatory line focuses on the viability of motor stage theory. Roberton (1977a) proposed that the notion of motor stages is actually a developmental theory and as such is open to testing. Rather than accepting stage theory as a developmental 'given,' Roberton proceeded to investigate its validity. Specifically, she examined the concepts of a universal sequence and intransitivity by adopting a two-phase 'within-time/across-time' methodological paradigm. In the first phase, Roberton (1977b) studied the stability of children's movements across trials at one point in time. With regard to forceful overarm throwing, hypothesized stage classifications for pelvic-spinal and arm movements were analyzed to determine if the same movements were consistently used from trial to trial. Initial data reduction suggested a new model of developmental stages based on components of movement rather than total body configuration. In essence, the 'component model of intratask development' posits that certain components of body action change while others do not. Thus, while the ideas of universality and intransitivity of 'intratask stages' would persist, one would not expect to find all individuals at the same point in all their components at the same time. Preliminary analysis of phase-two longitudinal data supported the model (Roberton, 1978), which will undoubtedly serve to stimulate and guide further motor stage research.

## Movement Product-oriented Research

Prior to the resurgence of movement process-oriented investigations in the 1960s, the bulk of motor development research was devoted to tracing patterns of change in mean achievement scores from early school years through adolescence. Age trends were charted for performance of fundamental skills and measures of basic skill elements, such as balance, strength, flexibility, agility, and reaction time. Sex comparisons were frequently the objective of these studies, which were usually cross-sectional and lacked uniformity in assessment procedures. The age-related changes have been fairly well documented for the years of childhood and adolescence, and the research is summarized in numerous sources (Cratty, 1970; Eckert, 1973; Espenschade and Eckert, 1967, 1973; Keogh, 1973; Rarick, 1961). There is, however, a conspicuous lack of information regarding changes during adulthood and, in particular, the later years of life. The relatively few studies available have involved comparing adult to old-age performance in measures of strength, reaction time, and movement time (e.g. Botwinick and Storandt, 1973; Hodgkins, 1963; Montoye and Lamphiear, 1977; Noble, Baker, and Jones, 1964). In spite of the problems in accounting for the confounding effects of mortality, occupational influences, motivation, and similar variables for elderly subjects, researchers are currently seeking to gain greater understanding of the deterioration in performance that takes place in old age.

A logical corollary of age-trend research involves attempts to determine the extent to which specific performance capabilities change in a systematic and predictable way over a period of years. Utilizing longitudinal strength and motor performance data, investigators addressed the question of whether there is consistency among children in development of these attributes as they advance in age, or if the magnitude of variability is so great that accuracy of prediction over time is precluded (Carron and Bailey, 1974; Clarke, 1971; Espenschade, 1940; Glassow and Kruse, 1960; Rarick and Smoll, 1967). Correlational analyses were used to assess the degree of individual stability in terms of relative position in the group as the children moved through childhood into adolescence. Valuable information has been provided on stability of within-group position (see Keogh, 1973; Rarick, 1973a), and yet many questions remain unanswered regarding factors that may potentially account for variability in performance with advancing age.

With regard to the structure of motor skills, it is commonly held that there are certain general factors which underlie successful performance. In determining the organizational structure of children's gross motor skills, numerous factor analytic studies have been devoted to identifying traits such as balance, strength, flexibility, agility, and co-ordination (e.g. Barry and Cureton, 1961; Chissom, 1971; Cumbee, Meyer, and Peterson, 1957; Ismail and Cowell, 1961; Neeman, 1972; Whitener and James, 1973; Peterson, Reuschlein, and Seefeldt, 1974; Rarick, 1973c). These studies not only provided considerable insight into the structure of children's motor abilities, but have aided in explaining individual differences in levels of performance on a broad range of tasks.

Studies of children's motor behavior generally have relied on measures of mean performance in their data analyses. Recognizing that an individual's performance scores systematically fluctuate across a series of trials, it is unfortunate that intraindividual variability had been ignored in earlier research. More recently, however, researchers (e.g. Dobbins and Rarick, 1977; Eckert, 1974; Eckert and Eichorn, 1977; McGowan, Dobbins, and Rarick, 1973; Smoll, 1975, 1976) have focused on variable error as a measure of the degree of children's motor response consistency. Information about this relevant aspect of motor behavior serves to enhance our understanding of developmental phenomena and thus merits continued empirical attention.

During the past two decades, the upswing in interest in the welfare of mentally retarded children has stimulated a considerable amount of research, some of which has improved our understanding of their motor functions and the potential role of physical activity and skill attainment in their overall development. A growing body of literature has led to the realization that mentally retarded children are motorically much more like their intellectually normal counterparts than they are unlike them, and that retarded children make substantial gains in physical proficiency as a result of participation in structured physical activity programs. As in the case of normal youngsters, however, the majority of research done on motor behavior of mentally retarded children has focused primarily on performance outcomes rather than on movement processes. Rarick (1973b) compiled an excellent review of what is known about the motor abilities of mentally retarded children and factors related to their motor proficiency, and Wickstrom (1975) synthesized the relatively sparse evidence available concerning motor pattern development of these children. It is apparent that a body of knowledge is being developed from which should come greater comprehension and practical techniques that will lead to improved programming for the mentally retarded.

**Endogenous Determinants of Motor Development**

With due regard for the mediating effects of environmental factors, one cannot, however, deny the primacy of certain intrinsic phenomena underlying motor development. Endogenous determinants will be considered separately in this section, yet it must be emphasized that in reality they form a complex network of interactions fundamental to motor development.

*Genetics*

Behavioral genetics has made significant advances in areas such as personality and intellectual development. Yet the study of motor behavior genetics is still in its infancy, and research reports are scattered in several fields of study. Bouchard's (1977) review of literature has drawn together information illustrating the contribution of genes in perceptual efficiency, motor learning, and performance. In this regard, cotwin studies (e.g. Dales, 1969; Freedman and

Keller, 1963; Illigworth, 1968; Marisi, 1977) have been used rather extensively to determine the degree of similarity in motor development among monozygotic and dizygotic twins, that is, the degree of correspondence in development of motor abilities between identical as compared to fraternal twins (see Malina, 1973a). It is virtually impossible to disentangle the role of the genetic blueprint from the impact that environmental experiences have on its expression. However, we can anticipate that scientists will strive to learn more about the critical role that genes play as determinants of motor development.

### Neural and Reflex Substrates

Empirical evidence has substantiated the association between neurological changes and development of overt motor behavior. The early work of Conel (1939, 1941), for example, established that development of neonatal prehensile abilities is accompanied by concomitant changes within the portion of the motor cortex that controls hand movements. Neurophysiologists have subsequently incorporated histological, biochemical, and electrochemical techniques to investigate neural structures and functions underlying development of motor behavior (see Herman *et al.*, 1976). Additionally, Taub (1976) recently used neurosurgery to study the development of the nervous system and behavior in nonhuman primates. Applying new surgical techniques, monkey fetuses were removed from the uterus; dorsal rhizotomies were performed; and the fetuses were replaced in utero. The effects of the forelimb deafferentation were then assessed after birth. These techniques have proven effective for obtaining direct knowledge of prenatal origins of mammalian motor behavior.

It is well known that the neurological status of the newborn and young infant is reflected by the presence of reflexes acquired during fetal life. During the normal course of central nervous system development, the gradual transition from subcortical to cortical control and inhibition is marked by diminution of certain reflexes. These observable changes provide the 'tools' necessary for screening pathological conditions. However, reflex responses are not only important in developmental diagnosis. There is general agreement that these mechanisms play a prominent role in development of volitional motor behavior. For example, Twitchell (1965) showed that reflex grasping is a vital precursor to voluntary prehension; Brown and Fredrickson (1977) examined the relationship of sucking and grasping reflexes as the basis of hand–mouth co-ordination; and Milani-Comparetti and Gidoni (1967) associated reflexive righting reactions with achievement of erect posture. Similarly, Knott and Voss (1968) and Shambes and Campbell (1973) emphasized that four inherent diagonal patterns form the common denominators upon which many motor skills are built. It seems reasonable to expect that future research will lead to

greater comprehension of neural-reflex substrates on which voluntary movement is elaborated.

## Growth and Biological Maturation

The processes of physical growth and biological maturation have long been
accepted as important determinants of motor development. Physical growth
and maturation may be viewed conceptually as two distinct processes of
biological change, that is, quantitative incremental change in the size of the
body and/or any of its parts *versus* qualitative increases in structural and
functional complexity. These processes are, however, inextricably interwoven
in reality and must therefore be considered in an integrated manner with regard
to their influence on motor development.

Numerous investigators have sought to ascertain the extent to which
differences in physical performance may be attributed to differences in body
size, body proportions, physique, body composition, and maturity status (see
Malina, 1975; Malina and Rarick, 1973). These studies utilized movement
product scores and were primarily correlational in nature, focusing on patterns
of relationships during middle childhood, adolescence, and young adulthood. It
is readily apparent that many biophysical factors are operating on performance
and that the differential relationships are not simple. Furthermore, because
relatively little is known about such associations during early childhood,
studies are needed of anthropometric dimensions relative to motor development across these earlier ages.

## Cognitive Processes

As previously noted, motor development research has been characterized
primarily by movement product and process-oriented approaches. Connolly
(1970), however, was among those who pointed out that 'in addition to asking
the question *when*, we must also ask *how*; what are the processes underlying
the observed changes which have been so elegantly described?' (p. 8). This
emphasis has stimulated interest in applying information-processing models to
derive insight into developmental aspects of cognitive processes subserving
motor behavior.

The information-processing approach, which has been the bailiwick of cognitive psychologists, focuses on determining and understanding the sequence of
a number of mental operations that occur between a stimulus and response. In
explaining information processing, Massaro (1975) noted that the presentation
of a stimulus, which has potential information, initiates a sequence of processing stages. Each stage operates on the information available to it, which takes

time. The transformed information is then made available to the following stage of processing. Although there is not total agreement among theorists as to the number of stages necessary to account for human information-processing behavior, Wickens (1974) presented the following four-stage conceptualization:

> The four stages consist of a preperceptual, or sensory store, which receives and stores for a brief duration all sensory stimulus information; a perceptual system, which receives and encodes the attended stimulus information; a decision and response selection mechanism, which, from the data received from the perceptual system, selects a response; and a response execution mechanism, which releases the selected response. The latter three stages have access to a memory system and are controlled by a central attention or processing mechanism. (p. 739)

Information processing has provided a framework for examining the roles of sensation, perception, memory, attention, and decision-making in the acquisition and performance of motor skills. Several of these components have received consideration with regard to implications for the study of motor development (see Clark, 1977; Rothstein, 1977; Todor, 1978; Williams, 1974). In addition, there are a number of recently proposed conceptual and theoretical formulations holding promise for elucidating mechanisms of motor development (see Keogh, 1977; Newell, 1977). However, although increasing interest has been expressed, there is a paucity of investigatory activity focusing on the processing and transformation of information directly relative to motor development. Hopefully, those who have adopted information-processing paradigms and research strategies will move from merely applying such approaches to children's motor behavior toward an emphasis on the study of cognitive operations underlying changes over time in motor behavior.

## Environmental Factors Influencing Motor Development

The human organism must adapt to a vast array of stresses imposed by its environment. The organism–environment interaction consequently has an impact on developmental processes, including, of course, motor development. In this section, consideration is given to several environmental factors which influence achievement of inherent motor ability potentialities.

### Nutrition

It has been recognized that nutrition is perhaps the most ubiquitous factor affecting physical growth and that undernutrition is undoubtedly the most common cause of retarded growth in childhood (Malina, 1972; Tanner, 1962). An abundance of evidence reviewed by Birch (1972), Lathem and Cobos (1971), and Scrimshaw and Gordon (1968) also indicates strongly that nutritional factors at a number of different levels contribute significantly to depressed intellectual level and learning failure. Moreover, detrimental effects of inadequate nutritional intake have been reported for motor development (see Malina, 1973a, 1974). Two processes, which may operate simultaneously, have been postulated as bases for affecting motor development. The first is that malnutrition causes irreparable alterations of the nervous system resulting in impaired intersensory functioning; that is, malnutrition directly causes defective information processing. The second is that malnutrition is accompanied by a combination of apathy and irritability which consequently results in unresponsiveness to surroundings and ultimately in lack of experience and stimulation. Researchers are currently probing these explanations and are seeking answers to questions concerning timing, severity, and duration of malnutrition and the possibility of a catch-up phenomenon following correction of the malady.

## Deprivation, Stimulation, and Environmental Intervention

In the seemingly age-old question of the respective roles of maturation and learning, the concept of critical periods occupies a central position. The effects of critical periods have been associated with various types of emotional development and the formation of basic social relationships. Our primary concern is with critical periods as applied to acquisition of motor skills. Outdated interpretations erroneously emphasized that motor behaviors emerge spontaneously with the invariable maturation of the nervous system. Current research supports the importance of neuroanatomical and neurophysiological maturation, but not as an immutable condition for motor skill acquisition. Rather, because of the plasticity of human development, the influence of sensory stimulation and enriching environmental conditions cannot be discounted in the promotion of optimal development. Thus, according to contemporary usage, the term *critical periods* implies that for any given motor skill, acquisition occurs most efficiently during certain intervals of time when the organism is more susceptible to the influence of environmental stimuli than at other times, and that the limits of these 'sensitive periods' are flexible (Connolly, 1972; Magill, 1978; Seefeldt, 1975).

In deference to the welfare of the subjects, experimental evidence relative to the effects of deprivation of sensory stimulation on motor development exists from studies on infrahuman subjects. These studies have consistently shown that stimulus deprivation or inhibition of opportunity to respond to stimuli is detrimental. Although preliminary evidence suggests that humans can make up for motor deficits incurred from sensory deprivation, little research information is available on either the limits of deprivation tolerance (intensity and duration) or the mechanisms underlying the catch-up phenomenon (Seefeldt, 1975).

Laboratory data for infrahuman organisms have indicated beneficial alterations in ontogenesis as a function of neonatal stimulation, as well as detrimental effects of excessive stimulation. Such evidence of the plasticity of the nervous system provided the impetus for studies of the effects of various forms of sensory stimulation during human infancy (e.g. Clark, Kreutzberg and Chee, 1977; Rice, 1977; Zelazo, Zelazo, and Kolb, 1972). Findings generally supportive of beneficial outcomes subsequently led to the advent of programs designed to accelerate infant motor development. While logical rationales exist for provision of early experiences (Seefeld, 1975), additional research should be directed to determining the strengths and limitations of such programs (Ridenour, 1978). In other words, greater realization of human capacities will ultimately accrue from research on the kinds and amounts of sensory stimulation necessary for optimal motor development.

Current concepts of readiness for acquisition of motor skills emphasize consideration of developmental status, provision of appropriate preliminary experiences, and acquisition of prerequisite or subordinate skills (Seefeldt, 1978). Some of the investigatory activity at Wisconsin's Motor Development and Child Study Center has focused on the effects of environmental settings on stimulating emergence and progress in motor pattern development. For example, researchers have examined the effects of guided practice, including setting of force goals, on development of kindergarten children's overhand-throw ball velocities (Halverson et al., 1977) and on motor pattern development (Halverson and Roberton, 1979). Future research will hopefully provide evidence on when the introduction of skills should occur (i.e. when optimal readiness exists for specific skills) and which antecedent experiences and environmental conditions enhance readiness and promote acquisition of specific skills.

## Cultural Factors

Various aspects of the cultural milieu are known to condition or modify the expression of underlying motor processes. Unfortunately, however, studies of culturally defined factors have been concerned primarily with child socialization, personality development, and cognitive development, and motor behavior data were of secondary interest. Because investigators have rarely focused on motor variables, we are essentially limited to specualtive interpretations of the influences of child-rearing practices, socioeconomic status, and ethnicity, or more specifically their ramifications relative to a permissiveness-restrictiveness continuum (see Malina, 1973b, 1973c, 1977).

As previously noted, movement product-oriented research provided normative data describing sex differences on selected motor skills. The patterns of change and magnitude of differences have been explained, to a certain extent, in terms of anatomical and physiological sex characteristics. Biophysical factors are influential indeed, yet cultural norms, expectations, and experiences play an important role in differentiation of performance levels between the sexes. Studies of sex differences in play behavior have indicated that cultural conditioning for specific sex-associated roles begins very early in life (see Lewko and Greendorfer, 1978). Moreover, the continued effects of sex-role socialization on performance have been shown in investigations of children's game preferences, their perceptions of sex-appropriate motor acts, and the influence of sex-typed labels on children's motor performances and preferences (Herkowitz, 1978a). Societal changes in female sex roles are being accompanied by encouragement and greater opportunities for participation in physical activities and sports. These changes hold heuristic promise for the study of motor development and clearly warrant the attention of researchers.

## Play Behavior and Environments

Rather than being viewed as a frivolous endeavor, play has long been regarded as a primary vehicle for preparing youngsters to participate in society. Numerous developmentalists, including Bruner (1975), Piaget (1952), and Sutton-Smith (1971), have emphasized that most of the early learning of children evolves through play and play situations. Yet relatively little research has focused on play behavior as it affects motor development or on the design of playspaces and equipment relative to enhancement of motor development. In this regard, Wade (1976) reviewed methodological procedures having implications for the study of chidlren's play, and Herkowitz (1978b) presented a theoretically based rationale for the design of playspaces and described techniques for evaluating playspaces. It is anticipated that future research will be directed toward investigating the relation of this relevant form of behavior to motor development.

## Sport Participation

In examining the nature of motor development, it was noted that complex motor skills are superimposed upon fundamental skills which should be acquired during preschool and early elementary school years. Children have always engaged in play and informal games as a way of practicing these skills. Furthermore, participation in organized sports programs affords additional opportunities for continued refinement and expansion of the child's motor repertoire. Since development of motor competencies is an objective of youth sports programs (Martens and Seefeldt, 1979), questions regarding the effects of participation are logical concerns of developmental kinesiologists. In fact, many of the research topics referred to earlier in this paper have been dealt with in youth sports settings. For example, researchers have investigated relationships among physical growth, biological maturation, and performance of young athletes (see Malina, 1978), and questions regarding critical periods and readiness to participate in youth sports have been addressed (see Magill, 1978; Seefeldt, 1978; Singer, 1978). Organized youth sport programs are a firmly established part of our society and will continue to grow in scope and popularity. The continuing involvement of developmental kinesiologists can serve to increase scientific knowledge in this previously neglected area.

**The Psychological Impact of Motor Development**

The issues considered in the three preceding sections have a basic commonality. Research conducted on these issues is oriented toward acquiring knowledge about motor development *per se*, including the manner in which it is affected by endogenous and environmental determinants. In this section, attention is directed to research concerning the influence of motor development on psychosocial variables.

*Cognitive Development and Academic Achievement*

During the 1960s, a national concern arose for providing appropriate educational opportunities for children with learning problems. This trend stimulated renewed interest in motor development, or more exactly, in examination of the role of movement experiences in the educational process. The utilization of motor activities to foster achievement of academic objectives became the trademark of 'perceptual-motor programs' which Seefeldt (1974b) described as '. . . those organized activities wherein locomotion or gross motor responses constitute an essential part of the training procedure designed to enhance the development of visual, auditory, verbal, tactile, and kinesthetic perceptions' (pp. 266–267). The rationale for programs intended to prevent, detect, and remediate learning disabilities is the notion that all learning has a motor foundation. As a result, the programs of Delacato (1963), Frostig (1964), Getman (1962), and Kephart (1960) have been highly influential as models from which the vast majority of existing perceptual-motor programs are descendent. These programs vary in content, but their proponents all subscribe to the idea that higher order cognitive functioning develops from basic perceptual-motor attributes and that progression occurs in stages through the establishment of sensory integrations. Heavy emphasis is thus placed on perceptual-motor training with the assumption that improvement will directly transfer to academic performance.

Abundant testimony and opinion has been issued on the value of perceptual-motor programs in the enhancement of academic achievement. Reviewers, however, unanimously agree that research in general has failed to substantiate their efficacy (Andrews, 1976; Goodman and Hammill, 1973; Hartman and Hartman, 1973; Myers and Hammill, 1976; Seefeldt, 1970, 1974b). Nevertheless, the perceptual-motor craze has had a positive impact in several ways. First, attention has been centered on the importance of early childhood education and the role of physical activities. Second, elementary school physical education has similarly derived benefits in the form of efforts directed toward curriculum development and ultimately toward improved program content and methodology. Third, researchers in different fields have become aware of the correspondence of their objectives and concerns, which has resulted in collaborative efforts in studying the whole child. Fourth, as Keogh (1977) pointed out, '. . . the naive and superficial linking of movement development and perceptual-cognitive development served to direct current research interests in the reverse direction of studying perceptual-cognitive aspects of movement development' (p. 78). Finally, while falling short of the objective of enhancing academic achievement, there is evidence that acquisition of skills directly related to program content does result from certain training programs (e.g. fine and gross motor co-ordinations and specific components of vision: Seefeldt, 1974b). Consequently, these programs will undoubtedly continue to provide the impetus for research activity.

## Psychosocial Development

A considerable amount of knowledge and information concerning the contribution of motor development to emotional and social development has resulted from examining psychosocial maladjustment in motor-impaired children (see Morris and Whiting, 1971; Rosenbloom, 1971; Smoll, 1974). In addition, motor prowess has long been recognized as an important determinant in gaining peer acceptance among normal children, particularly for boys in our culture. Consequently, numerous researchers have studied relationships between children's proficiency in physical activities and various aspects of personal–social adjustment (e.g. Anastasiow, 1965; Clarke and Green, 1963; Rarick and McKee, 1949; Thomas and Chissom, 1973; Yarnall, 1966). Investigations of psychosocial concomitants of motor development typically involve research designs that require correlational analyses. For example, Smoll, Schutz, and Keeney (1976) utilized canonical correlation analysis to study the relationships among children's attitudes, involvement, and proficiency in physical activities. While valuable information may be derived, such approaches preclude the drawing of causal inferences. On the other hand, the recent study by Duke, Johnson, and Nowicki (1977) illustrates the use of an experimental approach in which motor development was used as an independent variable. These investigators presented preliminary evidence indicating that improvement in children's physical skills promotes desirable changes in locus of control orientation. Incorporation of experimental designs in future research will hopefully serve to enhance our understanding of the impact of motor development on psychosocial development.

## SUMMARY

An examination has been presented of the nature and content of developmental kinesiology – a subdiscipline of the human movement discipline pursuing knowledge about motor development and its effects on associated behaviors and processes. Initially, motor development was defined, and its salient features were explored in relation to concepts that are characteristic of the total process of development. In this regard, consideration was given to the interaction of genotype and environment in the bipolar regulation of motor development; change in motor behavior as a function of time within a lifespan perspective; the sequential, hierarchical nature of the process as it proceeds toward greater complexity and precision of motor skill performance; the integration of simple motor patterns into smoother and more refined patterns of functioning; the concept of maturity relative to the lifespan view of motor development; and the reciprocal relationships among motor development and other aspects of development. Following this, a frame of reference was developed regarding the discipline of kinesiology. In so doing, emphasis was given to the distinction between disciplines and professions; the cross-disciplinary nature of kinesiology; and the relation of kinesiology to physical education. Next, the objectives of developmental kinesiology in expanding knowledge were identified, after which the subfield was described in terms of its focus of attention on motor development and associated effects; the uniqueness of its cross-disciplinary body of knowledge; and its empirical mode of inquiry. In commenting on research design and the relation of empirical and theoretical approaches, it was pointed out that future advances in developmental kinesiology will be dependent not only on soundly designed empirical investigations, but also on the concomitant development and testing of theoretical frameworks and models that can serve as a source of testable hypotheses. Finally, in delineating the content of developmental kinesiology, an overview was presented of traditional issues, research approaches, and some current investigatory lines. The subject matter was dealt with within the categories of overt motor behavior; endogenous determinants of motor development; environmental factors influencing motor development; and the psychological impact of motor development.

In closing, it can be concluded that developmental kinesiology constitutes a significant area of inquiry concerning human movement and it has enormous potential for researchers seeking to expand knowledge as well as professionals striving to implement such knowledge for realization of practical goals.

Hopefully, the conceptual ordering presented here will serve to facilitate communication among developmental kinesiologists and will promote their working together as members of a co-operative enterprise, which will ultimately bring more sophistication and depth to our body of knowledge. However, while conceptualization efforts are needed, we should be less concerned about describing ourselves and devote greater attention to conducting scientific inquiry. In other words, as Kenyon (1968) so aptly stated, 'while I believe our efforts from the armchair can make some contribution, they will never substitute for actual efforts to create new knowledge' (p. 35).

## NOTES

Appreciation is expressed to W. Robert Morford and Ronald E. Smith for commenting on an earlier draft of this paper.

1. This definition is an adaptation of one collectively developed by Wade *et al.* (1974).
2. While students of motor development are primarily concerned with the human organism, this orientation does not preclude implications derived from animal models and related research.
3. Some authors still use *kinesiology* in a traditional sense to describe the functional anatomical and mechanical analysis of movement. However, the term *biomechanics* is currently favored as a more appropriate designation (see Carr, 1978).
4. The term *developmental kinesiology* was used by Roberton (1972) and later by Wickstrom (1975) to refer to '. . . the application of kinesiological techniques to the study of motor development' (Roberton, 1972, p. 65). Given the contemporary usage of *kinesiology* in a disciplinary context, utilization of *developmental kinesiology* in a methodological sense is obviously dated and inappropriate. Furthermore, the term *motor development* has been applied incongruously by some writers both as an aspect of the process of development and as an area of study – a practice which is apt to create misunderstanding and confusion. In the present paper, the separate usages of *motor development* and *developmental kinesiology* are proposed with the intention of avoiding semantic ambiguity.
5. The reader is referred to the works of Baltes (1968), Schaie (1965), and Wohlwill (1970) for comprehensive analyses of the strengths and weaknesses of cross-sectional and longitudinal designs for studying age-functional relationships.
6. While a considerable body of knowledge exists concerning conditions of motor impairment, the present treatment of topical areas deals primarily with the 'normal' end of the skill continuum.

## REFERENCES

Abernathy, R., and Waltz, M. (1964). Toward a discipline: First steps first, *Quest*, **2**, 1–7.
Ames, L. B. (1937). The sequential patterning of prone progression in the human infant, *Genetic Psychology Monographs*, **19**, 409–460.
Anastasiow, N. J. (1965). Success in school and boys' sex-role patterns, *Child Development*, **36**, 1053–1066.
Anderson, J. E. (1957). Dynamics of development: System in process, in D. B. Harris

(ed.), *The Concept of Development*, Minneapolis, Minn.: University of Minnesota Press.

Andrews, R. J. (1976). The Doman–Delacato program: Review and comment, *The Exceptional Child*, **23**, 61–69.

Ausubel, D. P., and Sullivan, E. V. (1970). *Theory and Problems of Child Development* (2nd edn.), New York: Grune & Stratton.

Baltes, P. B. (1968). Longitudinal and cross-sectional sequences in the study of age and generation effects, *Human Development*, **11**, 145–171.

Baltes, P. B., and Schaie, K. W. (eds.) (1973). *Life-span Developmental Psychology: Personality and socialization*, New York: Academic Press.

Barry, J., and Cureton, T. K. (1961). Factorial analysis of physique and performance in prepubescent boys, *Research Quarterly*, **32**, 283–300.

Bayley, N. (1935). Development of motor abilities during the first three years, *Monographs of the Society for Research in Child Development*, **1**, 1–26.

Bayley, N. (1963). The life span as a frame of reference in psychological research, *Vita Humana*, **6**, 125–139.

Bijou, S. W. (1968). Ages, stages, and the naturalization of human development, *American Psychologist*, **23**, 419–427.

Birch, H. G. (1972). Malnutrition, learning and intelligence, *American Journal of Public Health*, **62**, 773–784.

Botwinick, J., and Storandt, M. (1973). Age differences in reaction time as a function of experience, stimulus intensity, and preparatory interval, *Journal of Genetic Psychology*, **123**, 209–217.

Bouchard, C. (1977). Genetics and motor behavior, in R. W. Christina and D. M. Landers (eds.), *Psychology of Motor Behavior and Sport – 1976, vol. II: Sport Psychology and Motor Development*, Champaign, Ill.: Human Kinetics.

Brown, J. V., and Fredrickson, W. T. (1977). The relationship between sucking and grasping in the human newborn: A precursor of hand–mouth coordination? *Developmental Psychobiology*, **10**, 489–498.

Bruner, J. S. (1973). Organization of early skilled action, *Child Development*, **44**, 1–11.

Bruner, J. S. (1975). Play is serious business, *Psychology Today*, **8**, 81–83.

Burnside, L. H. (1927). Coordination in the locomotion of infants, *Genetic Psychology Monographs*, **2**, 279–372.

Carr, J. A. (1978). The biomechanical perspective, in R. S. Rivenes (ed.), *Foundations of Physical Education: A scientific approach*, Boston: Houghton Mifflin.

Carron, A. V., and Bailey, D. A. (1974). Strength development in boys from 10 through 16 years, *Monographs of the Society for Research in Child Development*, **39**, 1–37.

Chissom, B. S. (1971). A factor analytic study of the relationship of motor factors to academic criteria for first and third grade boys, *Child Development*, **42**, 1133–1134.

Clark, D., Kreutzberg, J. R., and Chee, F. K. W. (1977). Vestibular stimulation influence on motor development in infants, *Science*, **196**, 1228–1229.

Clark, J. E. (1978). Memory processes in the early acquisition of motor skills, in M. V. Ridenour (ed.), *Motor Development: Issues and applications*, Princeton, NJ: Princeton Book Co.

Clarke, H. H. (1971). *Physical and Motor Tests in the Medford Boys' Growth Study*, Englewood Cliffs, NJ: Prentice-Hall.

Clarke, H. H., and Green, W. H. (1963). Relationships between personal-social measures applied to 10-year-old boys, *Research Quarterly*, **34**, 288–298.

Clouse, F. C. (1959). A kinematic analysis of the development of the running pattern of pre-school boys, unpublished doctoral dissertation, University of Wisconsin-Madison.

Conel, J. L. (1939). *The Postnatal Development of the Human Cerebral Cortex, vol I: The Cortex of the Newborn*, Cambridge: Harvard University Press.

Conel, J. L. (1941). *The Postnatal Development of the Human Cerebral Cortex, vol II: The Cortex of the One-month Infant*, Cambridge: Harvard University Press.

Connolly, K. (1970). Skill development: Problems and plans, in K. Connolly (ed.), *Mechanisms of Motor Skill Development*, New York: Academic Press.

Connolly, K. (1972). Learning and the concept of critical periods in infancy, *Developmental Medicine and Child Neurology*, **14**, 705–714.

Cratty, B. J. (1970). *Perceptual and Motor Development in Infants and Children*, New York: Macmillan.

Cumbee, F. Z., Meyer, M., and Peterson, G. (1957). Factorial analysis of motor coordination variables for third and fourth grade girls, *Research Quarterly*, **28**, 100–108.

Dales, R. J. (1969). Motor and language development of twins during the first three years, *Journal of Genetic Psychology*, **114**, 263–271.

Delacato, C. H. (1963). *The Diagnosis and Treatment of Speech and Reading Problems*, Springfield, Ill.: Thomas.

Department of Kinesiology, University of Washington (1979). Revised undergraduate curriculum, Seattle: Author, September. (Mimeographed).

Dittmer, J. (1962). A kinematic analysis of the development of the running pattern of grade school girls and certain factors which distinguish good from poor performance at the observed ages, unpublished master's thesis, University of Wisconsin-Madison.

Dobbins, D. A., and Rarick, G. L. (1977). The performance of intellectually normal and educable mentally retarded boys on tests of throwing accuracy, *Journal of Motor Behavior*, **9**, 23–28.

Duke, M., Johnson, T. C., and Nowicki, S. (1977). Effects of sports fitness camp experience on locus of control orientation in children, ages 6 to 14, *Research Quarterly*, **48**, 280–283.

Eckert, H. M. (1973). Age changes in motor skills, in G. L. Rarick (ed.), *Physical Activity: Human Growth and Development*, New York: Academic Press.

Eckert, H. M. (1974). Variability in skill acquisition, *Child Development*, **45**, 487–489.

Eckert, H. M., and Eichorn, D. H. (1977). Developmental variability in reaction time, *Child Development*, **48**, 452–458.

Elliott, J. M., and Connolly, K. J. (1974). Hierarchical structure in skill development, in K. J. Connolly and J. S. Bruner (eds.), *The Growth of Competence*, New York: Academic Press.

Espenschade, A. S. (1940). Motor performance in adolescence, *Monographs of the Society for Research in Child Development*, **5**, 1–126.

Espenschade, A. S., and Eckert, H. M. (1967). *Motor Development*, Columbus, Ohio: Merrill.

Espenschade, A. S., and Eckert, H. M. (1973). Motor development, in W. R. Johnson and E. R. Buskirk (eds.), *Science and Medicine of Exercise and Sports* (2nd edn.), New York: Harper & Row.

Eyler, M. H. (ed.) (1967). The nature of a discipline, *Quest*, **9**, December.

Forscher, B. K. (1963). Chaos in the brickyard, *Science*, **142**, 339.

Fraleigh, W. P. (1967). Toward a conceptual model of the academic subject matter of physical education as a discipline, *Proceedings of the 70th NCPEAM National Conference*, 31–39.

Freedman, D. G., and Keller, B. (1963). Inheritance of behavior in infants, *Science*, **140**, 196–198.

Frostig, M. (1964). *The Frostig Program for the Development of Visual Perception*, Chicago: Follett.

Garrett, C., and Widule, C. J. (1971). Kinetic energy: A measure of movement individuality, in C. J. Widule (ed.), *Kinesiology Review, 1971*, Washington, DC: American Association for Health, Physical Education, and Recreation.

Gesell, A. (1946). The ontogenesis of infant behavior, in L. Carmichael (ed.), *Manual of Child Psychology*, New York: Wiley.

Getman, G. N. (1962). *How to Develop your Child's Intelligence*, Luverne, Minn.: Author.

Glassow, R. B., and Kruse, P. (1960). Motor performance of girls age 6 to 14 years, *Research Quarterly*, **31**, 426–433.

Goodman, L., and Hammill, D. D. (1973). The effectiveness of the Kephart–Getman activities in developing perceptual-motor and cognitive skills, *Focus on Exceptional Children*, **4**, 1–9.

Goulet, L. R., and Baltes, P. B. (eds.) (1970). *Life-span Developmental Psychology: Research and Theory*, New York: Academic Press.

Halverson, H. M. (1931). An experimental study of prehension in infants by means of systematic cinema records, *Genetic Psychology Monographs*, **10**, 107–286.

Halverson, L. E., and Roberton, M. A. (1966). A study of motor pattern development in young children, paper presented at the national convention of the American Association for Health, Physical Education, and Recreation, Chicago, March.

Halverson, L. E., and Roberton, M. A. (1979). The effects of instruction on overhand throwing development in children, in G. C. Roberts and K. M. Newell (eds.), *Psychology of Motor Behavior and Sport – 1978*, Champaign, Ill.: Human Kinetics.

Halverson, L. E., Roberton, M. A., and Harper, C. J. (1973). Current research in motor development, *Journal of Research and Development in Education*, **6**, 56–70.

Halverson, L. E., Roberton, M. A., Safrit, M. J., and Roberts, T. W. (1977). Effect of guided practice on overhand-throw ball velocities of kindergarten children, *Research Quarterly*, **48**, 311–318.

Harper, C., and Struna, N. (1973). Case studies in the development of one-handed striking, paper presented at the national convention of the American Association for Health, Physical Education, and Recreation, Minneapolis, April.

Harris, D. B. (1957). Problems in formulating a scientific concept of development, in D. B. Harris (ed.), *The Concept of Development*, Minneapolis, Minn.: University of Minnesota Press.

Hartman, N. C., and Hartman, R. K. (1973). Perceptual handicap or reading disability? *The Reading Teacher*, **26**, 684–695.

Hellebrandt, F. A., Rarick, G. L., Glassow, R. B., and Carns, M. L. (1961). Physiological analysis of basic motor skills. I. Growth and development of jumping, *American Journal of Physical Medicine*, **40**, 14–25.

Henry, F. M. (1964). Physical education – An academic discipline, *Proceedings of the 67th NCPEAM National Conference*, 6–9.

Henry, F. M. (1978). The academic discipline of physical education, *Quest*, **29**, 13–29.

Herkowitz, J. (1978a). Sex-role expectations and motor behavior of the young child, in M. V. Ridenour (ed.), *Motor Development: Issues and applications*, Princeton, NJ: Princeton Book Co.

Herkowitz, J. (1978b). The design and evaluation of playspaces for children, in M. V. Ridenour (ed.), *Motor Development: Issues and applications*, Princeton, NJ: Princeton Book Co.

Herman, R. M.., Grillner, S., Stein, P. S. G., and Stuart, D. G. (eds.) (1976). *Neural Control of Locomotion*, New York: Plenum.

Hodgkins, J. (1963). Reaction time and speed of movement in males and females of various ages, *Research Quarterly*, **34**, 335–343.

Illigworth, R. S. (1968). Delayed motor development, *Pediatric Clinics of North America*, **15**, 569–580.

Ismail, A. H., and Cowell, C. C. (1961). Factor analysis of motor aptitude of pre-adolescent boys, *Research Quarterly*, **32**, 507–513.

Kenyon, G. S. (1968). On the conceptualization of sub-disciplines within an academic discipline dealing with human movement, *Proceedings of the 71st NCPEAM National Conference*, 34–45.

Kenyon, G. S. (1969). A sociology of sport: On becoming a sub-discipline, in R. C. Brown and B. J. Cratty (eds.), *New Perspectives of Man in Action*, Englewood Cliffs, NJ: Prentice-Hall.

Keogh, J. (1973). Fundamental motor task development: Individual changes, in C. B. Corbin (ed.), *A Textbook of Motor Development*, Dubuque, Iowa: Brown.

Keogh, J. F. (1975). Consistency and constancy in preschool motor development, in H. J. Muller, R. Decker, and F. Schilling (eds.), *Motor Behavior of Preschool Children*, Schorndorf: Hofmann.

Keogh, J. F. (1977). The study of movement skill development, *Quest*, **28**, 76–88.

Kephart, N. (1960). *The Slow Learner in the Classroom*, Columbus, Ohio: Merrill.

Knott, M., and Voss, D. E. (1968). *Proprioceptive Neuromuscular Facilitation*, New York: Harper & Row.

Kroll, W. P. (1971). *Perspectives in Physical Education*, New York: Academic Press.

Latham, M. C., and Cobos, F. (1971). The effects of malnutrition on intellectual development and learning, *American Journal of Public Health*, **61**, 1307–1324.

Lewko, J. H., and Greendorfer, S. L. (1978). Family influence and sex differences in children's socialization into sport: A review, in D. M. Landers and R. W. Christina (eds.), *Psychology of Motor Behavior and Sport – 1977*, Champaign, Ill.: Human Kinetics.

Locke, L. F. (1977). From research and the disciplines to practice and the profession: One more time, *Proceedings of the 80th NCPEAM/NAPECW National Conference*, pp. 34–45.

Magill, R. A. (1978). Critical periods: Relation to youth sports, in R. A. Magill, M. J. Ash, and F. L. Smoll (eds.), *Children in Sport: A contemporary anthology*, Champaign, Ill.: Human Kinetics.

Malina, R. M. (1972). The nature of physical growth and development, in R. N. Singer, D. R. Lamb, J. W. Loy, R. M. Malina, S. Kleinman, and J. Felshin (eds.), *Physical Education: An interdisciplinary approach*, New York: Macmillan.

Malina, R. M. (1973a). Physical development factors and motor performance, in C. B. Corbin (ed.), *A Textbook of Motor Development*, Dubuque, Iowa: Brown.

Malina, R. M. (1973b). Environmental factors and motor development, in C. B. Corbin (ed.), *A Textbook of Motor Development*, Dubuque, Iowa: Brown.

Malina, R. M. (1973c). Ethnic and cultural factors in the development of motor abilities and strength in American children, in G. L. Rarick (ed.), *Physical Activity: Human growth and development*, New York: Academic Press.

Malina, R. M. (1974). Motor development: Determinants and the need to consider them, in M. G. Wade and R. Martens (eds.), *Psychology of Motor Behavior and Sport*. Urbana, Ill.: Human Kinetics.

Malina, R. M. (1975). Anthropometric correlates of strength and motor performance, in J. H. Wilmore and J. F. Keogh (eds.), *Exercise and Sport Sciences Reviews* (Vol. 3), New York: Academic Press.

Malina, R. M. (1977). Motor development in a cross-cultural perspective, in R. W. Christina and D. M. Landers (eds.), *Psychology of Motor Behavior and Sport – 1976, vol II: Sport Psychology and Motor Development*, Champaign, Ill.: Human Kinetics.

Malina, R. M. (1978). Physical growth and maturity characteristics of young athletes, in R. A. Magill, M. J. Ash, and F. L. Smoll (eds.), *Children in Sport: A contemporary anthology*, Champaign, Ill.: Human Kinetics.

Malina, R. M., and Rarick, G. L. (1973). Growth, physique, and motor performance, in G. L. Rarick (ed.), *Physical Activity: Human growth and development*, New York: Academic Press.

Marisi, D. Q. (1977). Genetic and extragenetic variance in motor performance, *Acta Geneticae Medicae et Gemellologiae*, **26**, 197–204.

Martens, R. (1974). Psychological kinesiology: An undisciplined subdiscipline, paper presented at the annual meeting of the North American Society for the Psychology of Sport and Physical Activity, Anaheim, March.

Martens, R., and Seefeldt, V. (eds.) (1979). *Guidelines in Children's Sports*, Washington, DC: American Alliance for Health, Physical Education, and Recreation.

Massaro, D. W. (1975). *Experimental Psychology and Information Processing*, Chicago: McNally.

McGowan, C. M., Dobbins, D. A., and Rarick, G. L. (1973). Intra-individual variability of normal and educable retarded children on a coincidence timing task, *Journal of Motor Behavior*, **5**, 193–198.

McGraw, M. B. (1941). Development of neuro-muscular mechanisms as reflected in the crawling and creeping of the human infant, *Journal of Genetic Psychology*, **58**, 83–111.

Milani-Comparetti, A., and Gidoni, E. (1967). Routine developmental examination in normal and retarded children, *Developmental Medicine and Child Neurology*, **13**, 631–638.

Montagu, A. (1963). *Human Heredity* (2nd edn.), Cleveland, Ohio: World Publishing.

Montoye, H. J., and Lamphier, D. E. (1977). Grip and arm strength in males and females, age 10 to 69, *Research Quarterly*, **48**, 109–120.

Morford, W. R., and Lawson, H. A. (1979). A liberal education through the study of human movement, in W. J. Considine (ed.), *Alternative Professional Preparation in Physical Education*, Washington, DC: American Alliance for Health, Physical Education, and Recreation.

Morris, P. R., and Whiting, H. T. A. (1971). *Motor Impairment and Compensatory Education*, Philadelphia: Lea & Febiger.

Myers, P. I., and Hammill, D. D. (1976). *Methods for Learning Disorders* (2nd edn.), New York: Wiley.

Neeman, R. L. (1972). Perceptual-motor attributes of normal school children: A factor analytic study, *Perceptual and Motor Skills*, **34**, 471–474.

Nesselroade, J. R., and Reese, H. W. (eds.) (1973). *Life-span Developmental Psychology: Methodological issues*, New York: Academic Press.

Newell, K. M. (1977). Motor control: Developmental issues, *Proceedings of the 80th NCPEAM/NAPECW National Conference*, pp. 190–198.

Noble, C. E., Baker, B. L., and Jones, T. A. (1964). Age and sex parameters in psychomotor learning, *Perceptual and Motor Skills*, **19**, 935–945.

Norrie, M. L. (1977). Should basic knowledge paradigms provide the foundation for mission-oriented practice? *Proceedings of the 80th NCPEAM/NAPECW National Conference*, pp. 27–34.

Okamoto, T. (1973). Electromyographic study of the learning process of walking in 1- and 2-year-old infants, in S. Cerquiglini, A. Venerando, and J. Wartenweiler (eds.), *Medicine and Sport, vol 8: Biomechanics III*, Zurich, Switzerland: S. Karger.

Park, R. J. (1977). The perennial necessity: The future as theory and practice (or – hats are nice but they won't keep you warm in winter), *Proceedings of the 52nd WSPECW Annual Conference*, pp. 30–39.

Peterson, K. L., Reuschlein, P., and Seefeldt, V. (1974). Factor analyses of motor performance for kindergarten, first and second grade children: A tentative solution, paper presented at the national convention of the American Association for Health, Physical Education, and Recreation, Anaheim, March.

Piaget, J. (1952). *The Origins of Intelligence*, New York: International Universities Press.

Poe, A. (1973). Developmental change in movement characteristics of the punt, paper presented at the national convention of the American Association for Health, Physical Education, and Recreation, Minneapolis, April.

Poe, A. (1976). Description of the movement characteristics of two-year-old children performing the jump and reach, *Research Quarterly*, **47**, 260–268.

Rarick, G. L. (1961). *Motor Development during Infancy and Childhood* (2nd edn.), Madison, Wisc.: College Printing & Typing.

Rarick, G. L. (1973a). Stability and change in motor ability, in G. L. Rarick (ed.), *Physical Activity: Human growth and development*, New York, Academic Press.

Rarick, G. L. (1973b). Motor performance of mentally retarded children, in G. L. Rarick (ed.), *Physical Activity: Human growth and development*, New York, Academic Press.

Rarick, G. L. (1973c). Basic components in the motor performance of children six to nine years of age, paper presented at the national convention of the American Association for Health, Physical Education, and Recreation, Minneapolis, April.

Rarick, G. L., and McKee, R. (1949). A study of twenty third-grade children exhibiting extreme levels of achievement on tests of motor proficiency, *Research Quarterly*, **20**, 142–152.

Rarick, G. L., and Smoll, F. L. (1967). Stability of growth in strength and motor performance from childhood to adolescence, *Human Biology*, **39**, 295–306.

Renshaw, P. (1973). The nature of human movement studies and its relationship with physical education, *Quest*, **20**, 79–86.

Rice, R. D. (1977). Neurophysiological development in premature infants following stimulation, *Developmental Psychology*, **13**, 69–76.

Ridenour, M. V. (1978). Programs to optimize infant motor development, in M. V. Ridenour (ed.), *Motor Development: Issues and applications*, Princeton, NJ: Princeton Book Co.

Rivenes, R. S. (ed.) (1978). *Foundations of Physical Education: A scientific approach*, Boston: Houghton Mifflin.

Roberton, M. A. (1972). Developmental kinesiology, *Journal of Health, Physical Education and Recreation*, **43**, 65–66.

Roberton, M. A. (1977a). Motor stages: Heuristic model for research and teaching, *Proceedings of the 80th NCPEAM/NCPECW National Conference*, pp. 173–180.

Roberton, M. A. (1977b). Stability of stage categorizations across trials: Implications for the 'stage theory' of overarm throw development, *Journal of Human Movement Studies*, **3**, 49–59.

Roberton, M. A. (1978). Stability of stage categorizations in motor development, in D. M. Landers and R. W. Christina (eds.), *Psychology of Motor Behavior and Sport – 1977*, Champaign, Ill.: Human Kinetics.

Rosenbloom, L. (1971). The contribution of motor behavior to child development, *Physiotherapy*, **57**, 159–162.

Rothstein, A. L. (1977). Information processing in children's skill acquisition, in R. W. Christina and D. M. Landers (eds.), *Psychology of Motor Behavior and Sport – 1976, vol II: Sport Psychology and Motor Development*, Champaign, Ill.: Human Kinetics.

Roy, B., Youm, Y., and Roberts, E. M. (1973). Kinematics and kinetics of the standing long jump in 7-, 10-, 13-, and 16-year-old boys, in S. Cerquiglini, A. Venerando, and J. Wartenweiler (eds.), *Medicine and Sport, vol 8: Biomechanics III*, Zurich, Switzerland: S. Karger.

Schaie, K. W. (1965). A general model for the study of developmental problems, *Psychological Bulletin*, **64**, 92–107.

Scrimshaw, N. S., and Gordon, J. E. (eds.) (1968). *Malnutrition, Learning and Behavior*, Cambridge, Mass.: MIT Press.

Seefeldt, V. (1970). Perceptual-motor skills, in H. J. Montoye (ed.), *An Introduction to Measurement in Physical Education, vol 2: Growth, Development and Body Composition*, Indianapolis, Ind.: Phi Epsilon Kappa.

Seefeldt, V. (1971). Concerns of the physical educator for motor development, in M. D. Robb, C. L. Mushier, D. A. Bogard, and M. E. Blann (eds.), *Foundations and Practices in Perceptual-motor Learning – a Quest for Understanding*, Washington, DC: American Association for Health, Physical Education, and Recreation.

Seefeldt, V. (1974a). A researcher's view: Motor development, in L. E. Halverson and M. A. Roberton (eds.), *Elementary School Physical Education: Progress – problems – predictions*, Madison, Wisconsin: Women's Physical Education Alumnae Association, University of Wisconsin.

Seefeldt, V. (1974b). Perceptual-motor programs, in J. H. Wilmore (ed.), *Exercise and Sport Sciences Reviews* (Vol. 2), New York: Academic Press.

Seefeldt, V. (1975). Critical learning periods and programs of early intervention, paper presented at the national convention of the American Association for Health, Physical Education, and Recreation, Atlantic City, March.

Seefeldt, V. (1978). The concept of readiness applied to motor skill acquisition, in R. A. Magill, M. J. Ash, and F. L. Smoll (eds.), *Children in Sport: A contemporary anthology*, Champaign, Ill.: Human Kinetics.

Seefeldt, V., Reuschlein, S., and Vogel, P. (1972). Sequencing motor skills within the physical education curriculum, paper presented at the national convention of the American Association for Health, Physical Education, and Recreation, Houston, March.

Shambes, G. M., and Campbell, S. K. (1973). Inherent movement patterns in man, in C. J. Widule (ed.), *Kinesiology III*, Washington, DC: American Association for Health, Physical Education, and Recreation.

Shirley, M. M. (1931). *The First Two Years: A study of twenty-five babies. Vol I: Postural and Locomotor Development*. Minneapolis: University of Minnesota Press.

Singer, R. N. (1978). The readiness to learn skills necessary for participation in sport, in R. A. Magill, M. J. Ash, and F. L. Smoll (eds.), *Children in Sport: A contemporary anthology*, Champaign, Ill.: Human Kinetics.

Smoll, F. L. (1974). Motor impairment and social development, *American Corrective Therapy Journal*, **28**, 4–7.

Smoll, F. L. (1975). Variability in development of spatial and temporal elements of rhythmic ability, *Perceptual and Motor Skills*, **40**, 140.

Smoll, F. L., and DenOtter, P. (1976). Intraindividual variability in development of accuracy of motor performance, *Journal of Motor Behavior*, **8**, 195–201.

Smoll, F. L., Schutz, R. W., and Keeney, J. K. (1976). Relationships among children's attitudes, involvement, and proficiency in physical activities, *Research Quarterly*, **47**, 797–803.

Sutton-Smith, B. (1971). Child's play: Very serious business, *Psychology Today*, **5**, 66–69, 87.

Tanner, J. M. (1962). *Growth at Adolescence* (2nd edn.), Oxford: Blackwell Scientific Publications.

Taub, E. (1976). Movement in nonhuman primates deprived of somatosensory feedback, in J. Keogh and R. S. Hutton (eds.), *Exercise and Sport Sciences Reviews* (Vol. 4), Santa Barbara, Ca.: Journal Publishing Affiliates.

Thomas, J. R., and Chissom, B. S. (1973). Differentiation between high and low sociometric status for sixth-grade boys using selected measures of motor skill, *Child Study Journal*, **3**, 125–130.

Todor, J. I. (1978). A neo-Piagetian theory of constructive operators: Applications to percentual-motor development and learning, in D. M. Landers and R. W. Christina (eds.), *Psychology of Motor Behavior and Sport – 1977*, Champaign, Ill.: Human Kinetics.

Twitchell, T. E. (1965). The automatic grasping responses of infants, *Neuropsychologia*, **3**, 247–259.

Wade, M. G. (1976). Method and analysis in the study of children's play behavior, *Quest*, **26**, 17–25.

Wade, M. G., Keogh, J. F., Rarick, G. L., Seefeldt, V., Smoll, F. L., and Williams, H. G. (1974). Research directions in motor development, report submitted to the Scholarly Directions Committee of the National College Physical Education Association for Men and the National Association for Physical Education of College Women, November.

Whitener, S. F., and James, K. W. (1973). The relationship among motor tasks for pre-school children, *Journal of Motor Behavior*, **5**, 231–239.

Whiting, H. T. A. (1972). Sports psychology in perspective, in H. T. A. Whiting (ed.), *Readings in Sports Psychology*, London: Kimpton.

Wickens, C. D. (1974). Temporal limits of human information processing: A developmental study, *Psychological Bulletin*, **81**, 739–755.

Wickstrom, R. L. (1975). Developmental kinesiology: Maturation of basic motor patterns, in J. H. Wilmore and J. F. Keogh (eds.), *Exercise and Sport Sciences Reviews* (Vol. 3), New York: Academic Press.

Wickstrom, R. L. (1977). *Fundamental Motor Patterns* (2nd edn.), Philadelphia: Lea & Febiger.

Wilberg, R. (1973). The direction and definition of a field (sports psychology), *Proceedings of the 3rd World Congress of the International Society of Sports Psychology*, pp. 1–13.

Wild, M. R. (1938). The behavior pattern of throwing and some observations concerning its course of development in children, *Research Quarterly*, **9**, 20–24.

Williams, H. G. (1974). Perceptual-motor development as a function of information processing, in M. G. Wade and R. Martens (eds.), *Psychology of Motor Behavior and Sport*, Urbana, Ill.: Human Kinetics.

Wohlwill, J. F. (1970). Methodology and research strategy in the study of developmental change, in L. R. Goulet and P. B. Baltes (eds.), *Life-span Developmental Psychology: Research and theory*, New York: Academic Press.

Yarnall, C. D. (1966). Relationship of physical fitness to selected measures of popularity, *Research Quarterly*, **37**, 286–288.

Zeigler, E. F., and McCristal, K. J. (1967). A history of the Big Ten Body-of-Knowledge Project in Physical Education, *Quest*, **9**, 79–84.

Zelazo, P. R., Zelazo, N. A., and Kolb, S. (1972). 'Walking' in the newborn, *Science*, **176**, 314–315.

# Author Index

355

# Subject Index